Culturally Responsive Practices

in Speech, Language,
and Hearing Sciences

Culturally Responsive Practices

in Speech, Language, and Hearing Sciences

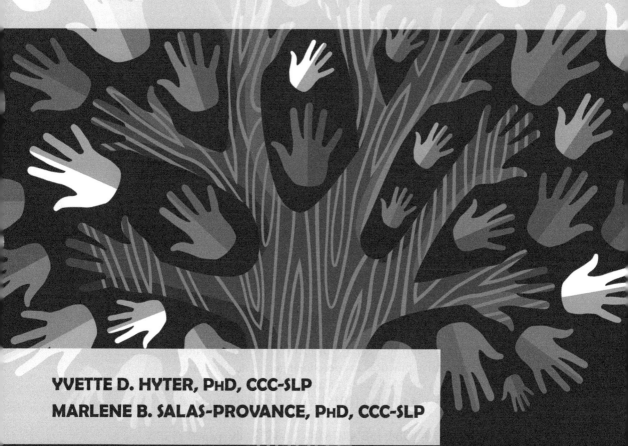

YVETTE D. HYTER, PhD, CCC-SLP

MARLENE B. SALAS-PROVANCE, PhD, CCC-SLP

PLURAL
PUBLISHING
INC.

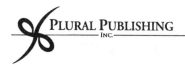

5521 Ruffin Road
San Diego, CA 92123

e-mail: information@pluralpublishing.com
website: https://www.pluralpublishing.com

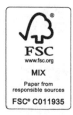

Typeset in 11/13 Adobe Garamond by Flanagan's Publishing Services, Inc.
Printed in the United States of America by McNaughton & Gunn
23 22 21 20   5 6 7 8

Library of Congress Cataloging-in-Publication Data

Names: Hyter, Yvette D., author. | Salas-Provance, Marlene B., author.
Title: Culturally responsive practices in speech, language, and hearing sciences / Yvette D. Hyter, Marlene B. Salas-Provance.
Description: San Diego, CA : Plural, [2019] | Includes bibliographical references and index.
Identifiers: LCCN 2017045983| ISBN 9781597568678 (alk. paper) | ISBN 1597568678 (alk. paper)
Subjects: | MESH: Speech Therapy—methods | Culturally Competent Care—methods | Language Therapy—methods | Hearing Disorders—therapy
Classification: LCC RC424.7 | NLM WL 340.3 | DDC 616.85/5—dc23
LC record available at https://lccn.loc.gov/2017045983

CONTENTS

FOREWORD

The globe provides us with many learning opportunities and challenges. As people move across the globe for one reason or another, many face insurmountable challenges. At the same time, they have experienced tremendous learning opportunities. The recent influx of refugees from Africa to Europe has become a hot topic for policymakers and leaders of many nations. The migration of people from place to place, the displacement of people from country to country and the habits of nomads who travel from border to border have all been interesting topics for people in multiple disciplines. It is about time that speech-language pathologists, audiologists, and researchers in speech-language pathology and audiology take a serious look at our shared responsibilities in understanding and serving such populations.

Take Asia, for example: countries such as Portugal, Spain, Great Britain, France, and the Netherlands had all been traveling to Asia establishing colonies, including Vietnam, Cambodia, Laos, India, Sri Lanka (Ceylon), Pakistan, Bangladesh, Malaysia, and Indonesia. Such colonization had created multiple contacts and multicultural challenges. Although the history of the United States (except for the First Nations) is comparably short, during this short period of time there have been forced migration of slaves, emancipation of slavery and also migration and immigration for many countries of the world. The concept of a socially and culturally responsible society is at the center of discussion in multiple educational forums. Further, the need to provide culturally and globally responsive practices should be the guiding principles for all professionals who uphold the notion that communication and education are human rights.

I applaud the efforts of the two esteemed colleagues, Yvette Hyter and Marlene Salas-Provance, for their groundbreaking work and research and their dedication in improving the quality of life of many.

The book has valuable content information relevant to the study and research of human behaviors and communication imperatives across the lifespan and across multiple cultures. Case studies have been provided to link theory to practice. As we are promoting interprofessional communication and studies, we need to also look at our responsibilities in interpersonal and intercultural communication.

The authors provided very extensive and comprehensive background information from the World Health Organization and related organizations. They have provided rationale for upholding our professional standards as well as ethics. Not only do the authors provide the clinical and theoretical background for understanding the challenges we face on a daily basis, they also provide reflective and learning opportunities for readers and students who participate in the exercise of self-discipline and self-improvement.

As the globe is becoming smaller, it is incumbent upon all of us to create a discourse that includes discussions about culturally and globally responsive practices. I offer my heartfelt congratulations to the efforts of Yvette and Marlene in making the daring journey into a topic that is not only worthwhile but thought provoking. By reading this book, you will find yourself digging into your consciousness and asking many questions. I believe you will come out a better person. Enjoy!

Li-Rong Lilly Cheng, PhD, CCC-SLP
Professor
School of Speech, Language and
    Hearing Sciences
San Diego State University

PREFACE

The authors have been teaching, researching, and implementing culturally responsive practices for more than 54 years between them. In this first edition of a text of this type in speech, language, and hearing sciences, we felt it important to address this topic from an angle that is not traditionally used in these professions. It is 2018, and we live in a world that has been changing exponentially, particularly since the 1980s.

OUR INTERCONNECTED WORLD

Globalization—*the interconnectedness and interdependence of nations, blurring of borders, and intermingled cultures, ecologies, economies, languages, politics, and technologies*—has uneven effects; that is, there are countries that often benefit from this increasing interdependence, and there are those that are frequently disadvantaged by them (Steger, 2010). Regardless of whether your country experiences the privileges or the hindrances of globalization, all of us perceive that the world is getting smaller.

In this 21st century, there have been major movements of groups of people across the world. Sometimes this movement is voluntary in search of diverse opportunities elsewhere. At other times people are forcefully displaced because of such issues as political instability, ethnic persecution, natural and environmental disasters, and wars. Nevertheless, because of this movement of groups of people, there are increasing opportunities for communication specialists, audiologists, educators, and health care providers to counsel, assess, diagnose, and provide services to people with cultures (*values, beliefs, assumptions transmitted from one generation to another that drive daily practices*) and who speak languages different from one's own. We are also in a time where there have been unprecedented examples of violations of civil and human rights, extrajudicial killings, and increasing expressions of racism, sexism, islamophobia, linguicism[1] (as per Phillipson, 1992), cultural exclusion, political domination, and economic exploitation in the United States, and abroad. For these reasons, the authors know that the time is right to "do a new thing," and that "business as usual" just will not suffice.

TOWARD A CRITICAL SPEECH, LANGUAGE, AND HEARING SCIENCES

In this regard, we approach culturally responsive practices from interprofessional, transdisciplinary and macro practice perspectives. To do this we have drawn from the literature of

---

[1]Linguicism is composed of "ideologies and structures that are used to legitimate, effectuate and reproduce an unequal division of power and resources between groups, which are defined on the basis of language" (Phillipson, 1992, p. 47).

several disciplines (e.g., economics, education, interdisciplinary health, nursing, political science, psychology, social work, and sociology) and integrated theoretical perspectives, conceptual frameworks, and concepts with the writings from the professions of speech-language pathology and audiology. Finally, as practicing clinicians, professors, administrators, and scholar-activists, we approach culturally responsive practices from a position of critical speech-language pathology—nomenclature first used by Claire Penn (2002) to imply "a detailed examination of biopsychosocial influences on our discipline" (p. 95). Hyter (2010) extends this concept to refer to the practice of "examining the relations between communication, speech, language development processes, and the historical, sociocultural, political, economic and ecological structures (conditions) that govern spoken and written language uses and cultural practices, and that shapes linguistic culture" (p. 1).

WHAT IS IN A NAME?

What is in a name? Everything! We have used well-thought-out decisions about what terms to use to refer to ethnic, cultural, and racialized groups in this text. It has been a detailed and difficult decision, but our goal was to be as accurate as possible, while being sensitive. There really are no good ways to refer to groups of people. Some terms are perceived as insensitive or disparaging, such as referring to the people who originated on U.S. soil as "Indians." We have chosen to refer to this group of people as *First Nations*. First Nations has been used to refer specifically to people living in Canada but has of late been generalized to replace the term *Indian* (Pinder, 2010).

Many people of African descent living in the United States prefer to be called Black or

African American. Watts Smith (2014) conducted a study of 3,374 African Americans in the United States and found that the majority (56%) preferred to refer to themselves as Black, and 34% preferred to call themselves as African American, but whether they referred to themselves as Black or African American was context dependent; that is, it depended on to whom they were talking. Immigrants of African descent or from Haiti or the Caribbean who were Black preferred to call themselves Black, but also used African American. In this text, we use both *African American* and *Black* interchangeably.

Spanish speakers in the United States have been referred to as *Hispanic* and *Latino*. But these terms are used to refer to people from Mexico, Puerto Rico, Cuba, Central America, Argentina, and the Dominican Republic who have a language in common but speak different variations of that language, come from different countries, and have diverse cultures. The U.S. government developed the category called "Hispanic," under which Spanish speakers were grouped (Mora, 2014). Also, the term *Hispanic* has been associated with Spanish ancestry, whereas *Latino* has been used to refer to groups of people with a colonized past "and history of oppression" (Mora, 2014, p. 78). In this text, we are using both *Latin@/Hispanic*. The "at" sign is used to refer to a gender-neutral version of Latino or Latina (Demby, 2013). We also use Arab American, Asian American, Pacific Islander, and White or European American but also realize that these terms do not adequately describe the diverse ethnic groups associated with these names. Typically, in the United States the word *minority*, has been used to refer to the groups of people mentioned above, with the exception of people who identify as White or European American. We deliberately have not used *minority*, as it carries a negative connotation. Also, *minority* is no longer used to refer to a numerical group but speaks more to the amount of power a group of people are perceived to hold.

In addition to trying to use sensitive names for groups, we struggled with what to call different regions of the world. We use the concepts of the *Global South* to refer to countries that have a history of colonialism and where access to resources is strained. This is the part of the world where a majority of the world's populations live, leading some to use the term *Majority World Countries*. *Global North* refers to countries with high incomes, such as the United States, Canada, and many countries in Europe, but also Australia, Israel, Japan, New Zealand, and South Africa (Freedman & Crépeau, 2017). The Global North is where a minority of the world's populations live, also referred to as *Minority World Countries*.

WHO WE ARE

We thought it important to share with the readers some information about our backgrounds.

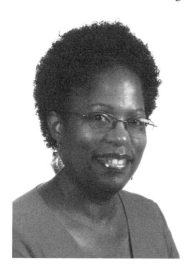

I am Yvette D. Hyter, PhD, CCC-SLP, and American Speech-Language-Hearing Asso-

ciation Fellow. I identify as Black. With the help of my parents, aunts, uncles, and cousins, and Ancestry.com, I have been able to trace my paternal family back to 1811, and maternal family back to 1856. My maternal great grandfather was a farmer who owned his own farm, outright, and was also literate. My investigation about my paternal great, great, great grandparents, who were also farmers, led me to Louisa, Virginia, but I lost track of them there because those who were enslaved were only counted in the "slave schedules," which provided the name of the slaver, the number of enslaved, the age of the enslaved, their gender, and color—but they were not given names. My parents were teenage sweethearts, married in their 20s and as of 2017 have been married for 63 years. They were part of the *The Great Black Migration* (see Reich, 2014 and Wilkerson, 2011), migrating from Alabama to Michigan in the 1950s. Although I was raised in Detroit, while growing up I (along with my siblings and parents) spent every summer in Alabama. My father, who wanted to be an architect, faced insurmountable obstacles to reaching that goal as a Black man in the south in 1950. Instead he taught science and math in Alabama, for a year before becoming a science teacher in Detroit. He later went to Cornell University, earned a master's degree in teaching in science, and when he returned to Detroit became science department head, and later served as the science supervisor for the Detroit Public Schools until he retired. My mother had two years of Registered Nurse (RN) education when they moved to Detroit, but was not able to continue her RN education in the late 1950s being told by the hospital nursing program, "we just don't accept Blacks." As an alternative, she became a Licensed Practical Nurse, and because the hours were difficult for raising a young growing family, she went back to school to obtain her bachelor's degree in sociology and for more than 20 years worked as a social worker for the state of Michigan. In this role, she worked with teens living in residential centers and in out-of-home placements until her retirement. My siblings and I had a front row seat to the challenges (some of it due to racism) and triumphs that my parents faced daily. They always had an alternative "story" for us, in that they told us about who we were, about our proud cultural and familial history, and assured us of what was possible when someone called us a disparaging name or told us what we could not aspire to be. All of this rich history, abbreviated quite significantly here, contributes to the fabric of who I am. Of course, I have had and continue to have my own challenges . . . but that is a story for another day. My last comment is about a dream I had in 1990 when enrolled at Temple University to earn a doctorate in Speech-Language Pathology, after having worked as a speech-language pathologist for several years. While obtaining my PhD, I was experiencing significant cognitive dissonance around the topic of assessments and interventions with "multicultural populations." I was trying to reconcile what I was learning with how I could have served children of color on my previous caseloads more effectively. I had a dream that all the children of color were locked in a barn, and I could not get them out. I had the key but the key did not work. I tried to break the barn door down but was unable. I had that dream repeatedly until I realized my purpose was to contribute to a change in the way children who are impoverished, who speak languages other than English, who speak variations of English, and who are marginalized are assessed and served by speech-language pathologists. That has been my sole focus since 1990. Writing a book with my friend and colleague Marlene Salas-Provance is just the next natural step for my contribution to the field of speech, language, and hearing sciences.

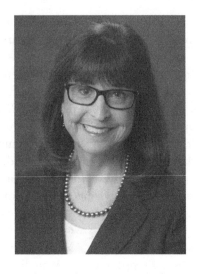

I am Marlene Salas-Provance, PhD, MHA, CCC-SLP, and American Speech-Language-Hearing Association Fellow. I was born and raised in Albuquerque, New Mexico, into a large Hispanic family, the youngest of seven children. I believe that my life experiences are similar to those of many Hispanic individuals who were raised in strong religious (Catholic) and extended families. Growing up, my family included many brothers, sisters, uncles, aunts, and cousins around whom our entire life revolved, full of the cultural and religious rituals of baptisms, confirmations, weddings, and funerals. My Salas name originates from my Conquistador grandfather of many generations past, Sebastian Salas, who crossed into New Mexico in the late 1500s having journeyed from Estonia, Spain, looking for a new world. My family has a Salas family shield that represents our long ancestry. New Mexico has many families similar to my own who have lived in the state for hundreds of years. My mother's father, Enrique Lopez, was a man ahead of his years in terms of educating his daughters. He took his daughters by horse and wagon from a small town, Torreon, New Mexico, to Santa Fe, New Mexico, to be educated at the Loretto School for Girls. Two of my aunts became teachers. My own mother, Cora, only went to eighth grade but was a passionate believer of education for her children. She was a volunteer for numerous causes as long as I can remember. My own passion for volunteering, I believe, was passed down. My father was a musician and a welder in the same job for 30 years. We learned the value of hard work, dedication to a cause, and the importance of family. I was the first in my family home to receive a college education, and there are numerous stories to tell about that journey. But I credit my mother, Cora, with instilling in me a belief that you never quit. That no matter the challenges, education is worth it. So educated I became. My early success in college began with the unending support of Dr. Edgar Garrett, chair of the Department of Communication Disorders at New Mexico State University. He supported me and continued to do so throughout my life. I truly believe that role models are critical to our success as individuals. My professional work in diversity began with the American Speech-Language-Hearing Association's Hispanic Caucus in 1994, and cultural issues have been a focus of my personal and professional life since that time. My friend and colleague Yvette Hyter and I hope that the years we spent thoughtfully preparing this book resulted in a comprehensive story that will allow you to improve the lives of your diverse students, patients, or clients, no matter their disability.

REFERENCES

Demby, G. (2013 January 7). "Latin@" offers a gender-neutral choice: But how to pronounce it? *Breaking News from National Public Radio.* Retrieved from http://www.npr.org/sections/thetwo-way/2013/01/07/168818064/latin-offers-a-gender-neutral-choice-but-how-to-pronounce-it

Freedman, R., & Crépeau, F. (2017). Supporting or resisting? The relationship between Global North states and special procedures. In A. Nolan, R. Freedman & T. Murphy (Eds.), *The United Nations special procedures system* (pp. 411–442). Leiden, The Netherlands: Koninklijke Brill NV.

Hyter, Y. D. (2010). *Critical speech-language pathology: A concept for communication sciences and disorders* (Unpublished document). Western Michigan University, Kalamazoo, MI.

Mora, G. C. (2014). *Making Hispanics: How activists, bureaucrats, and the media created a new American.* Chicago, IL: University of Chicago Press.

Penn, C. (2002). Cultural narratives: Bridging the gap. *Folia Phoniatrica et Logopaedica, 54*(2), 95–99.

Phillipson, R. (1992). *Linguistic Imperialism.* New York, NY: Oxford University Press.

Pinder, S. O. (2010). *The politics of race and ethnicity in the United States: Americanization and de-Americanization of racialized ethnic groups.* New York, NY: Palgrave Macmillan.

Reich, S. (2014). *The great Black migration: A historical encyclopedia of the American mosaic.* Santa Barbara, CA: Greenwood.

Steger, M. (2010). *Globalization: A very short introduction.* Oxford, UK: Oxford University Press.

Watts Smith, C. (2014). *Black mosaic: The politics of Black pan-ethnic diversity.* New York, NY: New York University Press.

Wilkerson, I. (2011). *The warmth of other suns: The epic story of America's great migration.* New York, NY: First Vintage Books.

ACKNOWLEDGMENTS

If it were not for God and my yielding to the Holy Spirit, I would not have had the ideas represented in this book. There are also many people, and circumstances, to acknowledge. First, I would like to thank the five people who served as the most influential mentors to me since the 1980s until today—Dr. Nickola W. Nelson, Dr. Ida Stockman, Dr. Aquiles Iglesias, Dr. Robert Mayo, and Dr. Carol Westby.

First, I met Dr. Nickola W. Nelson as an undergraduate in speech-language pathology at Western Michigan University (WMU). I remember wanting to go to another university for my master's degree because there was an African American professor at that university. Nicki encouraged me to examine my interests and the focus of other universities that I was considering for graduate school. WMU turned out to be the best fit for my interests (i.e., young children in educational settings). Nicki recognized, however, my desire and need to have African American speech-language pathologists as role models. She also recognized that I had abilities that were not recognized when I was an undergraduate. I became her graduate assistant, which was the real beginning of a 36-year mentor/mentee relationship and friendship between us. She has been a constant example and encourager throughout my career. Nicki has always told me (and other students, I am sure) to embrace cognitive dissonance because it is at that moment that you are beginning to learn something great. I have held on to that idea throughout my career.

It is through Nicki that I learned about and met Dr. Ida Stockman, whom I wanted to be like when I "grew up." Ida has been like a ray of light in an obscured context and has made and is continuing to make significant contributions to the field of speech-language pathology that are not always widely recognized. After I graduated with my master's, Ida and I became reacquainted through the National Black Association of Speech-Language-Hearing (NBASLH), where she mentored students conducting research. Years later when talking about a new idea I was trying to write about (i.e., speech-language pathology from a social justice perspective), Ida told me that to "do something new in the field, any field, you have to have a strong constitution." Then she looked at me directly, and said "and honey . . . YOU, need to get a strong constitution." It was so true at the time, as I was overly concerned about whether my ideas would be valued. As a result of Ida's advice, I no longer worry about whether my ideas will be valued; I already know they are valuable, but I stand behind these ideas with a "strong constitution" and the evidence to back them up.

After working as an itinerate speech-language pathologist and in a hospital for several years, I went back to school to earn a doctorate degree. I enrolled in Temple University in Philadelphia, under the supervision of Dr. Aquiles Iglesias (affectionately called AI). After every class with him, I had significant cognitive dissonance, so I had ample opportunity to employ Nicki's advice to embrace the dissonance. Through working with AI and learning to think critically and dialectically from him and through other courses at Temple, I realized my mission in life, which I mentioned in the preface of this text. I will be forever grateful to AI for lovingly challenging me to question long-held assumptions.

AI introduced me to Dr. Robert Mayo who was a professor at the University of North Carolina at the time. While I was working on my doctorate degree and throughout my early years as a young faculty member, Robert, his wife Carolyn, and I communicated regularly, where he asked questions that helped to guide my research, made suggestions about writing strategies, and encouraged me to think beyond traditional boundaries. I am grateful to Robert for the example of student mentorship that he extended to me, and to many others over the years.

Although I knew Dr. Carol Westby's work before I met her, I did not meet her until I was in my first faculty position at Wichita State University in the mid-1990s. We were hired on there at the same time. Carol is a master at teaching by using real-life examples and makes riveting, engaging professional presentations. From Carol I learned to make learning come to life for students, to engage them in real-life activities from which they can learn and apply what they learned in realistic ways.

In addition to mentors, I must thank my extended family and friends who were supportive of my work, whose critical suggestions helped to make the book better, and more engaging: my parents, Betty and Leroy Hyter, who literally read every word I wrote; my siblings and their families, Michael, Leroy Jr., Patricia Walker, and Pamela Lewis, who encouraged me at every turn; my "sister and brother," Angie and Macgregor Coleman, who asked questions that helped me clarify ideas, and whose council fortified me when I become discouraged with the writing; dear friends Dr. Jan Bedrosian and Steve Pifer, whose texts with "hugs" and encouragement to engage in self-care helped me take the time to rest when I was exhausted, and to continue writing after respite; Dr. Sarah Summy, who

offered to read chapters, and who picked up the slack during our study abroad course in Senegal, while Marlene and I were finalizing the last two chapters; to my family in Senegal who encouraged my book writing efforts and who taught me to see the world differently; and to all of the young children I have served over the years both in the United States and abroad who taught me, and continue to teach me about culturally responsive practices. Finally, I am indebted to my husband, partner (compañero), friend, and colleague, Dr. W. F. Santiago-Valles (Santiago) who is a big picture person but who looked after all the small minutia and details of life that I could not while pouring out words on the computer. In everything, "we are together."

—Yvette D. Hyter

I must begin by thanking my mother, Cora Lopez Salas, who believed that I could do anything. In fact, she made great sacrifices because she believed school was important and she believed I was 'special'. She would be proud of this textbook, even though it would be a challenge for her to read with her eighth grade education. She would probably frame it!

I want to acknowledge Dr. Edgar Garrett, my lifelong mentor. He was the head of the Speech and Hearing Department at New Mexico State University and I met him as a freshman at NMSU. He taught me to think critically and ask thoughtful questions. His support never waned and he propelled me to excel beyond what I thought was possible at the age of 18 when we first met.

I want to recognize the guidance of Dr. David Kuehn who made my doctoral experience pleasant and academically fulfilling. I was provided a lifetime of knowledge in a short three years. He, along with Dr. Joan Good Erickson, taught me to take my clinical writing into the academic arena. Dr. Erickson was my introduction and first taste of the power of diversity thinking, which became my passion. She lived it, breathed it and owned it. I could not have had a better role-model.

There are several important colleagues who were a special part of my academic life for the past 27 years and whose encouragement and support kept me moving toward the writing of this book. Dr. Janie Von Wolfseck was my first academic 'boss' and became my lifelong friend and confidant. More than anyone, she supported and validated my work in the classroom and love of teaching. Dr. Paul Fogle and his wife Carol Fogle cherished me and taught me so much about how to be successful in the broader arena of life.

I have shared more meetings, dinners, laughs, dances, and tears than I can count with my friend and colleague, Dr. Luis Riquelme. He changed my thinking about my role as a Hispanic professional in ASHA. The first Hispanic Caucus meeting in 1994 was a turning point in my life as I watched Luis speak the truth about diversity. I became a believer and loyal follower of his vision that soon became my vision for diversity. Other colleagues who were an important part of my diversity journey are Dr. Noma Anderson, Julie Bisbee, Dr. Carol Higdon, DeAnne Owre, Dr. Deborah Rhein, and Dr. Emily Tobey. Friends who have been supporters through more than the writing of this book are Billy and Cynthia Garrett, Jimmie Jinks, Tom and Linda Lindsay, Dr. Michael and Jan Morehead, Senator Mary Kay Papen, Dr. Mary Prentice, Ricardo Rel, Sandra Romero, J Paul Taylor, Lisa Warren and Clare Zeagler.

My sister, Jean, became my business associate in my medical interpreting company and steadfastly supported her 'little' sister through building and growing the business for the past 12 years. As an educator herself, she taught me from a young age, how to "do school". She reached the upper levels of public school administration and set the bar high. There was

never a moment that she did not believe in this book, its words, and in me. Both my Salas and Provance extended families have always been supportive of the richness of my career choices over the years. This sense of family has always been essential to my professional growth.

My best teachers were my thousands of students. I wish I could thank each one of them personally. You know who you are. Yes, you! They taught me so much, through the multicultural course and cleft lip and palate course at Fontbonne College, St. Louis University, Southern Illinois University at Edwardsville, University of the Pacific, University of Montevallo, and finally, New Mexico State University. I hope they can hear my words in this book and know that those words can become their words as well. They were so passionate, so excited, and so committed to diversity, to bilingualism, to changing the lives of others in a culturally responsive manner. They let me be their teacher, they let me fill them with knowledge and guide them into their careers. It was a joy for me.

I have international colleagues in Lima, Peru I would like to thank, especially Dr. Margot Escobedo, Dr. Margarita Marchino, and Dr. Umberto Escobedo who have expanded my world view sensitivities. They have taught me so much about embracing culture, embracing difference, embracing things you cannot change. To watch my students and these colleagues work together showed me that diversity is worth it, that we are all needed to improve the lives of others.

I want to thank my two sons Severin Alan Provance and William Hal Provance who knew their mother had a career to take care of and they were always there with their support and patience. I was fortunate to have such good and thoughtful children who became such wonderful men.

Finally, and most importantly, Bill, my best friend and partner in life, provided me the safety net that allowed me to try anything, to fully embrace and commit to the career I loved and to which I was completely dedicated. He read every word in my dissertation, helped input hundreds of thousands of data points into spreadsheets over the years, and believed in and listened thoughtfully to every single idea in this book.

—Marlene B. Salas-Provance

We both want to give a special thanks to Severin Provance who completed the original and adapted artwork for this textbook. Severin is a graphic designer in Chandler, Arizona (SeverinsDesigns.com). He is a graduate of the Herberger Institute for Design & the Arts at Arizona State University. He has completed design work for educational organizations and professional workshop presenters, marketing projects for public businesses and packaging designs for individual startups.

Also, we want to extend our gratitude to Melissa Ruthven, Carly Roell, and Carolyn Mooi, who conducted literature searches for topics covered in this text, and to Justin A. Gripentrog who helped to develop the power point slides provided in the PluralPlus companion website.

REVIEWERS

Plural Publishing, Inc., and the authors would like to thank the following reviewers for taking the time to provide their valuable feedback during the development process:

Shatonda S. Jones, PhD, CCC-SLP
Assistant Professor
Communication Sciences and Disorders
Rockhurst University
Kansas City, Missouri

Laura B. Willis, MCD, CCC-SLP
Associate Clinical Professor
Department of Communication Disorders
Auburn University
Auburn, Alabama

Grace E. McConnell, PhD, CCC-SLP
Assistant Professor
Communication Sciences and Disorders
Rockhurst University
Kansas City, Missouri

Janice M. Wright, MA, CCC-SLP
Assistant Clinical Professor
Hearing, Speech and Language Clinic
Ohio University
Athens, Ohio

Stacey Wallen, PhD, CCC-SLP
Clinical Associate Professor
Educational Psychology, Special Education,
    and Communication Disorders
Georgia State University
Atlanta, Georgia

"The idea that some lives (or cultures, beliefs, values, languages, world views, practices, theoretical perspectives . . .) matter less is the root of all that is wrong with the world."

—*Paul Farmer (text within the parentheses was added by Yvette D. Hyter)*

This book is dedicated to multiple people in my life.

First, I dedicate this book to the children around the world who continue to teach me how to be more culturally responsive.

Second, it is dedicated to my parents, Betty and Leroy Hyter, who are the best reflection of God's grace and selfless love that I've ever known. How can anyone fail with support like that?

Third, this book is for my husband, friend, and partner, W. F. Santiago-Valles, who continues to provide the best example of living a life consistent with one's principles, even when there is no "thank you" at the end of the day. Santiago, thanks for helping me understand that the *real story* is in what's missing, rather than in what's obvious for all the world to see.

In memory

When working on my doctorate, a dear friend, who passed away in 1998, regularly teased me about forgetting her when I published my first book. "Z," it took more than 20 years, but I remember.

—Yvette D. Hyter

This book is dedicated to Bill
The love of my life.
After 40 years together, this book is as much his as mine.
Thank you, Dear!

In memory

My Big Brother Henry Salas (1938–2017)
He was unabashedly proud of everything I did.

—Marlene B. Salas-Provance

Introduction

To live in the United States of today means to live with almost 325 million people (U.S. Census, 2017), where First Nations, African Americans, Latin@s/Hispanics, Pacific Islanders, and people from Asia and the Middle East represent 40.8% of that population (U.S. Census, 2013, 2017). The term that is usually used to refer to these groups of people is *minorities*; however, it is a term that is problematic, particularly since its use no longer typically refers to numbers of people. This is particularly important to think about since for children under the age of 5, the numerical majority of these children in many large cities are from those communities of color and diverse ethnicities. As of 2014, 52.2% of children in this age group were from an ethnic background other than European and a racialized background other than White or Caucasian (Colby & Ortman, 2015; U.S. Census, 2015) (Table 1–1).

The First Nations, African American, Asian, Latin@/Hispanic, and Pacific Islander populations combined are expected to rise to over 60% of the total population by 2060, compared with 38% in 2017. The United States is continuing along the path to becoming a plurality of racial and ethnic people. Part of this racial and ethnic plurality are those who

identify as European American, Caucasian, or White, who also have histories, cultures, and world views. One goal of this text is to help the readers produce the knowledge, and acquire skills and attitudes that will help you be able to engage, interact, and provide services to anyone from any racial or ethnic group in a responsive and equitable manner.

The diversity of languages spoken is wide with over 350 languages spoken in U.S. homes and approximately 35 of these languages spoken by at least 100,000 individuals over the age of 5. These data indicate that one out of every five children in the United States is speaking a language other than English (U.S. Census, 2015). A closer look across the United States's large metropolitan areas reveals that 185 languages are spoken in Los Angeles, 166 in Seattle, 145 in Houston, and 126 in Detroit. Figure 1–1 shows the number of languages spoken in the 15 most populated areas of the country. This tells only one side of the story, as there are a multitude of smaller pockets of linguistic diversity across the country, including languages of First Nations people, like Navajo, Cherokee, and Apache, and other smaller language groups such as Dutch, Indonesian, and Romanian, among others (U.S. Census, 2015).

TABLE 1–1. Populations by Race and Hispanic Origin: 2014–2060 (Population in Thousands)

Race and Hispanic Origin	2014		2060		Change, 2014–2060	
	Number	Percent	Number	Percent	Number	Percent
Total population	318,748	100.0	416,795	100.0	96,047	30.8
One race	310,753	97.5	390,772	93.8	80,020	25.8
White	246,940	77.5	285,314	68.5	38,374	15.5
Non-Hispanic white	198,103	62.2	181,930	43.6	–16,174	–8.2
Black or African American	42,039	13.2	59,693	14.3	17,654	42.0
American Indian and Alaska Native	3,957	1.2	5,607	1.3	1,650	41.7
Asian	17,083	5.4	38,965	9.3	21,882	128.1
Native Hawaiian and Other Pacific Islander	734	0.2	1,194	0.3	460	62.6
Two or more races	7,995	2.5	26,022	6.2	18,027	225.5
Race alone or in combination						
White	254,009	79.7	309,567	74.3	55,558	21.9
Black or African American	45,562	14.3	74,530	17.9	29,968	63.6
American Indian and Alaska Native	6,528	2.0	10,169	2.4	3,640	55.8
Asian	19,983	6.3	48,575	11.7	28,592	143.1
Native Hawaiian and other Pacific Islander	1,458	0.5	2,929	0.7	1,470	100.8
Hispanic or Latino Origin						
Hispanic	55,410	17.4	119,044	28.6	63,635	114.8
Non-Hispanic	263,338	82.6	297,750	71.4	34,412	13.1

Source: Reprinted from Colby, S., & Ortman, J. M. (2015, March 3). Projections of the size and composition of the U.S. population 2014–2060: Population estimates and projections. Retrieved from http://www.census.gov/content/dam/Census/library/publications/2015/demo/p25-1143.pdf.

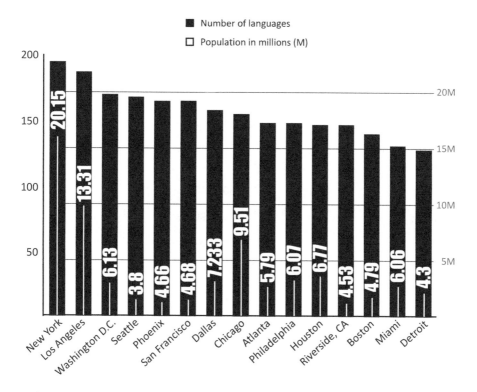

FIGURE 1–1. Number of languages spoken in the 15 largest U.S. metro areas. Reprinted from Colby, S., & Ortman, J. M. (2015). Projections of the size and composition of the U.S. Population 2014–2060: Population estimates and projections. Retrieved from http://www.census.gov/content/dam/Census/library/publications/2015/demo/p25-1143.pdf. Illustrated by Severin Provance.

English remains the predominant language spoken in the United States with almost 232 million speakers, followed by Spanish, with almost 38 million speakers (Ryan, 2013) (Table 1–2).

It is important to understand the racial, ethnic, and language diversity in this country, because the work of policymakers, researchers, educators, and service providers will be or "should be" influenced and dictated by this reality. These millions of diverse people build "ways" of living together. Their everyday lives are established as a result of shared experiences. There is collective problem solving among individuals and groups—and cultures are born. Chapter 2 is devoted to definitions, but we briefly define two of the primary concepts that occur throughout this text—culture and cultural responsiveness. We also discuss unconscious bias.

TABLE 1–2. Language Use in the United States: 2011

Detailed Languages Spoken at Home by English-Speaking Ability for the Population 5 Years and Over: 2011		
Characteristics	Population 5 Years and Over	Spoke a Language Other Than English at Home (%)
Population 5 years and over	291,524,091s	x
Spoke only English at home	230,947,071	x
Spoke a language other than English at home	60,577,020	100.0
Spanish or Spanish Creole	37,579,787	62.0
Other Indo-European languages		
French	1,301,443	2.1
French Creole	753,990	1.2
Italian	723,632	1.2
Portuguese	673,566	1.1
German	1,083,637	1.8
Yiddish	160,968	0.3
Other West Germanic languages	290,461	0.5
Scandinavian languages	135,025	0.2
Greek	304,928	0.5
Russian	905,843	1.5
Polish	607,531	1.0
Serbo-Croatian	269,624	0.4
Other Slavic languages	336,062	0.6
Armenian	246,915	0.4
Persian	407,586	0.7
Gujaranti	358,422	0.6
Hindi	648,983	1.1
Urdu	373,851	0.6
Other Indic languages	815,345	1.3
Other Indo-European Languages	449,600	0.7

TABLE 1–2. *continued*

Characteristics	Population 5 Years and Over	Spoke a Language Other Than English at Home (%)
Asian and Pacific Island languages		
Chinese	2,882,497	4.8
Japanese	436,110	0.7
Korean	141,277	1.9
Mon-Khmer, Cambodian	212,505	0.4
Hmong	211,227	0.3
Thai	163,251	0.3
Laotian	140,866	0.2
Vietnamese	1,419,539	2.3
Other Asian languages	855,303	1.4
Tagalog	1,594,413	2.6
Other Pacific Island languages	428,476	0.7
Other languages		
Navajo	169,369	0.3
Other Native American languages	195,407	0.3
Hungarian	93,102	0.2
Arabic	951,699	1.6
Hebrew	216,343	0.4
African languages	884,660	1.5
All other languages	153,777	0.3

Source: Reprinted from U.S. Census (2009–2013). American Community Survey. Retrieved from https://www.census.gov/data/tables/2013/demo/2009-2013-lang-tables.html

DEFINITION OF CULTURE

At its core, culture is a set of factors from multiple dimensions that can describe how one person or a group of people experience life, and engage in daily practices. Culture is learned and transmitted socially through patterns of behavior driven by such factors as problem solving strategies, value systems, beliefs, symbols, attitudes, religion, artifacts, and communication. We learn these practices over time, and they essentially "become" our culture. How we accept these variations, especially when they go well beyond our own personal preferences, speaks to our sensitivity level for other cultures. Yet, we can fit into a variety of cultures, and we do so, on a regular basis. Some cultural connections come more naturally than others. We continue to return to this concept of culture throughout the book.

In our daily interactions, we encounter cultures that are different from our own. It is up to us individually, and as part of a group, to decide who or what we accept or reject. We measure differences and similarities and then make choices. Some cultural practices we reject outright—sometimes consciously, but often unconsciously (Moule, 2009). There are degrees of this decision-making paradigm that are acceptable and unacceptable according to the laws of our country. For example, in employment, the Equal Employment Opportunity Commission (EEOC) rejects discrimination based on age, disability, pay, genetic information, sexual orientation, national origin, pregnancy, race/color, religion, among other characteristics (EEOC, n.d.; Yang, 2015). There are consequences when the line is crossed in these areas in our place of work. However, apart from the laws of this country, each person has a personal choice on how to live his or her life and how to treat others, and much of that is framed by what he or she has learned over time, that person's experiences, and that person's culture.

Let's read a story that may or may not be familiar to you. Interject yourself into this scenario and take the time to consider how you would decide to accept or reject some of these cultural practices. Are they something new and interesting to you, or are they too different so that you could not possibly adapt or consider this practice under any circumstances? Are you willing to say, "This is not for me, but I understand how these individuals may benefit from this experience?"

> **Box 1–1**
> **La Matanza**
> **(matar means "to kill" in Spanish)**
>
> You are invited to a family gathering of a colleague you know from work. You want to get to know him better, so you accept the invitation. You arrive at the home alone and are welcomed with hugs (*abrazos* in Spanish) from a number of people, similar to a receiving line. You are led to where your friend is sitting outside with a group of family members. You understood from the conversation that they are preparing to butcher a pig for the festivities. The family will gather to watch the *matanza* and then later partake in the meal. You learn that one of the best parts of the pig is the fat. It will be cooked into a delicacy that you can eat and enjoy as it is fried over the burning wood fire outside. They call this delicacy *chicharones* (fat rinds), and they can't seem to wait to start eating them.

As you think about the case in Box 1–1, ask yourself these questions:

- Do you stay or do you leave?
- Do you think what they are doing is right?
- Do you place a value judgment on this practice?
- Do you eat if you do stay?

- Do you ever accept another invitation from this colleague after this event?
- Was the culture of work (which was similar for the two of you) and the culture of home (your family does not eat meat) too different, so that you now see this colleague in a different (perhaps more negative) way?
- Should you accept all aspects of this new experience in order to be culturally sensitive or culturally responsive?

CULTURAL RESPONSIVENESS

The idea of cultural "competence" is difficult to conceptualize. It appears to be an all or nothing phenomenon. Either we are competent or we are not. But like with any other skill, being competent or responsive is *not* all or nothing, but an evolving process. Sometimes the term, *competence* itself causes confusion. Thus, throughout this text, we use another term. *Cultural responsiveness* provides us with a broader perspective from which to view our behaviors as they relate to our actions with individuals across a variety of cultures that are different from our own. In 1994, pedagogical theorist and educator Gloria Ladson-Billings talked about pedagogy that was relevant and responsive to the culture of the children being taught. Culturally responsive practices are those that take the client's cultural perspectives, beliefs, and values into consideration in all aspects of education or providing a service (Ladson-Billings, 1994, 1995).

Each person's degree of cultural responsiveness is a product of the fusion of their past experiences. Influences about how we feel and the decisions we make about our behavior toward others are not linear. Meaning, there is not one point in time where we can say that we are safely culturally responsive in every one of our interactions. It is, so to speak, always a work in progress. How we communicate with

our world stems from a more circular framework of decision making. It can be said that we go in and out of being culturally responsive at any point in time. What we hope for you as you read and reflect on the writings in this text, is that more often than not, your reaction to the people, families, and communities that you serve will become more and more responsive to their cultural world views, beliefs, and values.

Figure 1–2 shows a schematic based on Cross, Bazron, Dennis and Isaac's (1989), *Stages of Cultural Competence* neatly depicting six levels of development that we traverse from complete insensitivity shown at the bottom right side of the graphic, to behaviors which depict the highest levels of cultural

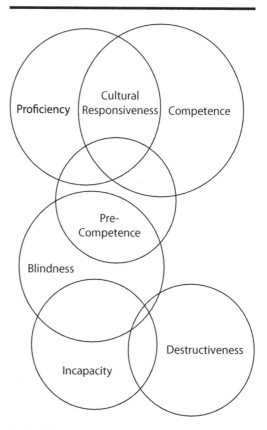

FIGURE 1–2. Schematic representing Cross, Bazron, Dennis, and Isaacs (1989) Stages of Cultural Competence. Illustrated by Severin Provance.

competence (or using the language of this text, cultural responsiveness). In these stages of cultural competence, we will start with cultural destructiveness, that reveals there is complete lack of empathy for anything or anyone that is outside the individual's belief system. At this level, individuals are willing to destroy others for self-serving purposes. The Tuskegee Experiments are a good example of cultural destructiveness. The Tuskegee experiments began in 1932 and were conducted by the US Public Health Service. The 600 men in the study (399 with syphilis and 201 without the disease) were not completely informed of the purpose or risks of the study, and "had been misled and had not been given all the facts required to provide informed consent" (CDC, 2016). Tragically, those with syphilis did not receive appropriate treatments, even as new cures became available over the 40-year period of the study. The researchers were, in the end, found to be "unethically justified" (CDC, 2016). In 1997, President Bill Clinton apologized to the families on behalf of the nation. The remaining men in the study, their spouses, widows and children were provided health benefits for life (CDC, 2016). This is a clear example of cultural destructiveness, and practices that had a lack of regard for the value of the life of another. Other examples of these types of atrocious practices are found throughout history in the treatment of the Jews by Hitler and the Germans, and the hostile removal of First Nations people from their lands throughout the United States, and the riot in Charlottesville, Virginia (August 2017) caused by the members of the KKK marching down the street carrying torches and guns, and yelling obscenities about Jews and other groups (read an article about this disturbance in the *New York Times* at https://www.nytimes.com/2017/08/11/us/white-nationalists-rally-charlottesville-virginia.html?mcubz=1).

In this graphic (see Figure 1–2), imagine the circles to be dynamic in that we can move within and among them in a circular way rather than linearly. Cultural destructiveness overlaps to some extent with cultural incapacity. If one is being culturally destructive they will not have the capacity to engage interculturally. Cultural blindness overlaps with incapacity and pre-competence. If one is culturally blind (seeing no differences among or between cultures) they do not have intercultural capacity. Cultural pre-competence is when a person begins to recognize that he/she needs more information and more skills with regard to interacting with cultural groups different than ones' own. Cultural competence is engaging in culturally responsive practices such as advocacy for others, and recurring self-education, and includes "respect" for cultural differences (National Center for Cultural Competence, 2004). Cultural proficiency is the ability to hold cultural diversity in high regard, and work within systems and organizations to make them more culturally responsive. In Figure 1–2, pre-competence overlaps with blindness, competence and proficiency. For those of us striving to become more culturally responsive, we are bound to have lapses from time to time, particularly when engaging with cultural groups with whom we have not previously engaged, meaning that we may inadvertently slip back into the pre-competence stage. Culturally responsive practices are comprised of Cultural Proficiency and Cultural Competence in this schema. There is a related extended learning activity available in the PluralPlus companion website.

There is no disagreement that cultural destructiveness is plain wrong. But what happens when the decisions are not so obvious? Are we always aware of how the phenomenon of culture impacts our decision making? When health care providers take the Hippocratic Oath that requires medical personnel to: (1) consider the well-being of the patient, (2) honor the profession and its traditions, (3) recognize limitations in the prevention and treatment of disease, (4) protect patient secrets, and (5) avoid abuse of the doctor-patient relationship (Chalmers, 2006, p. 83), what does it really mean? In short, this oath is commonly referred to as "First do no harm," which is the central doctrine of the oath. With this oath, health care providers are professing to abide by the highest levels of goodwill and practice toward others. In educational settings, the professional's code of ethics provides guidance as to how to treat others (see the American Speech-Language-Hearing Association's [ASHA's] code of ethics at http://www.asha.org/Code-of-Ethics/). There is an implied understanding that we take these oaths and partake in ethical practice to provide services to individuals from all walks of life, all ages, genders, gender identities, sexual orientations, and ethnicities; to those who speak languages other than English, practice different religions, whose parenting styles and child-rearing practices vary from our own, to name a few.

As we begin the journey to provide services, it is imperative to engage in critical self-reflection about our behaviors as they relate to culturally responsive practices. The journey to value those that think, act, and look different from ourselves never ends. In the end, it is not just stages that we pass through, but a life that we live, a culturally responsive life. Lives are messy, and we are constantly changing as we interact with others every day at school, work, home, in communities, in hospitals, and in clinics; as long as we are awake and there is another person in our experience, we are living culture, valuing that culture, and being responsive to that experience or rejecting that experience.

Opportunities for Reflection

Following are four stories to provide an opportunity to be reflective about your own thinking. We suggest that you read the stories, reflect on the questions, and then discuss your responses to the questions with others.

We are introduced to a small woman with whom we have a pleasant exchange and feel she is a "nice woman." We learn later that she is the Chief of Police for one of the largest metropolitan and crime-ridden areas in the country.

- Do we recheck ourselves and our impressions of this person now that we know some characteristics about her were not previously known?
- Is she smart enough, tough enough, and resolute enough to be the Chief of Police? And are we asking this question simply because she is a woman and this does not seem to be a typical woman's job?
- Do we like her or trust her as much now as we did when we first met her?
- Do our cultural values impact our impressions of others?

After only knowing this woman for 3 minutes, we now have a lasting impression of her, and based on our cultural experiences, it could be positive or negative.

Consider a situation where there is a nonverbal 4-year-old child in your summer preschool classroom who does not speak English. You know that he is in your classroom because his parents are migrant workers and that he will only be in your classroom for 3 months before moving on to the next school.

- Does the child's migrant status make a difference in the instruction you provide?
- If this nonverbal boy was the son of the superintendent, would you feel or think differently about putting in the work of developing and then carrying out a plan to support him?

- Does it make a difference if the child is there 1 day or 10 years?
- Is there some leeway to abiding by the code of ethics in this case?

There is the story of a Hmong child who has epilepsy, but the course of treatment puts the parents and doctors radically at odds (Fadiman, 2012). The parents, who do not speak English, believe there is a nonmedical explanation for the seizures. The medical doctors, who are sure they have the best medical procedures to offer, feel the parents are being negligent (Fadiman, 2012).

- If you will never see a Hmong child in your area of the country, should you even bother reading this book?
- Is there anything to learn from this story?
- Does cultural responsiveness come into play at all in a life-and-death medical situation?

Your cultural experiences will dictate your responses to these questions. There is one final story for self-reflection. On your caseload, you now have an individual who was once a male and is now a female named Jackie. Your role is to assist Jackie in creating a new voice and assisting her in using the paralanguage most suited for a woman. If there is an unconscious bias toward gender transitioning, this may be a difficult situation for you (without knowing it). Again, what in your cultural experiences has prepared you to deal with this type of encounter?

- Do you accept the case or do you pass it on?
- If you are the only therapist in the area that works in the area of voice, is it your ethical professional obligation to do this therapy?

- Should Jackie have to live with a low-pitched voice because the one therapist in the area would not see her?
- Are there other ways to manage this case?

Now that you reflected on the questions and on your responses to them, and have discussed your responses with others, what did you learn about yourself? How did these cultural vignettes challenge your own assumptions? Identify ways that you will strive to overcome those challenges.

Unconscious Bias

Unconscious bias is an automatic response (Moule, 2009). Just like we quickly draw back from a hot fire, we also make judgments immediately and without thought in many situations. In one story, a group of human resource staff members were reading resumes to hire someone for a management position in their company. They were provided with similar resumes. The only difference was that some had a female name and some had a male name. More males than females were accepted for the interview for the manager's position. This is an unconscious bias where these individuals perceived that a male would be more likely to do a better job in a managerial role. They were not aware of this bias and were surprised when they were appraised of the results of the study.

This textbook will be useful for persons in the field of communication sciences and disorders; however, cultural responsiveness is a far-reaching concept that goes well beyond any individual field. The cornerstones of this text are four building blocks that will be addressed in each chapter. These building blocks, presented in Figure 1–3, are theoretical foundations, concepts, connections, and

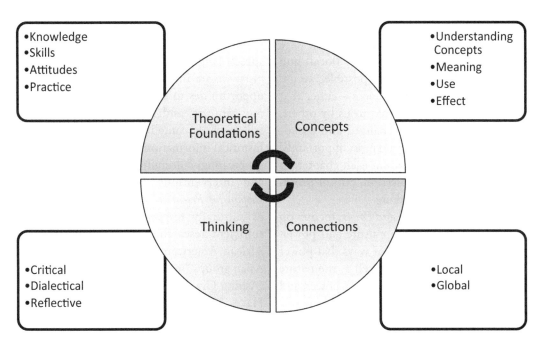

FIGURE 1–3. Building blocks of culturally responsive practices in speech, language, and hearing sciences.

thinking. After we discuss these building blocks, we provide a brief explanation of the content covered in the remaining chapters.

BUILDING BLOCKS OF THIS TEXTBOOK

Each chapter begins with a case study example to help contextualize the topic or situate the topic in real-life events. Although Chapter 3, *Theoretical Frameworks About Culture and Cultural Responsiveness*, is specifically devoted to *theoretical frameworks*, throughout the book, where appropriate, we incorporate the theories behind the ideas. Each chapter begins with a list of the knowledge, skills, and attitudes that can be learned and incorporated into your practice after reading about and reflecting

on the chapter. We are defining knowledge as having collectively produced information, as well as the interest in learning more about a topic (Hyter, Roman, Staley, & McPherson, 2017). Skills refer to the behaviors that one uses to act on what one knows, or has learned. Attitudes, which can be positive or negative, refer to a way of evaluating an event or person or situation (Hyter et al., 2017). Chapter 2, *Definitions*, focuses on **concepts**, where we go into depth defining concepts used throughout the text, and those that are related to cultural responsiveness in the literature. Additionally, at the beginning of each chapter is a list of key words that are defined and explained in the chapter. The goal is for those reading the text to gain an understanding of the meaning of the concepts, be able to use the concepts, and recognize the impact of the concepts within culturally responsive practice. We make **connections** between the material being covered in the text, and real events that have taken place in the United States (local) and in the world (global). When possible, we use personal stories and experiences—either that happened to us or were told to us by others. Names, of course, were changed and pseudonyms are used. Finally, and most importantly, we provide questions within each chapter, to promote critical self-reflection, critical **thinking**, and dialectical thinking.

Chapter 4, *Culture and Power*, focuses on the relationship between culture and power. In this chapter, the different ways that power is exerted are explained, as well as the nature of the relationship among culture, power, and communication. You will learn about the role of language in exerting power, and we underscore the importance of service providers, such as speech-language pathologists and audiologists, being conscious of the power we hold in relationship with those receiving our services. Chapter 5, *Culture and Language*, is about the role of language in transmitting culture from one generation to the next, and the relationship between culture and language. We also discuss linguistic culture—beliefs and values about and around languages—and language policy—how language is legislated, and what legislated language might mean for speakers of some languages. In Chapter 6, *Culture and Hearing Health*, the demographics of those who are hard of hearing or Deaf are reviewed, and the prevalence and incidence of hearing loss is discussed. This chapter includes a discussion about cultural and ethnic differences in the ways groups of people respond to hearing loss, or the extent to which they engage in help-seeking behaviors when they suspect or find out that they have a hearing loss. You will also learn about differences in the use and form of sign language between cultural and ethnic groups.

Chapter 7, *Building Ethnographic Skills*, includes information on ethnographic inter-

viewing, participant observation, and document and artifact analyses. In our role as speech-language pathologists and audiologists, we are in a unique position of having opportunities to engage with clients in various contexts, and these ethnographic skills will certainly come in handy when gathering historical information, and when engaging in (or creating) culturally responsive assessments and interventions. Chapter 8, *Culturally Responsive Research*, is about the importance of culturally responsive research. There is sufficient research published showing that African Americans, Latin@s/Hispanics, and Asian groups "received less and different care" (Ashing-Giwa & Kagawa-Singer, 2006, p. 33; Hayes & Smedley, 1999; Smedley, Stith, & Nelson, 2003). In this chapter, we provide information on processes and outcomes that are essential when conducting research with and about people of color or immigrants in the United States or with communities outside of the United States. We also discuss the importance of engaging in research that addresses all levels of interactions—micro level (individual), meso level (groups and communities, and local practices and policies), and macro level (organizations, institutions, and global practices and policies) (Wylie, 2013). Culturally responsive research will help to eliminate health disparities and better serve communities.

Chapter 9, *Working With Interpreters*, will help you build skills in working with interpreters. This activity is much more than putting words or conversations from one language into another. You will learn about the cultural nuances in interpretation, the proficiencies required of an interpreter, and the collaborative relationship that should exist between a service provider and an interpreter. Chapter 10, *Culturally Responsive Assessment*, and Chapter 11, *Culturally Responsive Intervention*, present information on assessment and intervention methods that are culturally responsive, and include discussions on assessment and intervention methods that can be used rather than or in addition to standardized assessment and treatment programs. We will review information on language differences and disorders, bilingual language development, and cultural aspects of sound production, among other topics.

Chapter 12, *Global Engagement, Sustainability, and Culturally Responsive Practices*, is a strong suggestion for the professions of speech-language pathology and audiology to look beyond the United States, to learn from and about speech, language, and hearing services provided abroad. Right now, as of 2017, there are large numbers of speech-language pathologists looking to work "overseas"; in fact, many from the United States and other countries already do work outside of their home country. There are also countries on every continent that provide speech, language, and hearing services. Additionally, as groups of people move around the world, for various reasons, those working in the service sector, such as educators, doctors, occupational therapists, speech-language pathologists, and audiologists, have multiple opportunities to meet and serve people and families who speak languages, and have world views, beliefs, and values that differ from one's own.

Read, engage with, and reflect on the material in this textbook. We hope that it serves you well as you strive to live a life and provide services that are increasingly culturally responsive.

REFERENCES

Centers for Disease Control and Prevention (CDC). (2016). *U.S. Public Health Service syphilis study at Tuskegee: The Tuskegee timeline.* Retrieved from https://www.cdc.gov/tuskegee/timeline.htm

Chalmers, D. (2006). International medical research regulation: From ethics to law. In S. A. M. McLean (Ed.), *First do no harm: Law, ethics and healthcare* (pp. 81–100). Burlington, VT: Ashgate.

Colby, S., & Ortman, J. M. (2015). *Projections of the size and composition of the U.S. population 2014–2016: Population estimates and projections. Report No. P25-1143.* Retrieved from http://www.census.gov/content/dam/Census/library/publications/2015/demo/p25-1143.pdf

Cross, T. L., Bazron, B. J., Dennis, K. W., & Isaacs, M. R. (1989). *Towards a culturally competent system of care: A monograph of effective services for minority children who are severely emotionally disturbed.* Washington, DC: Georgetown University Child Development Center.

EEOC. (n.d.). *Laws and guidance.* Retrieved from https://www.eeoc.gov/laws/index.cfm

Fadiman, A. (2012). *The spirit catches you and you fall down: A Hmong child, her American doctors and the collision of two cultures.* New York, NY: Farrar, Straus, and Giroux.

Kreps, G., & Kunimoto, E. (1994). *Effective communication in multicultural health care settings.* Thousand Oaks, CA: Sage.

Ladson-Billings, G. (1994). *The dreamkeepers.* San Francisco, CA: Jossey-Bass.

Ladson-Billings, G. (1995). Toward a theory of culturally relevant pedagogy. *American Educational Research Journal, 32*(3), 465–491.

Moule, J. (2009). Understanding unconscious bias and unintentional racism. *The Phi Delta Kappan, 90*(5), 320–326.

Ryan, C. (2013). *Language use in the United States: 2011.* American Community Survey Reports. Retrieved from https://www.census.gov/prod/2013pubs/acs-22.pdf

Smedley, B. D., Stith, A. Y., & Nelson, A. R. (Eds.). (2003). *Unequal treatment: Confronting racial and ethnic disparities in health care.* Washington, DC: National Academy Press.

U.S. Census. (2009–2013). *American Community Survey.* Retrieved from https://www.census.gov/data/tables/2013/demo/2009-2013-lang-tables.html

U.S. Census. (2013). *Arab households in the United States: 2006–2010.* Retrieved from https://www.census.gov/prod/2013pubs/acsbr10-20.pdf

U.S. Census. (2015). *Census Bureau reports at least 350 languages spoken in U.S. homes.* Retrieved from https://www.census.gov/newsroom/press-releases/2015/cb15-185.html

U.S. Census. (2017). *Population clock.* Retrieved from https://www.census.gov/popclock/

Wylie, K., McAllister, L., Davidson, B., & Marshall, J. (2013). Changing practice: Implications of the World Report on Disabilities for responding to communication disability in under-served populations. *International Journal of Speech-Language Pathology, 15*(1), 1–13.

Yang, J. R. (2015). *FY 2016 EEO policy statement.* Retrieved from https://www.eeoc.gov/eeoc/internal/eeo_policy_statement.cfm#fn1

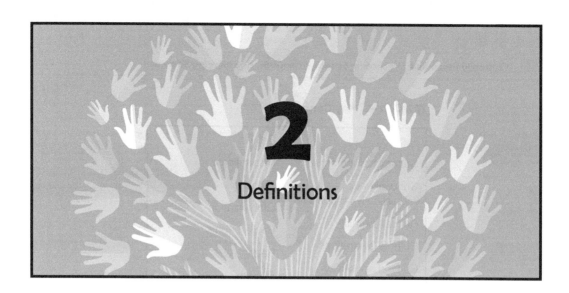

2
Definitions

There are several definitions of cultural responsiveness, and several viewpoints about it. When there are varied definitions of a concept, it is usually because the definitions are situated within diverse theoretical frameworks. The purpose of this chapter is to facilitate a common understanding of concepts pertaining to cultural responsiveness as they are used in different disciplines.

After reading, discussing, and processing the information presented in this chapter, you will be able to demonstrate the following knowledge, skills, and attitudes:

1. Knowledge
   a. Define key concepts relating to culture, cultural responsiveness, and diversity (see the Key Concepts table).
   b. Explain the importance of appropriate usage of the Key Concepts in course work and clinical practice.
2. Skills
   a. Correctly use the Key Concepts in responses to discussion questions and case studies.

   b. Identify important gaps in the literature pertaining to the Key Concepts.
   c. Explain the relationships (similarities and differences) among the Key Concepts.
   d. Recognize and synthesize inconsistencies among Key Concepts and their implementation, through dialogue with peers, professors, and the published literature being consumed.
3. Attitudes
   a. Demonstrate the ability to incorporate the Key Concepts into their daily thinking and writing as demonstrated through journals and portfolio entries of the work they have completed in a variety of courses.

KEY CONCEPTS

It is important for those of us learning about culturally responsive practices and those working in a service profession to have a collective definition of some concepts. The concepts in Table 2–1 serve as the basis for this text and

TABLE 2–1. Key Concepts

Culture	Beliefs
Cultural competence	Disparities
Culturally and linguistically responsive	Ethnicity
	Globalization
Cultural humility	Human rights
Cultural awareness	Race
Cultural sensitivity	Racism
Cultural reciprocity	Linguicism
Critical thinking	Linguistic human rights
Dialectical thinking	Values

will be defined in this chapter, and mentioned throughout the book.

As you review the following case example of a speech-language pathologist (SLP) interacting with the family of a school-age child, take note of

1. The **additional information** the graduate student SLP needs to know to be prepared to provide effective services to children and families in her or his clinical practicum placement.

2. The **professional and cultural knowledge, skills, and attitudes** that the SLP needs to have in her or his repertoire to be able to provide effective services to children and families in her or his clinical practicum placement. (You will have an opportunity to revise your entries at the end of this chapter.)

Box 2–1
Case: Mary Smith

Mary grew up in an upper middle class family in the state of Wyoming and is currently enrolled in the SLP master's program at Wayne State University in Detroit, Michigan. For her first practicum, Mary is assigned to a Head Start classroom, where she is expected to collaborate with the classroom staff in: (1) developing and implementing probes to acquire baseline information about the children's communication and language functioning; (2) developing and implementing classroom-based interventions to support children who present with concerns regarding their limited ability to participate fully in the activities and peer interactions in their classroom environment and beyond; and (3) facilitating the knowledge and utilization of some of these activities by the families of the children enrolled in the Head Start classroom.

Activity 2–1

Take a few minutes to brainstorm with two other classmates, and come up with a list of information that you can insert into both columns of Table 2–2—information, knowledge, skills, and attitudes needed to provide culturally, linguistically, and globally responsive services to the children and families in Mary's Head Start classroom. Keep this chart in mind as you read the remainder of this chapter. At the end of the chapter, once you have processed the Key Concepts and their definitions, you will revise the chart using a different color of ink.

THE CONTEXTS THAT GIVE MEANING TO CULTURE AND CULTURAL RESPONSIVENESS

All concepts need to be thought about in the context in which we live and work. Context is what gives meaning to anything and everything (Bruner, 1983). One of the most well-known theories that underscores the importance of context is Bronfenbrenner's (1979, 1986) Ecological Systems Theory (Figure 2–1). In this theory, Bronfenbrenner identifies the contexts that directly or indirectly influence child development and outcomes as occurring at multiple and reciprocal levels and within interdependent systems. For example, the microsystem, the context that is directly connected to or related to the child, could include the child's emotional or sensory regulation, or the child's family members. Interactions and structures that are part of the microsystem have a bidirectional influence; that is, the child can affect his or her parents, and the parents can influence the child (Bronfenbrenner, 2005). The exosystem refers to structures that indirectly affect the child, because they influence microsystem structures or relationships. An example of an exosystem is the work schedule of a parent, which directly affects the parent, but indirectly affects child (Bronfenbrenner, 2005).

These systems are at the micro level (e.g., internal influences that are often at the level of individuals, such as the cognitive development of a child or the relationship between sounds in a word produced by a child), meso level (e.g., external influences usually among or within groups, such as the interactions among immigrant children from Laos and their U.S. counterparts in Michigan), and the macro level (e.g., the farthest level of external

TABLE 2–2. Activity 2–1

Information Needed	Knowledge, Skills, and Attitudes Needed
•	•
•	•
•	•
•	•
•	•
•	•

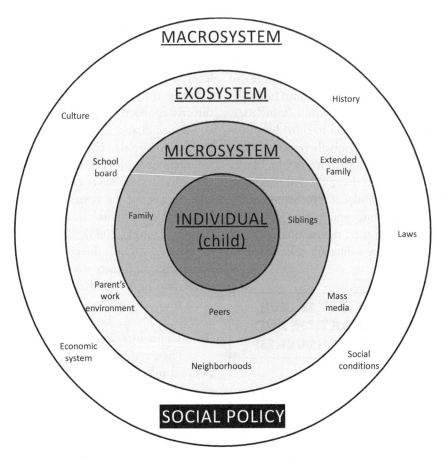

FIGURE 2–1. Bronfenbrenner's Ecological Systems. Based on Bronfenbrenner, 1979. Illustrated by Severin Provance.

influences, at the level of societies, as well as interactions among nation-states) (Blackstone, 2012; Hyter, 2014; Weiss, Kreider, Lopez, & Chatman, 2005; Wiley, McAllister, Davidson, & Marshall, 2013)

In this chapter, we discuss three primary contexts important for continuing to move along the continuum of cultural responsiveness: (1) the current phase and multidimensionality of globalization, which require SLPs and audiologists (AUDs) to be aware of how these processes affect economic, political, social/cultural, and ecological aspects of our clients' lives; (2) the changing demographics

of the world, the United States, and our professions in order to be prepared to be effective service providers consistent with this demographic change; and (3) the state of communication disabilities according to the World Health Organization (WHO) World Report on Disability (2011) and the WHO's International Classification of Functioning, Disability, and Health (WHO-ICF, 2002). It is important for SLPs and audiologists to be aware of multiple factors that facilitate and/or hinder clients' health, health concerns, and outcomes, as well as their ability to function and participate in daily living contexts.

Globalization and Its Multidimensional Effects

Globalization is most often defined as the process of increasing interdependence among countries due to more fluid borders and technological advances (Steger, 2010). This process has multiple dimensions such as economic, political, social/cultural, and ecological (see definitions, Table 2–3). Globalization is the intensification and expansion of these interdependencies across the globe (Steger, 2010). On the face of it, globalization sounds good —like a worthwhile and necessary advancement for humanity. There are also, however, bad and ugly sides to this process. Globalization is an uneven process that affects countries differently. For example, high-income countries (e.g., United States, countries in Europe) are often the beneficiaries of globalization, whereas low-income countries are frequently victimized by global processes (Akindele, Gidado, & Olaopo, 2002; Daouas, 2001; Gibson, 2004; Steger, 2010).

Let's consider Jamaica as an example. The negative consequences of globalization on the lives of the citizens of Jamaica are documented in a film by Stephanie Black (2001) called "Life & Debt" (http://www.lifeanddebt.org/). In this film, it is reported that Jamaican authorities needed to take on loans from the International Monetary Fund (IMF) and World Bank (WB) because when the British pulled out of the country in 1962, after a long and protracted history of slavery and colonization, the country was left impoverished, and many citizens were illiterate (Mordecai & Mordecai, 2001). One of the prime ministers of Jamaica (Michael Manley, 1972–1980 and 1989–1992) needed to take out loans from the IMF and WB, which were accompanied by several severe conditions, including liberalizing trade, privatizing public services, and deregulating the economy.

As a result of trade liberalization, potato companies and milk companies outside of Jamaica could import and sell their goods in Jamaica for less money than the Jamaican potato and dairy farmers could sell their goods within their own country (Black, 2001). As a result, several local (Jamaican) businesses were not able to compete on the international market, which caused job loss and impoverishment. Privatization of public services meant that public schools, hospitals, and utilities, for example, were sold to private companies or organizations, often resulting in lower wages or job losses for workers in those facilities, less accountability of the owners to the public, and higher costs for the services supplied by these privatized entities (Akindele et al., 2002). Deregulation usually goes hand in

TABLE 2–3. Definitions of Economics, Politics, Social, and Ecological

Term	Definition
Economics[a]	Access to resources (goods and services)
Politics[a]	Exercise of power in one's own interest and/or the interest of one's own group
Social[b]	A historical set of collective economic, political, and cultural experiences that shape current relationships
Ecological[c]	The relationship between groups of people and their local and global environment (i.e., air, climate, food, water)

Sources: [a]Hyter, 2014, p. 114. [b]Hyter, 2007, p. 131. [c]Begon, Howarth, & Townsend, 2014; Steger, 2010.

hand with privatization. Deregulation means that government laws were removed to reduce barriers to economic competition. Although more competition (the goal of deregulation) proposes to provide lower costs to consumers, this process can create problems with respect to how hazardous material is managed, for example, and could result in unregulated monopolies (Khan, 2016).

The consequences of globalization are uneven and frequently result in limited access to resources such as fresh and healthy food (Patel, 2008) and health care (Therborn, 2006), contributing to forced and voluntary movement of groups of people from their homeland across borders into other countries (Delgado-Wise, 2013; International Organization for Migration, 2011; Tenorino, 2013; UN News Center, 2013). As part of human nature, those migrating from one part of the world to another carry with them their economic, political, and cultural values, assumptions, and worldviews. It is important for speech-language pathologists and audiologists to be aware of the effects of these global processes on clients, as well as be able to integrate the diversity of cultural histories, values and worldviews into clinical practice (Hyter, 2014, p. 105). Globalization is one of the essential contexts of which SLPs and audiologists need to be aware. Another context pertains to the global and, therefore, local changing demographics, health disparities around the world and in the United States, and the World Health Organization's (2002) International Classification of Functioning, Disability, and Health. Each of these contexts is discussed below.

Changing Demographics Around the World

Demographics of the world are undergoing shifts and changes. As of the 2010 census in the United States, 50% of children younger than 5 years of age are African American and/or Latin@/Hispanic. It is estimated that in 4 years, by 2020, over half of the people in the United States under the age of 18 years will be people of color or people from ethnicities other than European (Colby & Ortman, 2015). Furthermore, the population in the United States is growing older, meaning that the working age of the population will decrease over the next several years. By 2030, one in five citizens of the United States are projected to be over 65 years of age. Additionally, the number of people living in the United States who were born in another country is projected to increase. The U.S. Census projects that by 2060, the "native born" population is expected to decrease by 22%, and the "foreign born" population will increase by 85% (Colby & Ortman, 2015, p. 2). Population growths and changes also are occurring in other parts of the world. As only one example, the population of the second largest continent in the world, Africa, is projected to double by 2050, while at the same time Europe's population is projected to decrease (Bish, 2016). Although the demographics of the United States are becoming more diverse, the fields of SLP and audiology are predominately White, female, and monolingual. According to the Member and Affiliate Counts of the American Speech-Language-Hearing Association (ASHA, 2016a), in 2015, there were 173,530 SLPs, audiologists, speech scientists, and hearing scientists registered as members of ASHA. There are 468 international affiliates, meaning that these are individuals living outside of the United States but who are associated with ASHA. Males comprise only 4.8% of the ASHA members, people of color only 7.8%, and Latin@s/Hispanics only 4.7% of the membership. Six percent of the membership qualify to provide bilingual services (ASHA, 2016b). These changing demographics around the world and in the United States urge SLPs and audiologists to be prepared to serve a more culturally and linguistically diverse population, and to make connections linking local and global concerns.

Health Disparities and the Goal of Health Equity

Health disparities occur when there are differences in health outcomes between groups of people (CDC, 2013). Health disparities are often associated with economic, social, and environmental disadvantages. Health disparities negatively affect groups of people "who have systematically experienced greater obstacles to health," due to some social characteristic such as race, gender, age, sexual orientation, language use, or others typically linked with exclusion (HHS, 2008). The goal for health care providers and others in the service sector, including SLPs and audiologists, is to strive for health equity for the people and families with whom we work. **Health equity** is the realization of the highest level of health for everyone, which requires professionals and government offices to make "ongoing societal efforts to address avoidable inequalities, historical and contemporary injustices, and the elimination of health and health care disparities" (CDC, 2010).

World Health Organization's International Classification of Functioning Disability and Health (WHO-ICF)

The WHO-ICF is an international system that provides a standardized language and way of classifying functioning and disability in relationship to health (Threats, 2006, 2010). The WHO-ICF model (Figure 2–2) is composed of two sections. The first section includes the health condition (e.g., com-

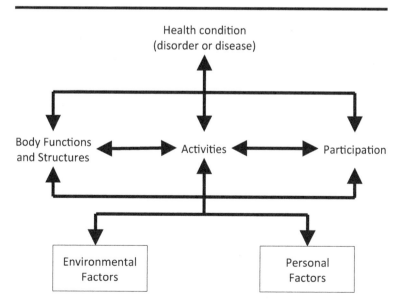

FIGURE 2–2. WHO-ICF Framework. Reprinted with permission from World Health Organization. (2007) *International Classification of Functioning, Disability, and Health: Children and Youth Version: ICF-CY.* Geneva, Switzerland: WHO Press.

munication disorder), body functions (the functions of the human biological systems and psychological functions), body structures (physical components of the body such as articulators), and activities and participation, referring to the daily living activities in which people engage. The second section of the WHO-ICF model focuses on the contextual factors that can facilitate or hinder health outcomes or full participation in daily life (Howe, 2008). These contextual factors are composed of every aspect of life. Contextual factors include environmental and personal aspects of life. Environmental factors occur at the individual and societal levels but are not necessarily within the control of the person but are vital to communication (Howe, 2008; Threats, 2000). Individual environmental factors include such issues as one's living, learning (e.g., school) or work environment, and access to resources such as technology; whereas the societal environmental factors consist of service, health, and educational systems and the policies within these systems (Howe, 2008; WHO, 2002). Personal factors include a person's health status, and other characteristics such as race, gender, sexual orientation, or age. It is important for SLPs and audiologists to have a significant understanding of how contextual factors may contribute to, facilitate, or prevent one's full functioning and participation in daily life.

In a local context affected by global issues—there are increased interdependencies among nations—it is essential for SLPs and audiologists to engage in macro practice (Hyter, 2012, 2014; Worrall, 2010). Macro practice is the ability to incorporate work at the societal level rather than only at the individual or familial level (Netting, Kettner, McMurtry, & Thomas, 2012). To be prepared for providing effective services across multiple levels, multiple cultures, and worldviews, SLPs

and audiologists need to continue to move along the continuum of cultural responsiveness. This text will facilitate that movement.

World Report on Disability

The World Report on Disability (WHO & World Bank, 2011) was designed to report on the prevalence[1] of disabilities in the world. In this report, it is estimated that approximately 15% of the world's populations (~1 billion people) has some form of a disability. This report, as wonderful as it is, may not have accurately made an account of people with communication disabilities (Wiley, McAllister, Davidson, & Marshall, 2013). Wiley and her colleagues call for SLPs and audiologists to understand and tackle communication disabilities across populations rather than only individually (p. 2).

DEFINING CONCEPTS

Essential Concepts and Their Definitions

In this next section of Chapter 2, we are going to define several concepts that will be used throughout the text. We believe it is important for SLPs and audiologists to have a shared vocabulary or shared notion of concepts. The concepts are listed as key words at the beginning of the chapter but are repeated here: culture, cultural competence, culturally and linguistically responsive, cultural humility, cultural awareness, cultural sensitivity, cultural reciprocity, critical thinking, dialectical thinking, beliefs, disparities, ethnicity, globalization, human rights, race, racism, linguicism, linguistic human rights, and values. Definitions for some

---

[1]Prevalence and incidence are defined in Chapter 6.

of these concepts will be discussed together, but the concepts will be written in bold text, and many will appear again throughout the text.

We begin by defining culture. **Culture** is a word frequently used in a variety of educational and clinical settings, although how culture is defined is widely variable. We like to use the definition of culture highlighted in the writings of Ting-Toomey and Chung (2012) in communication studies. In general, they compare culture to an iceberg. While looking at Figure 2–3, take a minute to think about an iceberg. What do you know about an iceberg? How is it constructed?

Like with an iceberg, there are visible or external as well as invisible or internal aspects of culture. These visible or external aspects of culture include such things as rituals, traditions, religious practices, language use, forms of dress, and hairstyles. The invisible or internal aspects of culture, in our professional opinion, are what truly make up culture, and include underlying values, beliefs, assumptions, and worldviews held by a person and his or her group. It is these internal, invisible, and often unconscious aspects of culture that drive the visible aspect of culture—the external behaviors and practices. It is difficult to name these aspects of culture because we do

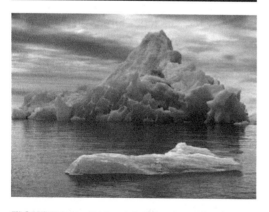

FIGURE 2–3. Iceberg. Image courtesy of Leroy Hyter, Sr., 1997.

not consciously think of why we do what we do, and from where certain beliefs and behaviors come. Let's try a little activity that will facilitate your understanding of these visual and invisible aspects of culture.

Activity 2–2

- First, make a list of the visible, conscious, and obvious aspects of your own culture.
- Second, next to the list of visible behaviors or practices, write what is the underlying value and belief maintained in that behavior or practice.

Being able to use critical self-reflection and to identify your own cultural values, beliefs, and assumptions is a critical first step in moving toward cultural responsiveness. Values are derived from cultural histories and realities (shared experiences) and indicate what practices or behaviors comprise a group's shared and deeply rooted ideals about the way things should be (Martin & Nakayama, 2000). If we examine the U.S. Declaration of Independence, the preamble written by Thomas Jefferson (one of the primary writers of the U.S. Declaration of Independence, and served as President of the United States in early 1800s) states, "We hold these truths to be self-evident, that all men are created equal, that they are endowed by their Creator with certain unalienable rights, that among these are life, liberty and the pursuit of happiness" (U.S. National Archives and Records Administration, 2016). The deeply rooted ideal about the way things should be is indicated in the phrase, "all men are created equal." What we do know, however, is that, in reality, at that time (and even now) not all men (or women) are *treated* equally. Jefferson enslaved people of African descent, which shows that although he penned the words "all men are created equal," he did not live up to that value. Another value evident in that first sentence of the U.S. Declaration of Independence is that these equally created men were "endowed with certain unalienable rights." "Unalienable" or inalienable rights are those rights of each U.S. citizen, such as the right to practice religion, or to have equal protection of laws, or to have freedom of speech. We know that these rights are the ideal that should exist but do not exist for many citizens in the United States. For example, in 2017 alone, 16 or more state legislative sessions' bills were introduced that would discriminate against the lesbian, gay, bisexual, transgender, intersexual, and asexual community, and recent anti-Muslim sentiment has been expressed in several ways including attempts by the current government to ban Muslims from traveling and/or immigrating to the United States (ACLU, 2017; Oxborrow, 2017). A **belief** is an idea that something is true or real, or that something is not true or real. In this vein, beliefs can be positive as well as negative. Some in the United States believe that all men have equal rights; others, based on their cultural history and shared historical experiences, do not hold that belief, although they may hold that value. An **assumption** is an unquestioned belief—that is, the belief in something to be true even when there is no proof of its truth. In the field of SLP in the United States, we often have the assumption that parents need to talk to their child from infancy for the child to develop language skills. There are data showing that this assumption might be true; however, in other parts of the world, parents do not talk directly to their child; yet, the child develops language adequately. Keep in mind that there are multiple definitions of culture, some of which are discussed in Chapter 3 when we examine some of the cultural frameworks developed by anthropologists, ethnographers, educators, intercultural communication scholars, sociologists, and speech-language pathologists.

Like culture, **culturally responsive practices** are defined in multiple ways (Srivastava,

2007). The concept of cultural competence itself is controversial and often misunderstood. We discuss the controversy later in this chapter. The term, culturally responsive was coined by educator Gloria Ladson-Billings (1994, 1995), but it is in the field of nursing where many advances in culturally responsive practices have been made in the health-related fields. The nursing literature defines culturally responsive care as "explicit use of culturally based care and health knowledge in sensitive, creative, and meaningful ways" (Leninger, 2002, p. 84). Burchum (2002) states that culturally responsive practice is the ability to apply learned knowledge and acquired skills in an effective manner. The most frequently quoted definition of culturally responsive practice, however, comes from Cross, Bazron, Dennis, and Isaacs (1989), who write in the domain of mental health services. They use the term *cultural competence* and define it as "a set of congruent behaviors, attitudes, and policies that come together in a system, agency or among professionals and enable that system, agency or those professions to work effectively in cross-cultural situations" (p. 7). Cross et al. (1989) emphasize that "competence" implies having the capacity to be effective. They also state that there are five "essential elements" that facilitate increasing culturally responsive practices, and these elements should be institutionalized at all levels of an organization/system, which includes hiring practices, policy making, administrative duties, and service provision. The five elements are: (1) valuing diversity, (2) having the capacity for cultural self-assessment, (3) being conscious of the dynamics inherent when cultures interact, (4) having institutionalized culture knowledge, and (5) having developed adaptations to service delivery reflecting an understanding of cultural diversity (Cross et al., 1989, p. 8). The Cross et al. definition also has been adapted and amended to some degree by the National Center for Cultural Competence

(NCCC, n.d.). The NCCC emphasizes that cultural competence is not a location but is a developmental and dynamic process where an organization, individual, or group of professionals go through various levels of awareness, knowledge, and skills along a cultural continuum. This idea of a cultural continuum is also inherent in the Cross et al. definition; NCCC underscores this idea. This discussion about cultural competence occurring on a continuum is also the source of a great deal of discussion in the literature on cultural competence and cultural humility.

Some scholars reject the concept of cultural competence stating that it sets up a false expectation that one arrives at a single point of competence (e.g., I know I need to learn more about other cultures; therefore, I am now culturally competent). This rejection of the concept of cultural competence is due to a misunderstanding of the term. We believe that inherent in the concept of cultural competence is its dynamic, ever-developing, nature. One never completely reaches a point of cultural competence, but rather continues to evolve over time to move along a cultural competence continuum. Campinha-Bacote (2011) state that one is "*becoming* culturally competent rather than *being* culturally competent." Rather than risking the readers' misunderstanding of the foundation of this text, we are using the term **culturally responsive practices** rather than cultural competence. The model of culturally responsive practices that we use includes several components, or steps if you will, which helps us move along the continuum of becoming more effective in providing services across cultures. This movement is not a linear direction but is more akin to a circular and iterative process (Figure 2–4).

The continuum of culturally responsive practices can be likened to a circular staircase, where each step is another stage on the continuum (Figure 2–5). The first step on the continuum of culturally responsive practice[2]

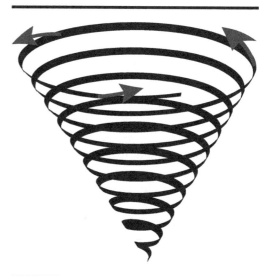

FIGURE 2–4. The iterative process of cultural responsiveness. Illustrated by Severin Provance.

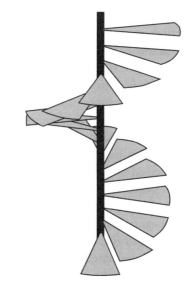

FIGURE 2–5. A circular staircase of cultural competence. Illustrated by Severin Provance.

---

[2]The continuum of culturally responsive practice is adapted from the continuum of global competence from Hyter (2014, pp. 115–116).

is cultural humility—the ability to recognize that there are diverse and valuable cultures, and the willingness to learn from others (Ortega & Faller, 2011). Approaching service provision from a position of cultural humility puts service providers in a position to be humble enough to learn from their clients and their clients' families—to learn their perspectives, needs, concerns, and material conditions that affect their clients' daily lives.

The second step on the continuum is self-awareness, the ability to engage in critical self-reflection, to deconstruct your own cultural assumptions, and to identify your own cultural values (Campinha-Bacote, 1991). To be able to employ this type of self-reflection, one needs to be able to think critically and dialectically. **Critical thinking** is the ability to see what is not there, and to challenge the status quo. Brookfield (2012) explains that critical thinking is when you can: (1) identify assumptions that support long-held beliefs and values, (2) challenge your own assumptions, (3) recognize the context that shapes and/or maintains those assumptions, and (4) identify alternatives to those assumptions. Critical thinking is closely related to dialectical thinking. **Dialectical thinking** deals with resolving contradictions and recognizing that the "truth" is dynamic or fluid rather than fixed. To think dialectically, one must be able to turn what seems like the truth on its head. In other words, you would need to separate what is perceived to be reality, to then think in a different manner (Calincos, 2007), negating what already seems to exist, which allows room for imagining another reality (Kellner, 1991; Marcuse, 1991).

Cultural knowledge is the third step, and this means to make consistent efforts to learn about the cultures, cultural histories, and worldviews of groups of people who are culturally different from you. Campinha-Bacote (2002, 2011) suggests that this cultural knowledge should be acquired through educational sources, which we translate into

documentaries and published and vetted literature. Moreover, others emphasize that this cultural knowledge should focus on learning the cultural beliefs, values, and behaviors of others, as well as the incidence and prevalence of communication disorders (Lavizzo-Mourey, 1996).

The fourth step is cultural reciprocity. Cultural reciprocity is a concept that comes out of the field of special education (Kalyanpur & Harry, 2012). Cultural reciprocity is the capacity to use critical and dialectical thinking to collaborate with clients and their families to develop intervention options that are consistent with their cultural values. To provide services from a posture of reciprocity, you would need to be able to identify the underlying assumptions of the intervention approaches you propose, identify the inconsistencies between those approaches and the family's cultural values, and discover how to modify those approaches to be more consistent with the family's cultural values and with the cultural values of your profession (Hyter, 2014).

The ultimate goal of moving along the culturally responsive practices continuum is the ability to provide culturally and globally responsive services that are effective for families receiving the services. Again, responsive services refer to a continuous and "ongoing process of self-reflection and reciprocity" (Hyter, 2014, p. 115), allowing service providers to move toward the goal and inching closer to the ideal of engaging in clinical practice in a manner that is in harmony with the cultural histories, beliefs, values, and worldviews of our clients and their families.

In addition to defining culturally responsive practices, we define other concepts that are essential for understanding and communicating across cultures, and for providing culturally and globally responsive services. Those concepts are ethnicity, race, racism, linguicism, human rights, and linguistic human rights.

People often confuse the meanings of ethnicity and race. Sometimes when defining culture, some will identify race or ethnicity as an aspect of culture. As with the other concepts discussed in this chapter, **ethnicity** has several definitions. Most define ethnicity as a social group with shared nationalities and traditions, such as "kinship, family rituals, food preferences" and celebrations (Srivastava, 2007, p. 12). Sometimes ethnicity is conflated with race. **Race**, however, refers to biological attributes, and ethnicity is associated with cultural or national attributes. Let us be more clear here. Ethnicity and culture are not the same thing, but groups who share ethnicity may also share culture. Let's get back to race. Race typically refers to physical attributes of a group of people, such as skin color, hair texture, and body shape. Race has been used as a tool to justify the abuse, exploitation, domination, inequality, and marginalization of some groups and the unwarranted privilege of others.[3] In this way, race is considered to be socially constructed (e.g., Omi & Winant, 1994)—that is "understandings of race are . . . social constructions imposed by dominant groups . . . " (Elias & Feagin, 2016, p. 133) that shape how people think about and respond to groups with physical characteristics different than their own. Using race to justify inequality leads to racism. Race is often perceived as a factor about persons who are of African, Asian, First Nations, and Latin@/Hispanic descent, but it is also a social construction of people who are White. The concept of "whiteness" was created when the "colonists who sought to view First Nations and Blacks as physically (*as well as intellectually and morally*) different (*inferior*)[4] from themselves." (Pinder, 2012, p. ix). To this day, whiteness organizes the social, political, economic, and cultural experiences of all people living in the United States (Pinder, 2012).

Racism is often defined as racial prejudice plus power (Crossroads Anti-Racism Organizing and Training, 2017). Prejudice means to pre-judge something (or someone) and refers to an "attitude, emotion or behavior towards members of a group, which directly or indirectly implies some negativity or antipathy toward that group" (Brown, 2011, p. 7). We all have prejudices or biases, even if we consciously do not act on them. It is the combination of racial prejudice plus *power* that is really detrimental. **Power** is when a group dominates another and then makes decisions in the interest of one's own group (Hyter, 2014). There are also structural systems (e.g., economic, political, and social) that work together to convince the dominated group(s) to act *against* their own interests. Racism still has a strong hold in the United States and refers to a group of practices that result in a hierarchical relationship among people of differing races.

Racism usually occurs in multiple forms including institutional and structural racism, as well as linguistic racism. **Institutional racism** is the privilege and power of some groups of people, and the disadvantage of other groups based on race that occurs when racial inequities take place within institutional policies and practices such as during college admissions policies or hiring practices. Because institutional racism operates with the sanction of the institution, it is not overtly noticeable, particularly by those who are not negatively affected by those practices. One example of institutional racism occurs in the schooling system in the United States. Although Black children comprise 18% of the preschool population, they are 50% of the preschoolers who are suspended (Nesbitt, 2015). There are similar disproportionate representations of children of color in special education, and in the judicial

---

[3]To truly understand race and its construction in the United States, one needs to understand the history of the country in relationship to slavery. These topics, of course, are beyond the scope of this chapter. Suggestions for further reading are listed at the end of the chapter.
[4]The italicized text was added by Hyter and Salas-Provance.

institutions. **Structural racism**, on the other hand, is the "interaction of multiple institutions in an ongoing process of producing racialized outcomes" (powell, 2008, p. 791).[5] For example, various institutions or systems (e.g., schooling, housing, judicial, transportation, health care) interact resulting in some groups profiting and receiving privileged outcomes and others paying the costs. For example, public schools in urban areas are often underfunded (i.e., housing policy is schooling policy according to powell, in that low-income housing results in lower tax monies available to fund some neighborhood schooling systems [Turner, Khrais, Lloyd, Olgin, Isensee, Vevea, & Carsen, 2016]). In addition to underfunded schools for some children, their neighborhoods are heavily patrolled by police, and typical childhood behavior is often criminalized resulting in young children being arrested or ending up with criminal records simply because of the institutional structures. Structural racism can be implicated in disparate infant mortality rates (Wallace, Crear-Perry, Richardson, Tarver, & Theall, 2017), school to prison pipeline (Reynolds, 2015), and health disparities (Benson & Yeun, 2014) among other issues. When there are persistent disparities among groups across multiple systems, that is structural racism (Hinson, Healey, & Weisenberg, n.d., p. 15). Racism is not only relegated to the color of a person's skin, or to a neighborhood where one grows up; it can also be applied to language.

Linguistic racism was called **linguicism** by Robert Phillipson (1992). Specifically, he defines linguicism as attributing positive characteristics to a desired language (e.g., English) and negative characteristics to a dominated language (e.g., Hmong). A type of linguicism is **linguistic imperialism**—that is, when there is "an imperialist structure of exploitation of one society by another" (p. 55), such as when the French language was imposed on the colonies of France in West Africa dur-

ing the 19th century. Much like racism, linguicism infringes on the basic human rights of people.

Human rights are attributed to every single human being regardless of one's race, gender, sexual orientation, ethnicity, nationality, religion, economic status, educational attainment, or any other position (OHCHR, 1996–2016). Having the right to your own language, to be educated in your own language, to have your language respected, and to have the right to learn another language are all aspects of **linguistic human rights** (Skutnabb-Kangas & Phillipson, 1994). An example of a family's linguistic human rights being violated can be found at the link in Box 2–2. Please note that the video presents xenophobia at its worst and may be very unsettling. In the following example, a mother and her college-age son wait for a table at a local restaurant in California and are engaged in a private conversation when they are berated for speaking Spanish. The woman doing the berating seems to be operating from the assumption that speaking a language other than English is un-American. John McWhorter (2015), professor of linguistics at Columbia University and who has published several books on languages of the world including English, says that the fear of other languages taking over English is unfounded. English is not under threat, but in reality, it is a global or world language—a language that is increasingly used for international communication, business interactions, and publications of scientific research (Ammon, 2010; Phillipson, 2008).

Box 2–2
Link to Example of Violation of Linguistic Human Rights

http://www.nbclosangeles.com/news/local/IHOP-English-Spanish-Rant-320609602.html

---

[5]john a. powell does not capitalize the first initials in his name.

Being able to communicate and having opportunities to communicate are also human rights. In 2014, over 38 professional associations of SLPs and audiologists around the world joined together to develop the **International Communication Project** (ICP). This advocacy project is based on the premise that communicating is a human right. Specifically, on the ICP website it states that "communication is vital to life, but largely ignored as a disability" (see http://www.internationalcommunicationproject.com/about-icp/).

As future communication sciences and disorders professionals, it is imperative for us to understand the relationship between human rights, language, and communication opportunities. Part of increasing our cultural competence is based on our recognizing and acting on our responsibility to advocate for the rights of individuals, groups of individuals who have communication disabilities and limited opportunities to communicate in their strongest language or using their most proficient communication mode.

CHAPTER SUMMARY

Ambiguous definitions of concepts related to culturally responsive practices can make it difficult to conceptualize and implement the knowledge one learns, as well as acquire the skills and attitudes necessary to be culturally responsive. For this reason, this chapter focused on the important task of defining concepts that will be used throughout this text and showing how these concepts are related to culturally responsive practices. To understand cultural responsiveness, it is essential to understand the context in which we currently live, and how that context affects service delivery. We discussed the contexts of globalization, demographic changes in the United States and abroad, communication disabilities in the

world, and the WHO's International Classification of Functioning, Disability, and Health. Engaging in culturally responsive practices is much more than being "respectful" of others. It includes, "challenging systemic barriers and changing the existing structures, practices, (and policies[6]) that perpetuate intolerance, oppressing and inequity" (Srivastava, 2007, p. 23). Learning and using clearly defined concepts while engaging in culturally responsive practices will help minimize confusion about culture, race, ethnicity, linguistic imperialism, and human rights.

EXTENDED LEARNING

Below are a few activities that are designed to highlight the knowledge, skills, and attitudes you should have acquired and developed from reading this chapter. Completing the following activities will help you begin to utilize the concepts explained in this chapter in your daily interactions with your peers, as well as clients and their families.

- Think of yourself as a cultural being

    We have adapted and then extended this activity from our colleague, Dr. Bea Staley, who is currently a SLP and lecturer in Education at Charles Darwin University in Australia. This activity is designed to facilitate your conscious and continual thinking about your own cultural assumptions, beliefs, and values.

- Make a drawing about how you perceive yourself as a cultural being.
    □ Make sure you include in your drawing pictures that exemplify your underlying cultural assumptions, beliefs, and values.
    □ Review this drawing once per month, and add to it (or delete from it) pictures

---

[6]The parenthetical phrase was added by Hyter and Salas-Provance.

as you gain clarity about your own cultural assumptions, beliefs, and values. This iterative editing process is essential for being a critically reflective lifelong learner.

A recent example of such a drawing, although the purpose of the drawing is not the same, is a drawing of a tenth-grade high school student in Washington, DC, who drew an award-winning doodle for Google. You can read more about the student and her drawing here (http://www.usatoday.com/story/tech/news/2016/03/21/google-4-doodle-winner-honors-black-heritage-akilah-johnson/8203 0582/). Also, refer to Figure 2–6 as an example of one of Hyter's drawings.

Figures 2–7A and B, 2–8A and B, and 2–9A and B are six drawings from three graduate students in Dr. Hyter's course on culturally responsive practices. Drawing A was completed on the first day of class, and drawing B was completed on the final day of class. You can see the changes in the way the students understood themselves as cultural beings over the course of the semester.

■ Engaging in critical and dialectical thinking

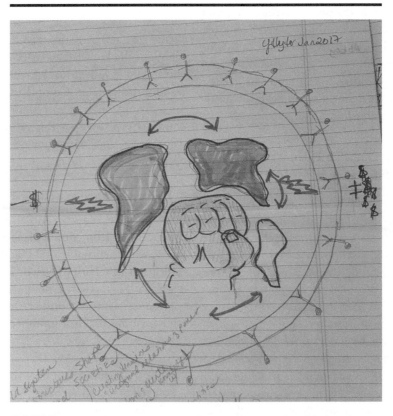

FIGURE 2–6. Hyter's illustration of herself as a cultural being. Image courtesy of Hyter, 2017.

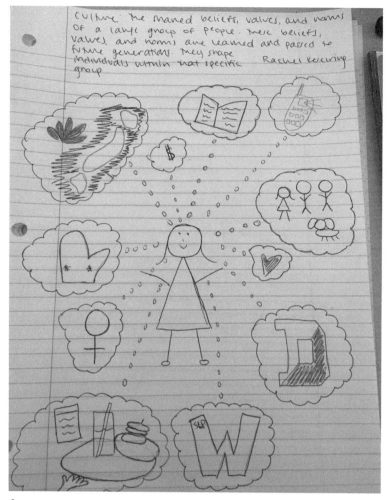

A

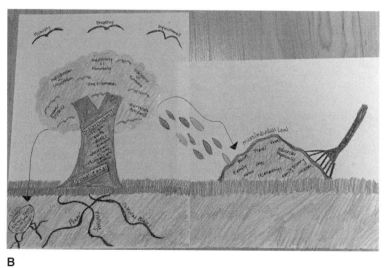

B

FIGURE 2–7. Cultural being example. Images courtesy of Rachel Margaret Keselring.

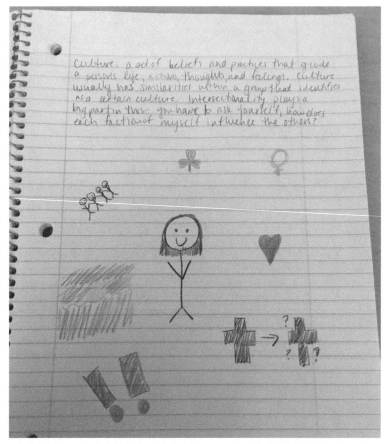

A

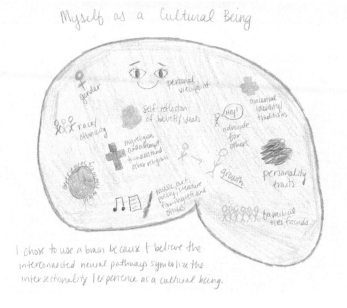

B

FIGURE 2–8. Cultural being example. Images courtesy of Jennifer Elise Otwell.

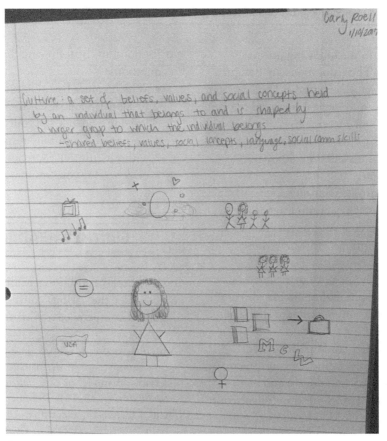

A

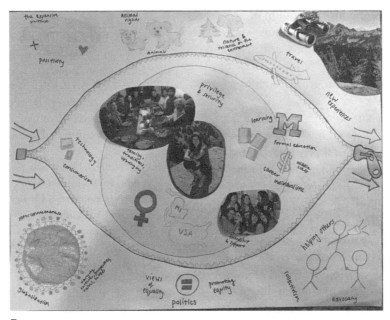

B

FIGURE 2–9. Cultural being example. Images courtesy of Carly MacKay Roell.

□ Respond to the following journal prompts. These questions are designed to challenge your long-held beliefs. You should plan to journal (respond to one question) on a weekly basis. Utilize your responses to write a critical self-reflection paper that includes the following components:

● Demonstrate your increased awareness of yourself as a cultural being, by

○ identifying your own cultural assumptions and where those assumptions came from,

○ how they may be interpreted by your peers and/or clients who are from a culture different than your own,

○ how they could positively and negatively influence your practice as a SLP or audiologist, and

○ how those assumptions affect your skills as a SLP or audiologist, and your relationship with others.

□ Develop an initial plan for continuing to move along the continuum of cultural competence (e.g., how you will modify your assumptions, attitudes, and behaviors).

● Evidence of your growth should include

○ an evolution of your cultural worldview—how it came to be, what historical events facilitated this worldview, and an ability to include a critique of long-held cultural assumptions;

○ your conceptual framework of practice including concepts and their connections, even if it is still under development; and

○ a discussion of cultural dimensions and macrostructure contexts, including Key Concepts in this text (definitions and connections).

□ Respond to the following discussion questions:

● Which comes first, Cultural Responsiveness or Cultural Humility? Provide evidence for your response.

● Can one be culturally responsive without cultural awareness? Provide evidence for your response.

FURTHER READING

You may find the additional readings helpful as you consider the various concepts pertaining to cultural competence in SLP and audiology.

Campinha-Bacote, J. (2002). The process of cultural competence in the delivery of healthcare services: A model of care. *Journal of Transcultural Nursing, 13,* 181–184.

Chengu, G. (2015, December 18). How slaves built American capitalism. *Counterpunch.* Retrieved from http://www.counterpunch.org/2015/12/18/how-slaves-built-american-capitalism/

Hyter, Y. D. (2014). Conceptual frameworks for responsive global engagement in communication sciences and disorders. *Topics in Language Disorders, 34*(2), 103–120.

Kalyanpur, M., & Harry, B. (2012). *Cultural reciprocity in special education: Building family-professional relationships.* Baltimore, MD: Paul H. Brookes.

Pinder, S. O. (2012). *Whiteness and racialized ethnic groups in the United States: The politics of remembering.* Boulder, CO: Lexington Books.

National Center for Cultural Competence: Website of Georgetown University Center for Child and Human Development. Retrieved from http://nccccurricula.info/culturalcompetence.html

Ortega, R. M., & Faller, K. C. (2011). Training child welfare workers from an intersectional cultural humility perspective: A paradigm shift. *Child Welfare, 90*(5), 27–49.

REFERENCES

Akindele, S. T., Gidado, T. O., & Olaopo, O. R. (2002). Globalisation, its implications and consequences for Africa. *Globalization, 2*(1). Retrieved from http://globalization.icaap.org/content/v2.1/01_akindele_etal.html

American Civil Liberties Union (ACLU). (2017). *Legislation affecting LGBT rights across the country.* Retrieved from https://www.aclu.org/other/legislation-affecting-lgbt-rights-across-country#antitrans

American Speech-Language-Hearing Association. (2016a). *ASHA summary membership and affiliation counts, year-end 2015.* Retrieved from http://www.asha.org

American-Speech-Language-Hearing Association. (2016b). *Demographic profile of ASHA members providing bilingual services, March 2016.* Retrieved from http://www.asha.org

Ammon, U. (2010). English and other international languages under the impact of globalization. *Neuphilologische Mitteilungen, 111*(1), 9–28.

Begon, M., Howarth, R. W., & Townsend, C. R. (2014). *Essentials of ecology* (4th ed.). Hoboken, NJ: Wiley.

Benson, L., & Yuen, L. (2014, January 30). "Structural racism" blamed for some of state's severe health disparities. *All things considered with Tom Crann, MPRNews.* Retrieved from https://www.mprnews.org/story/2014/01/29/structural-racism-blamed-for-states-health-disparities

Bish, J. (2016, January 11). Population growth in Africa: Grasping the scale of the challenge. *The Guardian.* Retrieved from https://www.theguardian.com/global-development-professionals-network/2016/jan/11/population-growth-in-africa-grasping-the-scale-of-the-challenge

Black, S. (Producer and Director). (2001). *Life and debt* [Motion picture]. Jamaica: Tuff Gong Pictures.

Blackstone, A. (2012). *Sociological inquiry principles: Qualitative and quantitative methods v. 1.0.* Retrieved from sociological-inquiry-principles-qualitative-and-quantitative-methods.pdf

Brofenbrenner, U. (1979). *The ecology of human development: Experiments by nature and design.* President and Fellows of Harvard College.

Bronfenbrenner, U. (1986). Ecology of the family as the context for human development: Research perspectives. *Developmental Psychology, 22*(6), 723–742.

Bronfenbrenner, U. (2005). The bioecological theory of human development (2001). In U. Bronfenbrenner (Ed.), *Making human beings human: Bioecological perspectives on human development* (pp. 3–15). Thousand Oaks, CA: Sage.

Brookfield, S. (2012). *Teaching for critical thinking: Tools and techniques to help students question their assumptions.* San Francisco, CA: John Wiley & Sons.

Brown, R. (2011). *Prejudice: Its social psychology* (2nd ed.). Malden, MA: Wiley-Blackwell.

Bruner, J. (1983). *Child's talk: Learning to use language.* New York, NY: W.W. Norton.

Burchum, J. L. (2002). Cultural competence: An evolutionary perspective. *Nursing Forum, 37*(4), 5–11.

Callinicos, A. (2007). *Social theory: A historical introduction* (2nd ed.). Malden, MA: Polity Press.

Campinha-Bacote, J. (2002). The process of cultural competence in the delivery of healthcare services: A model of care. *Journal of Transcultural Nursing, 13*(3), 181–184.

Campinha-Bacote, J. (2007). *The process of cultural competence in the delivery of healthcare services: The journey continues* (5th ed.). Cincinnati, OH: Transcultural CARE Associates.

Campinha-Bacote, J. (2011). Delivering patient centered care in the midst of a cultural conflict: The role of cultural competence. *The Online Journal of Issues in Nursing, 16*(2), manuscript 5. Retrieved from http://www.nursingworld.org/MainMenuCategories/ANAMarketplace/ANAPeriodicals/OJIN/TableofContents/Vol-16-2011/No2-May-2011/Delivering-Patient-Centered-Care-in-the-Midst-of-a-Cultural-Conflict.html

Centers for Disease Control and Prevention (CDC). (2013). CDC health disparities and inequalities report—United States 2013. *MMWR 2013; 62*(Suppl. 3), 1–187.

Colby, S., & Ortman J. M. (2015 March 3). *Projections of the size and composition of the U.S. population 2014–2016: Population estimates and projections. Report No P25–1143*. Retrieved from http://www.census.gov/content/dam/Census/library/publications/2015/demo/p25-1143.pdf

Cross, T., Bazron, B., Dennis, K., & Isaacs, M. (1989). *Towards a culturally competent system of care: A monograph on effective services for minority children who are severely emotionally disturbed.* Washington, DC: Georgetown University Child Development Center, CASSP Technical Assistance Center. Retrieved from http://files.eric.ed.gov/fulltext/ED330171.pdf

Crossroads Anti-Racism Organizing and Training (2017). *Dismantling racism, building racial justice institutions.* Retrieved from http://crossroadsantiracism.org

Daouas, M. (2001). Africa faces challenges of globalization. *Finance and Development, 38*(4). Retrieved from http://www.imf.org/external/pubs/ft/fandd/2001/12/daouas.htm

Delgado-Wise, R. D. (2013). The migration and labor question today: Imperialism, unequal development, and forced migration. *Monthly Review, 64*(9). Retrieved from http://monthlyreview.org/2013/02/01/the-migration-and-labor-question-today-imperialism-unequal-development-and-forced-migration

Elias, S., & Feagin, J. R. (2016). *Racial theories in social science: Systemic racism critique.* New York, NY: Routledge.

Gibson, N. C. (2004). Africa and globalization: Marginalization and resistance. *Journal of Asian and African Studies, 39*(1–2), 1–28.

Hinson, S., Healey, R., & Weisenberg, N. (n.d.). *Race, power and policy: Dismantling structural racism.* Retrieved from http://www.racialequitytools.org/resourcefilesrace_power_policy_workbook.pdf

Howe, T. J. (2008). The ICF contextual factors related to speech-language pathology. *International Journal of Speech-Language Pathology, 10*(1/2), 27–37.

Hyter, Y. D. (2007). Pragmatic language assessment: A pragmatics-as-social practice model. *Topics in Language Disorders, 27*(2), 128–145.

Hyter, Y. D. (2012). Making cultural connections across the professions. *SIG 17 Perspectives on Global Issues in Communication Sciences and Disorders, 2*(2), 49–58.

Hyter, Y. D. (2014). A conceptual framework for responsive global engagement in communication sciences and disorders. *Topics in Language Disorders, 34*(2), 103–120.

Hyter, Y. D. (2017). *Hyter's illustration of herself as a cultural being.* Unpublished document. Western Michigan University, Kalamazoo, MI.

International Communication Project (ICP) (2014–2016). *About.* Retrieved from http://www.internationalcommunicationproject.com/about-icp/

Kalyanpur, M., & Harry, B. (2012). *Cultural reciprocity in special education: Building family–professional relationships.* Baltimore, MD: Brookes.

Kellner, D. (1991). Introduction to the second edition. In H. Marcuse (Ed.), *One-dimensional man* (2nd ed., pp. xi–xxxix). Boston, MA: Beacon Press.

Khan, H. A. (2016). *The idea of good governance and the politics of the Global South: An analysis of its effects.* New York, NY: Routledge.

Ladson-Billings, G. (1994). *The dreamkeepers.* San Francisco, CA: Jossey-Bass.

Ladson-Billings, G. (1995). Toward a theory of culturally relevant pedagogy. *American Educational Research Journal, 32*(3), 465–491.

Lavizzo-Mourey, R. (1996). Cultural competence: Essential measurements of quality for managed care organizations. *Annals of Internal Medicine, 124*(10), 919–921.

Leininger, M. (2002). Theory of culture care and the ethnonursing research method. In M. Leininger & M. R. McFarland (Eds.), *Transcultural nursing: Concepts, theories, research and practice* (pp. 71–98). New York, NY: McGraw-Hill.

Lewis, M. P., Simons, G. F., & Fennig, C. D. (Eds.). (2016). *Ethnologue: Languages of the world* (19th ed.). Dallas, TX: SIL International. Retrieved from http://www.ethnologue.com

Marcuse, H. (1991). *One-dimensional man* (2nd ed.). Boston, MA: Beacon Press.

McWhorter, J. (2004). *The story of human language.* Chantilly, VA: The Teaching Company.

McWhorter, J. (2015, September 13). What Sarah Palin's "speak American" is all about. *CNN Opinion.* Retrieved from http://www.cnn

.com/2015/09/06/opinions/mcwhorter-palin-speak-american/

Mordecai, M., & Mordecai, P. (2001). *Culture and customs of Jamaica*. Westport, CT: Greenwood Press.

National Center for Cultural Competence. (NCCC). (n.d.). Washington, DC: Georgetown University. Retrieved from http://www.ncccurricula.info/culturalcompetence.html

Nesbit, J. (2015, May 6). Institutional racism is our way of life. *US News*. Available from http://www.usnews.com/news/blogs/at-the-edge/2015/05/06/institutional-racism-is-our-way-of-life

Netting, F. E., Kettner, P. M., McMurtry, S. L., & Thomas, M. L. (2012). *Social work macro practice* (5th ed). Boston, MA: Allyn & Bacon.

Nettle, D., & Romaine, S. (2000). *Vanishing voices: The extinction of the world's languages*. Oxford, UK: Oxford University Press.

Office of the High Commissioner of Human Rights. (1996–2016). *What are human rights?* Retrieved from http://www.ohchr.org/EN/Issues/Pages/WhatareHumanRights.aspx

Omi, M., & Winant, H. (1994). Racial formation. In M. Omi & H. Winant (Eds.), *Racial formation in the United States* (2nd ed., pp. 9–15). New York, NY: Routledge.

Ortega, R. M., & Faller, K. C. (2011). Training child welfare workers from an intersectional cultural humility perspective: A paradigm shift. *Child Welfare*, *90*(5), 27–49.

Oxborrow, I. (2017, January 29). *Trump ban on Muslim travelers entering US—live updates.* Retrieved from https://www.thenational.ae/world/trump-ban-on-muslim-travellers-entering-us-live-updates-1.85074

Patel, R. (2008). *Stuffed and starved: The hidden battle for the world food system*. New York, NY: Melville House.

Phillipson, R. (1992). *Linguistic imperialism*. Oxford, UK: Oxford University Press.

Phillipson, R. (2008) The linguistic imperialism of neoliberal empire. *Critical Inquiry in Language Studies*, *5*(1), 1–43.

Pinder, S. O. (2012). *Whiteness and racialized ethnic groups in the United States: The politics of remembering*. Boulder, CO: Lexington Books.

powell, j. (2008). Structural racism: Building upon the insights of John Calmore. *North Carolina Law Review*, *86*, 791–816.

Reynolds, A. (2016, September 9). The school-to-prison pipeline is institutional racism. *The Blog*. Retrieved from http://www.huffingtonpost.com/alexander-reynolds/school-to-prison_b_8108068.html

Skutnabb-Kangas, T., & Phillipson, R. (1994). Linguistic human rights, past and present. In T. Skutnabb-Kangas & R. Phillipson (Eds.), *Linguistic human rights: Overcoming linguistic discrimination* (pp. 71–110). Berlin, Germany: Mouton de Gruyter.

Srivastava, R. H. (2007). *The healthcare professionals guide to clinical cultural competence*. Toronto, Canada: Elsevier Canada.

Steger, M. (2003). *Globalization: A very short introduction*. New York, NY: Oxford University Press.

Steger, M. B. (2010). *Globalization: A brief insight*. London, UK: Sterling.

Tenorino, R. (2013, September 17). 232 million people left their countries for new ones—Where did they go? *The Atlantic*. Retrieved from http://www.theatlantic.com/international/archive/2013/09/232-million-people-left-their-countries-for-new-ones-where-did-they-go/279741/

Therborn, G. (2009). *Inequalities of the world: New theoretical frameworks, multiple empirical approaches*. London, UK: Verso.

Threats, T. (2000). The World Health Organization's revised classification: What does it mean for speech-language pathology? *Journal of Medical Speech-Language Pathology*, *8*, xiii–xvii.

Ting-Toomey, S., & Chung, L. C. (2012). *Understanding intercultural communication*. Oxford, UK: Oxford University Press.

Turner, C., Khrais, R., Lloyd, T., Olgin, A., Isensee, L., Vevea, B., & Carsen, D. (2016, April 18). Why America's schools have a money problem. *NPR*. Retrieved from http://www.npr.org/2016/04/18/474256366/why-americas-schools-have-a-money-problem

UNESCO. (2003). *Education in a multilingual world: Position paper*. Paris, France: Author.

UN News Centre. (2013, December 20). *2013 witnessed some of the highest levels of forced dis-*

placement ever—UN report. Retrieved from http://www.un.org/apps/news/story.asp/html/story.asp?NewsID=46792&Cr=displace&Cr1=#.UvafQUJdUR8

U.S. Department of Health and Human Services (HHS). (2008). *The Secretary's Advisory Committee on National Health Promotion and Disease Prevention Objectives for 2020. Phase I report: Recommendations for the framework a format of Healthy People 2020. Section IV: Advisory Committee findings and recommendations.* Retrieved from https://www.healthypeople.gov/sites/default/files/PhaseI_0.pdf

U.S. National Archives and Records Administration. (2016). *The Declaration of Independence.* Retrieved from https://www.archives.gov/founding-docs/declaration

Wallace, M., Crear-Perry, J., Richardson, L., Tarver, M., & Theall, K. (2017). Separate and unequal: Structural racism and infant mortality in the US. *Health Place, 45,* 140–144.

Weiss, H. B., Kreider, H., Lopez, E., & Chatman, C. M. (Eds.). (2005). *Preparing educators to involve families: From theory to practice.* Thousand Oaks, CA: Sage.

Wiley, K., McAllister, L., Davidson, B., & Marshall, J. (2013). Changing practice: Implications of the World Report on Disability for responding to communication disability in under-served populations. *International Journal of Speech-Language Pathology, 15*(1), 1–13.

World Health Organization (WHO). (2002). *International classification of functioning, disability, and health* (ICF). Geneva, Switzerland: Author.

World Health Organization (WHO) and World Bank. (2011). *World report on disability.* Malta: World Health Organization.

Worrall, L. (2010, August). *Discussant to Main Report 2: The complexity of social/cultural dimension in communication disorders.* Presented at the Triennial Congress of the International Association of Logopedics and Phoniatrics, Athens, Greece.

3

Theoretical Frameworks About Culture and Cultural Responsiveness

The focus of Chapter 3 is on theoretical frameworks for developing skills and engaging in culturally and linguistically competent care. The expected outcome of this chapter is the ability to begin to develop your own conceptual framework for providing culturally and globally responsive services. After reading this chapter and engaging in the learning activities outlined here, you will achieve the following learning objectives.

LEARNING OBJECTIVES

After reading, discussing and processing the information presented in this chapter, you will be able to demonstrate the following knowledge, skills, and attitudes:

1. Knowledge
   a. Explain four major social theories.
   b. Define cultural responsiveness from the perspective of four theoretical frameworks.
2. Skills
   a. Use each of the four major social theories to guide decisions about working with individuals and groups from cultural and linguistic

backgrounds different than your own.
   b. Begin to develop a conceptual framework for providing effective and sustainable services in the United States and abroad.
3. Attitudes demonstrated through journaling
   a. Show a positive regard for the role that theory places in service provision.
   b. Exhibit a commitment to thinking about culturally responsive services from a theoretical frame, as you would for providing any other service.

KEY CONCEPTS

Key concepts addressed in this chapter are presented in Table 3–1.

OVER-THE-COUNTER HEARING AIDS—A PROBLEM OR A SOLUTION?

We are introducing a case below. Read through it and then keep it in mind as you review the

TABLE 3–1. Key Concepts

Theory	Concepts
Social theory	Conceptual framework
Ideology	
Common sense	Premises
Social structures	Assumptions

remainder of the chapter. At the end of the chapter, we ask you to respond to it from the perspective of each of the theoretical perspectives discussed in this chapter. The case you will read now is a current event taking place in the U.S. government and playing out in the back pages of newspapers.

Box 3–1

In December 2016, U.S. Senators Elizabeth Warren (D-MA) and Charles Grassley (R-IA) introduced the Over-the-Counter Hearing Aid Act of 2016 (S.9, 2016), which requires the Food and Drug Administration (FDA) to let individuals purchase over-the-counter (OTC) hearing aids. The goal, we believe, is to allow hearing aids to be more accessible to persons with the need for them. These OTC hearing aids would only be provided to adults with mild to moderate hearing loss, but a concern is that individuals may self-diagnose and/or may purchase a hearing aid that is not tempered for their particular type of loss. The American Speech-Language-Hearing Association (ASHA) writes

ASHA opposes S.9 and believes that current federal and state requirements related to professional involvement are important consumer safeguards. Additionally, to assist in the positive outcomes of adapting to a hearing aid, audiologists and other hearing health professionals must be involved to determine the nature and severity of hearing loss in order to provide the proper diagnosis, fitting, and follow-up necessary to manage the individual's hearing health care needs. The legislation is also premature—FDA is currently evaluating its hearing aid regulations and should have the opportunity to complete this review

without a Congressional mandate. (ASHA, 2016)

The Academy of Doctors of Audiology (ADA) supports S.9 for the "foresight in introducing and advancing this legislation, which if enacted, will remove unnecessary and burdensome barriers to hearing care for millions of Americans" (ADA, 2017).

How do you determine what is best in this situation of the OTC hearing aids? Some will believe that it is best to allow OTC hearing aids to provide greater access to hearing aids for those who may need them but do not have the insurance to pay the high prices (e.g., thousands of dollars) for them. Others will think that OTC hearing aids will provide the opportunity for consumers to be taken advantage of —that is, purchasing a device that may not work at all with their type of hearing loss. Still others may say that ASHA does not support the S.9 because it will cut into the profits of audiologists and may put some professionals out of business altogether. What do you say? What do you think?

One way to navigate this conundrum of issues is to approach it systematically from a theoretical framework. As you read through the theories, and their corresponding assumptions, contemplate on how you would think about OTC hearing aids from each theoretical position.

THEORY AND SOCIAL THEORY

At the mere mention of the word "theory," your eyes may glaze over. In a certain way, however, everyone is already a "theorist" in that we all have some concept, beliefs, or opinions about the world and how it works (Gramsci, 1971, p. 323; Jones, Bradbury, & Le Boutillier, 2011). These types of common or folk theories are often unexamined ideas about reality (Monette, Sullivan, & DeJong, 2011). A higher level of theorizing is the awareness, critical reflection, and analysis of the history and effects of social events on the world. This higher level of thinking is the approach we take in this chapter.

When we speak of theory, we mean an abstract, systematic way of explaining and predicting phenomena (Baert, 1998; Elliott & Lemert, 2014; Monette et al., 2011, p. 29). In Social Development Theory (i.e., Vygotsky, 1978), as an example, the phenomenon to be explained is how development happens. The explanation is that child development and cognition are dependent on social interactions between the learner (e.g., a child) and more knowledgeable others (e.g., parents, older siblings, teachers, and interventionists).

Social theories include ideas regarding "how societies change, how social behavior is organized," and about roles that social structures play in the world (Harrington, 2005, p. 1). More specifically, a social theory is a school of thought or a set of intellectual ideas—a scientific model, used to describe, explain, and/or predict how the social world works. Social theory provides a description or explanation of totality (Baert, 1998; Dillon, 2010; Monette et al., 2011). Totality refers to the links that exist between social structures in society. Social structures refer to interconnected systems that form the social environment (Agger, 2006; Dillon, 2010; Hyter, 2014), which include

the systems of economics (i.e., access to and control of resources); politics (i.e., relations of power); state control (i.e., military and the state's arm of coercion such as the judicial system); and culture (i.e., assumptions and beliefs that drive daily practice), which includes race (i.e., socially constructed reference to skin color), gender identity (e.g., internal feeling of being male, female, cisgender[1] or transgender), as well as family and religious structures (Gramsci, 1971; Hyter, 2014; Santiago-Valles, 1998).

Social theory is not an opinion or uncritical judgements about social reality. In this way, social theory differs from ideology. Ideology is composed of unquestioned assumptions or unexamined beliefs about the way the world works (Brookfield, 2012; Verschueren, 2012). Ideology leads to "commonsense" arguments about the ways the world is organized (Brookfield, 2012). Common sense refers to the general widespread ideas about what is "normal," but this sense of normality differs among groups that have different levels of power, have competing interests, or have differing allegiances (Herman & Chomsky, 2012). A commonsense proposition, for example, might be that "it is 'common sense' to wear a helmet when riding a motorcycle." This argument is aligned with the interests of those who think it is "normal," to protect one's head. This commonsense argument is supported by legislation in some states in the United States; but, it also competes with the views of those who think it is "normal" to ride unimpeded by a helmet. A more difficult ideology to pinpoint could be the notion of democracy. In the United States, for example, one might think it is common sense that "democracy" is equated to the public having the opportunity to cast votes for officials who will make decisions on behalf of the public. Voting in the United States is always scheduled

---

[1] Cisgendered refers to identifying with the sex in which you are born. Transgendered refers to one's identity not conforming to the sex in which he or she was born.

on a weekday, which is a workday for many, minimizing the number of people who can participate in the voting process. In other regions of the world, it is considered common sense that democracy means that each person equally and directly participates in decision making in their communities. In many other countries, on voting day work is suspended or voting takes place on a Sunday when most people are not working, increasing the number of people who can participate in this direct decision-making process.

Since much of our existence and communication as humans are inherently social, being knowledgeable about social theories is useful regardless of one's field of study. Knowledge of social theories is particularly important for professionals and/or service providers who want to provide services in a culturally responsive manner. Social theories include information about social behavior, the structure of society, relationships among people in the society, and the way social structures affect individuals and/or groups of people (Dillon, 2010; Elliott, 2008). Thus, social theories explain social events and behaviors. Social theory can help facilitate what research questions to ask, which variables are important to examine, how to provide services, and how to predict the outcomes of practices and client responses (Chitty & Black, 2010). The primary point here is that social theories can be used to guide teaching, research, and practice. Several published theories of cultural responsiveness[2] exist in the fields of communication (Ting-Toomey & Chung, 2012), special education (Kalyanpur & Harry, 2012), health care and nursing (Campinha-Bacote & Campinha-Bacote, 2009; Campinha-Bacote, 2007;

Leininger, 2004; Munoz, Conrad DoBroka, & Mohammad, 2009; Purnell, 2002; Suh, 2004; Tervalon & Murray-Garcia, 1998), and social work (Ortega & Coulborn Faller, 2011).

To date, however, there are no published theories of cultural responsiveness in the field of speech, language, and hearing sciences[3]; yet, a few models (hypothetical representations of conceptual relations) do exist, such as those developed by the authors, Hyter (2014) and Salas-Provance (2010), as well as Stockman, Boult, and Robinson (2004), Bellon-Harn and Garrett (2008), and Horton-Ikard, Munoz, Thomas-Tate, and Keller-Bell (2009). After discussing the components of a theory, we review some of the existing theories and models of cultural responsiveness in various fields, and end with our effort to develop a cohesive theory of cultural responsiveness for speech, language, and hearing sciences.

Components of a Theory

Theories contain different parts. One aspect of a social theory is the conceptual framework consisting of concepts (terms), their definitions, and how they are related to each other. Another aspect of social theory is its premises. Premises are statements on which some belief is based (e.g., if statement one is true, then the conclusion is also true). Premises differ from assumptions in that assumptions are opinions and unquestioned beliefs—that is, the belief that something is true even without evidence of it being true or even when faced with evidence to the contrary. Conceptual frameworks and the premises of several theories are addressed in the next section of this chapter.

---

[2]Many disciplines have used the concept of cultural competence in the past but are moving beyond the concept of competence to those that are inherently dynamic—that is, terms that suggest a process rather than an outcome, such as reciprocity, sustainability, and responsiveness.

[3]This field is also known as Speech, Language, and Hearing Sciences; Speech-Language Pathology and Audiology; and Communication Sciences and Disorders.

Conceptual Frameworks

Concepts are ideas that are expressed as words. "Play" for example, is a concept, and so is "gender." Although we use concepts all the time in our daily interactions, concepts used within social theories are often defined in a specific manner that connects to the premises of the theory.

Let's again turn to Vygotsky (1978) and examine his Theory of Cognitive Development as an example of identifying premises and concepts. One premise of this theory is that social interaction contributes to cognitive development. Another premise is that imaginative play facilitates a child's ability to make sense or meaning of his or her social world. Concepts that correspond to these premises are the Zone of Proximal Development (ZPD) and problem solving. ZPD is the distance between a child's current developmental level (what he or she can do alone) and level of potential (what he or she can do with the assistance of a more knowledgeable other) (Vygotsky, 1978). In other words, ZPD is the zone in which a child is ready to learn something new. That learning takes place in the context of interacting with another more experienced person. Problem solving, the ability to work out solutions to difficulties, is learned in the context of imaginative play while children are engaged in dialogue with peers or with their selves.

A framework is like a map (Sinclair, 2007, p. 39); it provides a guide for decision making (Hyter, 2014). This map can help make clear connections among various concepts, providing an order to these concepts, and can be used to produce new knowledge (Hyter, 2014; Kirst-Ashman, 2013). Figure 3–1 shows a model of the relationship between ZPD and problem solving mentioned in the previous paragraph.

Imagine for a moment that you are a recent graduate of Millstone Wonderful University (MWU) with a master's degree. You have been offered an opportunity of a lifetime to travel to Kati, Mali, to provide speech-language services for 1 year, and to "build the capacity of personnel in Kati to address communication disorders." Specifically, your job will be to work with local community members, educators, and family members to conduct speech-language and hearing screenings and assessments, and to provide communication intervention when warranted. You must have a million questions! Take some time to look up Kati, Mali, using the Internet. Approaching this assignment using a social theory, and a conceptual framework—a cognitive map—will help guide your practice, whether you end up in Kati, Mali; Portland, Oregon; Kalamazoo, Michigan; or Huntsville, Alabama.

Although there are several social theories or schools of thought, in this chapter we focus on four different paradigms. A paradigm is a worldview that can be used to guide choices in one's conceptualization of reality, scope of knowledge, and methods of practice. The four theoretical paradigms discussed in this text are positivism, interpretivism, critical perspectives, and postmodernism (Hyde, 2004; Hyter, 2014; Mukherji & Albon, 2014; Neuman, 2006). Table 3–2 summarizes the main ideas of each of these four theoretical perspectives.

Positivism is often considered "real science" or the only legitimate form of science, although we strongly disagree with this notion. Some premises of positivism are that: (1) things in the world exist separately from perceptions of those things; (2) "science" is the use of "objective" practices to discover what exists in the world (Monette, Sullivan, & DeJong, 2011, p. 39); and (3) knowledge is observable, measureable, and value free (i.e., free from one's judgement of what is important, and what is right or wrong) (Jones, Bradbury, & Le Boutillier, 2011; Neuman, 2003).

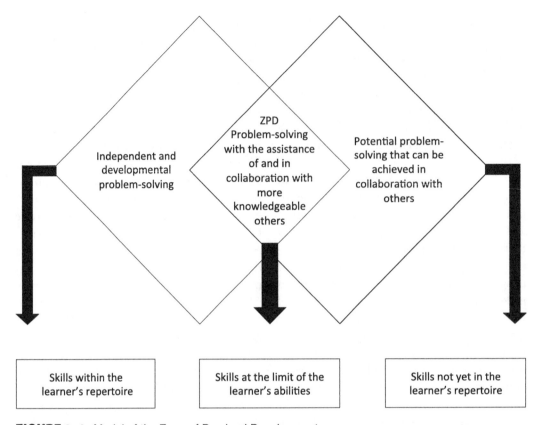

FIGURE 3–1. Model of the Zone of Proximal Development.

Positivists use a deductive process to measure observed behavior to identify consistencies allowing future behavior to be predicted (Neuman, 2003).

Let's revisit the case presented in the beginning of this chapter—the young professional having an opportunity to live and work in Kati, Mali. A positivist would say that this young person can learn about life in Kati, Mali, by observing what people do.[4] He or she would go on to say that people do things in their own self-interest and based on some external reason. What people are observed to do is ultimately more important and more telling than what they think, or believe, or desire. One determines observations to represent truth (reality) if there are no common-sense alternatives, and if conclusions drawn are consistent with behaviors that were observed. If observations can be agreed upon by others, then they were objective, not subjective.

Interpretivism refers to another scientific method and is an overarching term used to refer to several types of social theories including ethnography (e.g., Geertz), ethnomethodology (e.g., Garfinkel, Sacks), hermeneutics (e.g., Habermas), phenomenology (e.g., Husserl), and symbolic interactionism

---

[4]Note that the examples of positivism, interpretivism, and critical perspectives were adapted from Neuman, 2003, pp. 68–92.

TABLE 3–2. Summary of Four Social Theories

	Positivism	Interpretivism	Critical	Post-Modernism	Excluded Intellectual Traditions[a]
Some premises	Reality is composed of what is observable and measureable. Things in the world exist separately from perceptions of those things. "Science" is the use of "objective" practices to discover what exists in the world (Monette, Sullivan, & DeJong, 2011,[b] p. 39). Knowledge is observable, measureable, and value free.	Reality is socially constructed and is based on how people perceive it (Monette et al., 2011). There are cultural and historical bases for the way the world operates (Dillon, 2010; Neuman, 2003, 2006). Humans "attach subjective meaning" to behaviors, interactions, and communicative acts (Dillon, 2010, p. 118[c]).	Reality is continually changing—it is dynamic. Reality is based on conflicting interests and unequal distributions of power, which manifest as unequal distributions of capital, resources, land, and property. Critical and dialectical thinking are repressed by cultural institutions and by the arms of the state.	Reality is not explainable. Be wary of all-encompassing worldviews (e.g., Christianity, capitalism, feminism, etc.). A single universal worldview no longer exists. Rigid disciplinary boundaries are questioned. Truth is dynamic (diverse and always changing). Reject conventional forms of discourse.	Ideology and cultural institutions manufacture consent among the populace. Exploitation is worldwide and is part of Imperialism (Sivanandan, 2005[d]). Class and gender are racialized and used to justify exploitation (Robinson, 1983[e]).
Key focus	Search for the variables that cause an event or action.	Search for underlying meaning of behavior or text.[f] Focus on the way people make sense of and meaning out of daily life.	Search for underlying assumptions and ideologies that exploit, dominate, and/or exclude people/groups, and that maintain the status quo within any system. Identify causes, consequences, and ways to transform policies and practices that serve to exploit, dominate, or exclude.	Search for how the world is perceived and described.	Social Justice Economic Justice Human Rights Anti-Colonialism Anti-Imperialism

continues

TABLE 3–2. *continued*

	Positivism	Interpretivism	Critical	Post-Modernism	Excluded Intellectual Traditions[a]
Goal	Uncover facts and truth using quantitative methods.	Understand social life and the meaning that people ascribe to it, and the reasons that people act as they do.	Uncover the systemic conflicts, and transform reality.	Express the subjective self; stimulate others (Neuman, 2003, p. 91).	To recuperate the history and rights of exploited, dominated, and excluded peoples, and to gain socioeconomic redistribution (Fraser & Honneth, 2003), and equity for marginalized people.
How to explain reality	Valid, reliable, and precisely measured decontextualized variables.	Valid and reliable descriptions of events that may read like a novel (Neuman, 2003, p. 79).	Valid and reliable ways of identifying the underlying causes and consequences of problems, and the role that social structures have in maintaining or exacerbating those problems.	Valid and reliable ways to analyze and understand the discourses used.	Valid and reliable ways of identifying the underlying causes and consequences of problems, and the role that social structures have in maintaining or exacerbating those problems.
How to determine if the explained reality is true	If it can be replicated	If it is reality to those who experience it. If the person explaining reality demonstrates reality as others experience it	If it helps people understand the historical context of their problems, and provides them with ways to change their reality	Individual's notions about what is true are shaped by our cultural context. No one explanation is true—all are true (Neuman, 2003, p. 91)	If it transforms material conditions, and creates equity

	Positivism	Interpretivism	Critical	Post-Modernism	Excluded Intellectual Traditions[a]
Research methods	Experiments, questionnaires, secondary data analysis Quantitatively coded documents Regression Likert scaling Structural equation modeling	Ethnography Participant observation Interviews Conversational analysis Case studies; conversational and textual analysis	Field research Critical historical analysis Dialectical analysis Textual analysis Transdisciplinary praxis (Hyter, 2014)	Discourse analysis using deconstruction and interpretation of text	Participatory Action Research Conversation groups Resistance via social movements and networks intersecting across race, class, gender, nationality, and territory (Santiago-Valles, 2006)
Level of Objectivity (Hyde, 2004, p. 50)	Assumes objectivity Subjectivity has no place in positivism Positivism is objective and value free	Subjectivity is essential to social life No one's subjective experience is any better (or worse) than anyone else's Objectivity is not possible	All researchers approach a problem with a specific point of view, meaning that nothing is value free "Knowledge is power" (Neuman, 2003, p. 86) The critical social theorist's role is to engage in transformative research and political action	Objective knowledge is not possible Social reality is superior to scientific knowledge (Neuman, 2003, p. 91)	Objectivity is not possible

continues

TABLE 3–2. *continued*

	Positivism	Interpretivism	Critical	Post-Modernism	Excluded Intellectual Traditions[a]
Some key terms	Cause and effect Hypothesis Measureable Observable facts Reliability Validity	Intersubjectivity Reification Self-reflective Social construction	Dialectical thinking Domination Exploitation Hegemony Praxis Transdisciplinarity	Agency De-centering Deconstruction Discourse Hyperreality Narrative Privileged	Exploitation Human rights Anti-Imperialism Anti-Colonialism Ideology Hegemony
Some proponents	Auguste Comte, Emile Durkheim B.F. Skinner John Stuart Mill	Max Weber, Wilhelm Dilthey Harold Garfinkel Jürgen Habermas Edmund Husserl Jean-Paul Sartre Dorothy Smith	Karl Marx Theodor Adorno Pierre Bourdieu Herbert Marcuse Angela Davis Jürgen Habermas	François Lyotard Roland Barthes Jean Baudrillard Zym Bauman Jean-Jacques Derrida Michel Foucault Jürgen Habermas Martin Heidegger Julia Kristeva	Ella Baker Amilcar Cabral Ruth First Claudia Jones Kwame Nkrumah Cedric Robinson Walter Rodney Shlomo Sand Robert Allen Warrior

Sources: [a]Santiago-Valles, W. F. (2006). [b]Monette, D. R., Sullivan, T. J., & DeJong, C. R. (2011). [c]Dillon, M. (2010). [d]Sivanandan, A. (2005). [e]Robinson, C. (1983). Text as used here is broadly defined to include writings, modes of discourse, world events, pictures, etc.

(e.g., Blumer, Goffman) (Hyter, 2014; Neuman, 2003; Prasad, 2005). These theories approach scientific inquiry from an inductive process. Some of the primary premises that these theories have in common are that (1) there are cultural and historical bases for the way the world operates (Dillon, 2010; Neuman, 2003, 2006); (2) humans "attach subjective meaning" to behaviors, interactions, and communicative acts (Dillon, 2010, p. 118); and (3) reality is based on how people perceive it (Monette et al., 2011). The point here is that theories that fall within the interpretivist epistemology share a focus on understanding the "subjective reality" and how it is constructed in the social lives of persons from all walks of life (Prasad, 2005).

Keeping our focus on the young professional headed to Kati, Mali, we present an example of interpretivism in action. If this young professional was an interpretivist, she would head to Mali wanting to learn what was important to the people in Kati. She would become involved in the Kati community, volunteering where possible and conducting systematic observations of the people, their relationships with one another, and belief systems, for example. She would likely conduct some ethnographic interviews to learn people's reasons for doing what they do in given contexts. She would listen for key words that are used by members of the Kati community and ask them for explanations about those words, saying something like, "I heard you use the word 'denbaya.'[5] Please tell me what a 'denbaya' does, or Please tell me what a 'denbaya' looks like." Her ultimate goal would be to find out from the people in Kati, Mali, what their daily life is like and what is important to them from their own perspectives.

Critical social theories are used to examine and understand reality within historical, economic, political, and cultural contexts (Hyter, 2014, p. 108). Proponents of these theories have often been excluded from the theoretical "canon" particularly in the U.S. (Santiago-Valles, 2005, 2011), and especially in the fields of speech-language pathology and audiology. Critical social theories are composed of various theories including orthodox Marxism (e.g., Marx, Hegel), to which anarchism (e.g., Kropotkin) is attached; structural Marxism (e.g., Althusser); cultural or Western Marxism (e.g., Gramsci, Davis), including the Critical Social Theory of the Frankfurt School (i.e., Adorno, Davis, Horkeimer, Marcuse, Benjamin); Black Marxism (e.g., Robinson); radical feminism (e.g., hooks, Smith); Queer theory (Browne & Nash, 2016), and cultural studies (Hall, Williams) (Hyter, 2014; Prasad, 2005). Although there are differences in these theoretical approaches, they have some of the same premises, including their focus on the economic exploitation, political domination, and sociocultural exclusion of a variety of groups, and on changing their reality. Some premises of critical epistemologies are that: (1) reality is continually changing—it is dynamic; (2) reality is based on conflicting interests and unequal distributions of power, which manifest as unequal distributions of capital, resources, land, and property; and (3) critical and dialectical thinking are repressed by cultural institutions such as the media and schooling, and by the arms of the state, such as the law, the police, and the military (Dillon, 2010; Herman & Chomsky, 2002; Marcuse, 2012).

If the young professional mentioned earlier in the chapter heading to Kati, Mali, was a critical social theorist, she would focus on examining the causes and consequences of problems faced by people living in that town, such as fragile security, extreme impoverishment,

---

[5]Denbaya is a Bambara word for family (English–Bambara dictionary available from http://www.bambara.org/lexique/index-english/main.htm).

and food insecurity (United Nations, 2016). Her goal would be to reveal the ideologies that cause, maintain, and benefit from the problems there. Her role would be to collaborate with the people in Kati, as they bring about the changes in their town and lives that they know they need.

The last theory that we address is *postmodernism*. Sometimes, poststructuralism is explained as being related to postmodernism (Prasad, 2005). Some link these theories into one category called *antifoundational theories* referring to epistemologies that are against foundational ideas. As with the other theoretical frameworks, postmodernism (e.g., Lyotard, Coudrillard, Guatarri) and poststructuralism (e.g., Foucault, Derrida) are connected in that some of the same intellectual traditions were their antecedents (Callinicos, 1989; Prasad, 2005). What these theories have in common are their focus on deconstructing most aspects of Western thinking and science that occurred after the 18th century. The proponents of the *post–ism* theories also are informed by intellectual traditions from majority world countries (i.e., the Global South) including those on the continents of Africa, Asia, and Latin America. Postmodernist do not agree with grand narratives (also called meta-narratives and refer to cultural stories) because they are usually told based on assumptions and values of one group at the expense of other groups.

The remainder of this chapter focuses on the different frameworks that have been used to make sense of culture, and how cultures are similar and different. These frameworks emerged from a range of disciplines. We start with the World Health Organization's World Report on Disability (WHO, 2011) which provides a larger context for culturally responsive practices. Following our discussion of the World Report on Disability, we present a summary of other frameworks from a variety of disciplines, in-cluding those from speech, language, and hearing sciences. We end this chapter with the conceptual frameworks developed by the authors (Yvette D. Hyter and Marlene Salas-Provance), which serve as the foundation for this textbook.

WORLD REPORT ON DISABILITY

In a joint report of the WHO and the World Bank (WHO and World Bank, 2011), it was reported that 15% of the world's population has a disability. This percentage amounts to approximately one billion people; however, its number underestimates individuals with communication impairments. People are migrating in record numbers right now due to a variety of reasons such as natural disasters, unequal access to food, unemployment, impoverishment, political upheaval, and military interventions that decrease safety, increase violence, and make human rights fragile commodities (Delgado-Wise, 2013; Hyter, 2014; Tenorino, 2013). Because of the migration of people in several places around the world, it is more likely now than ever before for professions in the speech, language, and hearing sciences to have individuals from diverse cultural and linguistic backgrounds be referred for services, and possibly on caseloads. Wherever people are moving from or to, they carry with them their culture—beliefs, values, assumptions, and world views pertaining to "health, wellness and disability" (Hyter, 2014, p. 105).

MEANING OF ILLNESS, DISEASE, AND DISABILITY (Scheper Hughes and Kleinman)

Nancy Scheper-Hughes and Margaret Lock (1987) stressed that it was important to consider the human body as not just a physical one. They argue that it is important to deconstruct the assumptions about the relationship between the mind and the body, which influence health care planning and delivery, particularly in "Western societies." They described the body as being three bodies: (1) the phenomenally experienced body or how we experience our own bodies; (2) a social body, in that the body can be used as an example or symbol of nature or societal events; and the (3) body politic referring to the ways society regulates the body and determines how much control one has over his or her own body (Scheper Hughes & Lock, 1987, p. 7). Scheper Hughes and Lock state that how one experiences his or her body is cultural. Kleinman (1989) makes a similar argument in that he differentiates the patient's experiences within his or her body from the doctors' treatment of the symptoms reported by the patient. (We talk more about Kleinman's ideas in Chapter 6.) In other words, culture can affect beliefs about illness, health, and wellness behaviors, as well as diagnosis and treatment (Kleinman & Benson, 2006).

THE TIP OF THE ICEBERG

Culture has been compared to an iceberg in the writing of communication scholar Ting-Toomey in 1999 and then updated by Ting-Toomey and Chung in 2012. Figure 3–2 shows a picture of an iceberg, and below it is our version of a sketch of an iceberg showing the major aspects of culture as discussed by Ting-Toomey (1999) and Ting-Toomey and Chung (2012). There are visible and invisible aspects of culture. The invisible parts are beneath the surface of the water—they are what truly make up the construct of culture. The visible aspects of culture are at the tip of the iceberg; we see these expressions of people's cultural values, beliefs, and assumptions every day. The visible aspects of culture are cultural artifacts

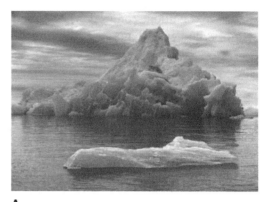

A

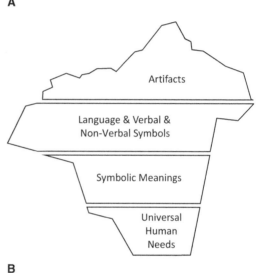

B

FIGURE 3–2. A. An iceberg. **B.** Our version of a sketch of an iceberg showing the major aspects of culture as discussed by Ting-Toomey (1999) and Ting-Toomey and Chung (2012). *(A)*: Image courtesy of Leroy Hyter, Sr., 1997. *(B)*: Illustrated by Severin Provance.

(objects and behaviors), such as music, hairstyles, and jewelry choices. These aspects of culture refer to underlying beliefs, values, and assumptions that drive the visible aspects of culture. These authors also say that to "understand commonalities between individuals and groups, we have to dig deeper into the level of universal human needs" (Ting-Toomey, 1999, p. 10). These universal human needs include such things as the need for safety, inclusion, dignity, recognition, connections, meaning, creativity, and well-being.

DIMENSIONS OF CULTURE (Hofstede)

Hofstede (2010, 2011), a psychologist, after a great deal of research, developed a model of culture described as including cultural dimensions. He created a survey that was administered to over 100,000 people in over 70 countries, including in Europe, United States, Latin America, Sub-Saharan Africa, and Western, Eastern, and Southern Asia (Hofstede, 1984, 2010, 2011). The six cultural dimensions are power distance, uncertainty avoidance, individualism collectivism, masculinity femininity, time orientation, and indulgence restraint, which occur on a continuum (Hofstede, 2010, 2011). Some groups will be closer to one end of the continuum than others, but these are cultural values that may occur in any cultural group.

Power Distance

Power distance refers to the extent to which people in a cultural group believe that there *should* be unequal relations and distributions of power in their society, and whether institutions and/or people in power should be contested or accepted (Hofstede, 1984, 2010, 2011). Cultural groups that have tendencies toward the small end of the power distance dimension will work to minimize inequalities and believe that it is appropriate to contest or challenge people and systems in power. A cultural value for those with small power distance is equity. Conversely, cultural groups with a large power distance will be less likely to question people perceived as having authority, and may believe that it is "natural" for there to be stratifications in a society, and therefore will not necessarily question them.

Review the continuum illustrated in Table 3–3. This table and those that follow simply summarize some of the characteristics listed by Hofstede. Where would you say that your cultural group falls on this dimension of power distance? Is your cultural group more likely to identify with a small power distance or a large power distance? What evidence do you have to support your responses?

According to Hofstede's research on 50 countries and three regions of the world (East Africa, West Africa, and Arab countries), he found differences in cultural groups on either end of the continuum. (We pause here to strongly caution against generalizing. As we discussed in Chapter 2, cultural groups

TABLE 3–3. Dimension of Power Distance

Small Power Distance	Large Power Distance
← ——————————————————→	
Members of a society should question their leaders, and oppose them to reduce or eliminate social, economic, or political inequities in society.	Members of a society should not question their leaders; it is acceptable for there to be social, economic, or political inequities in a society.

Source: Based on Hofstede, 2011.

are *not* homogeneous. Some members of the same cultural group will be similar in some beliefs and values; others will be dissimilar.) The country with the largest power distance index (PDI) was Malaysia with a PDI of 104. Austria had the smallest PDI (i.e., 11), and the United States fell somewhat in the middle of the continuum with a PDI of 40. Remember that these data were collected in the early to mid-1980s—country and cultural responses to Hofstede's survey may well be quite different now.

Uncertainty–Avoidance

The dimension of uncertainty–avoidance deals with how well the culture of a society or group is comfortable with unstructured contexts and uncertain outcomes (Hofstede, 2011). Cultural groups vary based on their relationship with ambiguity. Cultural groups with strong uncertainty avoidance may attempt to prevent uncertainty by enacting laws and rules that outline specific ways to behave, and these societies are often resistant to change. Con-sider the worry about immigration around the world. Based on the responses of different countries around the world to the immigration crisis, which countries seem to be closer to the strong end of the uncertainty avoidance con-tinuum and which ones seem to be closer the weak end of this continuum? Countries with weak uncertainty avoidance may see ambigu-ity as a natural part of life. Members of groups on the weak end of the uncertainty avoidance continuum have a high tolerance for unpre-dictability and, therefore, may be perceived as being more "laid back," and "relaxed" about events in their lives. Think about your own cultural group for a moment. Which end of the continuum would some members of your cultural group fall on the uncertainty–avoid-ance dimension? Table 3–4 identifies some of the primary characteristics of the weak and strong uncertainty–avoidance continuum.

Individualism–Collectivism

This cultural dimension focuses on the extent to which members of cultural groups see

TABLE 3–4. Continuum of the Uncertainty Avoidance Cultural Dimension

Weak Uncertainty Avoidance	Strong Uncertainty Avoidance
Uncertainty is a part of daily life and is acceptable.	Uncertainty is threatening and should be controlled as much as possible.
Comfortable with unpredictability	Need clarity, structures, laws, and rules to minimize unpredictability
Tolerant of diverse worldviews	Lack of tolerance of diverse perspectives
In religion, philosophy, and science: relativism and empiricism	In religion, philosophy, and science: belief in ultimate truths and grand theories

Source: Based on Hofstede, 2011, p. 10.

themselves as individuals and independent on one hand, and part of a larger collective group or society on the other (Hofstede, 2011). Cultures that are closer to the individualistic end of the continuum value independence, view themselves as being accountable to themselves, and make their own decisions individually. Members of cultural groups that are closer to the collectivistic end of the continuum see themselves as part of a larger society and are accountable to that society. Hofstede (2011) states that cultures on the "collectivist side . . . in which people from birth onwards are integrated into strong, cohesive in-groups, often extended families . . . that continue protecting them in exchange for unquestioning loyalty" (p. 11). Think about your own experiences. Are members of your cultural group more individualistic or collectivistic? Some of the primary characteristics of the individualism–collectivism continuum are presented in Table 3–5.

Masculinity–Femininity

These characteristics refer to the types of gender characteristics that are valued predominantly within a society or cultural group. Masculine characteristics include assertiveness, competitiveness, and the preference of facts over feelings. Feminine characteristics include modesty, sensitivity, and caring for others. For cultures that value feminine characteristics, the men and women will exhibit modesty and nurturing, have work–life balance, and sympathize with those who are suffering. Similarly, if a cultural group leans more toward the masculine end of the masculinity–femininity continuum, both the males and females will display characteristics that are perceived as "masculine," such as ambitiousness, work prevailing over family, beliefs that men deal with facts and women with feelings, and so on (Table 3–6).

Long-Term–Short-Term Orientation

This cultural dimension focuses on how groups of people think about goals and challenges. Groups that present with short-term orientation hold on to traditions and have the tendency to perceive changes in society as problematic or disconcerting. These groups also focus on past and present events or issues. Groups with long-term orientation are inclined to adapt to changing society, be

TABLE 3–5. Continuum of Individualism and Collectivism

Individualism	Collectivism
←	→
Everyone is socialized to take care of himself or herself and his or her immediate family.	Members of cultural groups are socialized that they are part of extended families and cohesive societies.
Independence and privacy are valued.	Relationships have more precedence than tasks.
Use of "I" is indispensable.	The use of "I" is avoided.
Tasks prevail over relationships.	Relationships prevail over tasks.

Source: Based on Hofstede, 2011, p. 11.

persistent, and have an outlook in life that focuses on preparation for the future. Some of the characteristics of groups with long-term and short-term focus are listed in Table 3–7.

Indulgence–Restraint

The indulgence–restraint dimension is about the way groups control or delay desires or happiness. The formulation of this dimen-

sion was based on "happiness research" (Hofstede, 2011, p. 15). Groups on the indulgent end of the continuum will more frequently engage in enjoyable pleasures than groups on the restraint end of the continuum. These groups will often focus on individual gratification, personal freedom, and the importance of leisure time. Restraint refers to those groups or societies that delay social pleasures, which are often managed through social norms, and where self-gratification and personal

TABLE 3–6. Continuum of Femininity and Masculinity

Femininity	Masculinity
← ──────────────────────────────── →	
Men and women should be modest and nurturing.	Men should be and women may be assertive and ambitious.
There should be a balance between family and work.	Work prevails over family.
Both fathers and mothers deal with facts and feelings.	The strong are admired.
Boys and girls may cry but should not fight.	Girls cry, boys do not cry; boys should fight back, but girls should not fight at all.

Source: Based on Hofstede, 2011, p. 12.

TABLE 3–7. Dimension of Time

Short-Term Orientation	Long-Term Orientation
← ──────────────────────────────── →	
Most important events occurred in the past or are taking place now.	Most important events in life will occur in the future.
A good person is always the same.	A good person adapts to the circumstances.
Traditions are revered.	Traditions are changeable depending on the circumstances.
There is pride in one's country.	Try to learn from other countries.

Source: Based on Hofstede, 2011, p. 15.

freedoms are not as highly valued as groups on the indulgence end of the continuum (Table 3–8).

MODELS FROM SPEECH, LANGUAGE, AND HEARING SCIENCES

Five models of culturally responsive practices from speech, language, and hearing sciences are reviewed here. These include The VISION Model (Bellon-Harn & Garrett, 2008), pedagogical frameworks proposed by Stockman, Boult, and Robinson (2004) and Horton-Ikard, Munoz, Thomas-Tate, and Keller-Bell (2009), a hierarchical model of cultural knowledge (Salas-Provance, 2010), and a conceptual framework for globally (and we add here culturally) responsive service (Hyter, 2014).

The VISION Model

Bellon-Harn and Garrett (2008) developed a model of cultural responsiveness for speech-

language pathologists working in family partnerships. This model was designed to aid in the awareness of cultural and linguistic difference among one's constituents. This model is composed of the following six components:

- (V) Values and belief systems of the family and professional refer to the cultural experiences that influence both the professional and the family with whom the professional is working. The professional must become conscious of his or her personal values, cultural biases, and assumptions, and be able to identify how his or her cultural experiences and worldview affect those values and assumptions.

- (I) Interpretation of experience of families with clinical process refers to the ability of the professional to be aware of and identify how a family may be interpreting experiences within the clinical process. This component of the model focuses on the ways that people within cultural groups may interpret relationships among others, and their environment. One example of this was exhibited in a novel called, *The spirit catches you and you fall down* (Fadiman, 1997) which focused on the story of a

TABLE 3–8. Dimensions of Indulgence Versus Restraint

Indulgence	Restraint
Individuals have control of their own lives and destiny.	Much of what happens in life is beyond one's individual control.
Many people indicate that they are very happy.	Fewer people express that they are happy.
Freedom of speech is seen as an important value.	Freedom of speech is not a primary value.
Educated people have higher birth rates.	Educated people have lower birth rates.

Source: Based on Hofstede, 2011, p. 16.

young Hmong child with epilepsy, and how this child's family interpreted the need for their child's medical treatment. It was a cultural belief that the soul of children with this disease, referred to as "the spirit catches you and you fall down," had left the child's body. In this story based on true events, the child's family believed that the child's seizures made her unique, and she was chosen to be a shaman. Although the family implemented both Western medical practices and their traditional cultural medical practices, they were concerned that the Western medicine would negatively affect their child's ability to be healed spiritually. The point being made here is that it is imperative for professionals to understand the perspectives of the families with whom they are working, and how the family members may interpret illnesses and intervention.

- (S) Structuring the relationship between the professional and family focuses on the importance of making sure the appropriate family members are engaged in the child's care. Specifically, Bellon-Harn and Garrett (2008) state that it is important to determine "who should be included in the clinical process and, . . . the degree of family participation in the clinical process" (p. 144).

- (I) Interaction style refers to the style of communication that is preferred by the family and by the clinician. The professional must be able to communicate with family members in ways that are perceived as respectful and responsive to those family members. To be successful with this skill, it is necessary to be aware of nonverbal cues as well as verbal ones. For example, there may be differences in the use of eye contact between the child and the professional. Some members of some cultural

groups believe that direct eye contact is disrespectful; whereas, other cultural groups believe it is a sign of respect.

- (O) Operational strategies refer to the manner in which selecting and addressing goals is carried out. Bellon-Harn and Garrett (2008) discuss the importance of the professional recognizing, addressing, and incorporating issues that are important to the family members into the assessment and treatment plan. One method of engaging in this culturally responsive process for carrying out an assessment or intervention plan is to collaborate with family members in determining how these activities will be implemented.

- (N) Need (Perceived) focuses on the outcomes agreed upon by the family members and the professional (p. 147). One way to identify outcomes important to family members is to conduct an ethnographic interview[6] where family members are asked about their hopes for the outcome of the assessment and/or intervention in general, and specifically about their hopes and plans for their child.

These components are like the skills discussed in the pedagogical framework developed by Stockman et al. (2004).

Proposed Pedagogical Frameworks

Stockman et al. (2004) described strategies for ways to teach multicultural content in speech, language and hearing courses, and for providing effective services across multiple cultures. There are several tasks that SLPs and audiologists engage in regardless of who they are serving. These tasks include, referring, scheduling appointments, collecting a history, assessment and intervention, making recommendations

---

[6]The method for conducting and analyzing an ethnographic interview is discussed in detail in Chapter 7.

for additional services or an action plan, and terminating intervention (Stockman et al. 2004). There are other tasks the SLPs and audiologists do that can be affected by cultural influences. Those skills include, having a similar history or shared experiences with the client, worldviews, traditions, use of technology, learning styles, language, social interaction styles, and family organization. These authors write that, "A mosaic of cultural variation is created by the patterning of similarities and differences among groups" (p. 7). In other words, it is important to keep in mind that cultural groups may be similar regarding some cultural variables (e.g., language or social organization) but dissimilar with respect to others (e.g., learning style). The point here is that when providing services to individuals and/or families from cultural backgrounds different than ones' own, it is necessary to recognize that there may be cultural beliefs, values, and worldviews that are shared within as well as among cultural groups, and there are other aspects that are unique to cultural groups. We will not know everything about every cultural group, but "instruction should expose students to enough examples to prime their expectations that cultural differences do matter in their professional work" (p. 20).

Horton-Ikard and colleagues (2009) also published a pedagogical framework for teaching a multicultural course in communication sciences and disorders. This pedagogical framework focused on three dimensions of cultural "competence," which were awareness, knowledge, and skills. We highlight the "competencies" that Horton-Ikard et al. (2009) suggest that speech-language pathologists and audiologists should be learning to become more culturally responsive.

The first component of this framework is cultural awareness, including self-awareness, examination of personal biases, and awareness of diverse worldviews. This first component of the Horton-Ikard et al. model (2009) is similar to the "V" component in the Bellon-Harn and

Garrett (2008) model discussed earlier, in that the knowledge of one's own cultural values, beliefs, and assumptions is an important first step in becoming more culturally responsive.

The second component is acquiring knowledge about "theoretical perspectives, research frameworks, ASHA position papers, and the assessment and treatment literature" addressing practice with populations from diverse cultural and linguistic backgrounds (Horton-Ikard et al., 2009, p. 197). The theoretical perspectives highlighted by these authors focused on the historical context leading the field of speech, language, and hearing sciences to require "multicultural competence," research methods used to assess the communication abilities of individuals from diverse cultural and linguistic backgrounds, and frameworks for "describing disability in minority groups" (p. 197).

The third component of this framework focused on skill development, particularly in the ability to differentiate cultural communicative differences from disorders. In Figure 3–3, we provide a visual representation of the outcomes of the Horton-Ikard et al. framework (2009).

Salas-Provance's (2010) Hierarchy of Cultural Knowledge

Salas-Provance has developed a model, presented in Figure 3–4, to organize knowledge and move systematically from a basic level of *knowledge of cultural stereotypes* to an advanced level of *knowledge of cultural value*. At the *stereotypical level*, we are influenced by and limited to the information provided from the media such as the news, advertising, television, or movies. The information provided at this level may not only be biased but untrue and hurtful. Most of the time it represents stereotypes, an overgeneralization of an individual trait to the entire group (Salas-Provance, 2010), such as the idea that Asian Americans

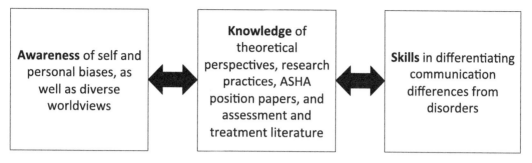

FIGURE 3–3. Visual representation of outcomes of a pedagogical framework for a multicultural course in communication sciences and disorders. Based on Horton-Ikard et al., 2009.

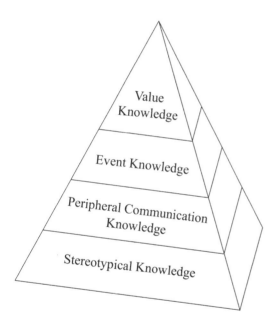

FIGURE 3–4. Visual representation of the Hierarchy of Cultural Knowledge Model. Republished with permission of Delmar Learning, a division of Cengage Learning, from Salas-Provance, M. B. (2010). Counseling in a multicultural society: Implications for the field of communication sciences and disorders. In L. Flasher and P. Fogel (Eds.), *Counseling skills for speech-language pathologists and audiologists* (pp. 159–189). Clifton Park, NY: Delmar; permission conveyed through Copyright Clearance Center, Inc.

It is important to stop here and remind you of approaching this information using a dialectical approach as mentioned in Chapter 2.

At the *peripheral level*, the information we receive about individuals from diverse groups is limited to our own personal experiences, such as a passive acknowledgment through a wave or smile to neighbors or coworkers ethnically different from us. For example, we observe that the African American family that lives down the street has many family members coming and going, and they have many family gatherings on the outdoor patio. We can then interpret what we wish from this limited knowledge, but keep in mind that our own interpretations come from our own cultural values, assumptions, and biases. We may decide that the family seems like a good family with strong family values, or that they are disruptive to the community with their outdoor gatherings.

As we move up the ladder of knowledge, we reach the *event knowledge* stage. At this level, we have an appreciation of other ethnic groups and their culture, but not a deep understanding. At the event stage, we may attend a First Nations dance, a Latin@/Hispanic Day festival, or a Chinese New Year parade and truly enjoy the event. This is the stage where many well-meaning individuals remain, because they may believe that attending events organized by groups from a cultural background different

do not maintain eye contact. While this may be true for some Asian Americans, it is not true for all individuals from this ethnic group.

than their own makes them culturally sensitive and knowledgeable. The cultural groups organizing these events, however, may end up being objectified[7] by the participants.

The top level, the *value stage*, is the highest stage of cultural responsiveness where we are most equipped to meet the needs of culturally and linguistically diverse clients. Clinicians at this stage value the diversity of clients and make a commitment to expanding their knowledge through additional training or readings. Because organizations value the contributions of individuals from diverse ethnic groups, they may make monetary commitments to improve medical and educational research or to train interpreters. At the national level, the government passes laws and expands programs to improve the lives of individuals from various cultural/ethnic groups.

Finally, the knowledge and skills for providing services to clients from diverse ethnic/racial/cultural backgrounds will best be developed through a combination of education and direct experience. Although we attempted to share some general values and behaviors that can be attributed to different cultural groups, there may be more differences than similarities within each group. It is important to consider each client and family as unique individuals who will present their own distinctive set of beliefs and behaviors in the clinical or educational process.

Hyter's (2014) Conceptual Framework for Responsive Global Engagement

Hyter, working from a critical social science perspective, proposed a conceptual framework for providing responsive services in a culturally diverse and globalized world (Hyter, 2014). She emphasizes the importance of approaching speech, language, and hearing services from a macro level perspective, incorporating a focus on policies and practices and other contextual factors (e.g., economics, politics) that affect communication outcomes. Hyter also emphasized the importance of having a conceptual framework for providing culturally (and globally) responsive services. A conceptual framework emerges from a theoretical position, and the concepts associated with that stance are organized into a framework or structure that can serve to guide decisions and practices. Table 3–9 shows the components of Hyter's framework, and how they manifest in the areas of research, curriculum, teaching, and clinical practice.

CHAPTER SUMMARY

There are diverse ways of thinking about culturally responsive practices, and each of these ways of thinking comes from a theoretical paradigm. In this chapter, we discussed only four paradigms of social theories—positivist, interpretivist, critical theories, and postmodernism—which can serve as a way of explaining and predicting phenomena. To build your own conceptual framework (philosophy of practice), which will serve as your guide for providing culturally responsive services, start with a social theory that will guide your thinking about your conceptual framework. (Note that very few people are theoretical purist these days. Sometimes you may find that operating from more than one theoretical framework best serves your work. As an example, first author, Dr. Hyter, is a critical social theorist but also values what knowledge can be constructed when using interpretivist social science methods such as ethnographic interviewing, participant observations, as well as document and artifact analyses.)

---

[7]Reducing the cultural group to an object with no other value than to engage in cultural events.

TABLE 3–9. Hyter's Conceptual Framework for Responsive Global Engagement

Conceptual Framework Components	Domains and Example Applications			
	Research	Curriculum	Teaching	Clinical
Transdisciplinary praxis	Questions emerge from dialogue among transdisciplinary team members. Activities are carried out in transdisciplinary teams that include local and global members.	Courses include explanations of social theories; material/readings pertaining to macro-level factors affecting diverse groups are incorporated into course content; students engage in critical reflection and collective practice of skills	Teaching strategies include case-based and team-based learning requiring dialectical thinking and critical self-reflection.	Clinicians partner with other disciplines (e.g., anthropology), as well as clients and their families (as a transdisciplinary team), to understand the cultural history of persons on their caseloads; they incorporate new knowledge into existing knowledge, alter practices based on new knowledge, and then critically reflect on those altered practices and their outcomes, revising as necessary.
World system	Research questions focus on explaining language and literacy processes, development, and disorders in the context of world system(s).	Courses include explanations of world systems and the relationships among them, including how these relationships affect communication, language, and literacy development and practices.	Case-based and team-based learning activities focus on groups from diverse world systems that are both in harmony and in conflict with one another.	Clinical services are implemented with consideration of the client's worldview, cultural assumptions, and practices. These factors are incorporated into assessment and/or intervention processes.
Effects of social structures	Social structures are considered when constructing research questions, as well as when collecting and interpreting data.	Courses include explanation of social structures and their impact on diverse groups of people from different world systems.	Case-based and team-based learning activities consider consequences of social structures on lives of potential client-partners.	Contextual factors are considered, including social structures, when planning, engaging in, and interpreting assessment and intervention.

continues

TABLE 3–9. *continued*

Conceptual Framework Components	Domains and Example Applications			
	Research	Curriculum	Teaching	Clinical
World literacy	Researchers use a dialectical and critical approach to construct research questions, and when collecting and interpreting data.	In addition to discussing various levels of print literacy, multiple courses include explanations of world literacy, and opportunities for students to engage in these forms of literacy.	Standard classroom and course topics include information about diverse communities inside and outside of one's country; opportunities occur to engage in critical inquiry of speech-language pathologist research and clinical strategies.	Clinicians demonstrate an understanding of the causes of problems faced by their clients, benefits and losses, and in collaboration with clients identify ways to overcome obstacles that hinder full participation in daily life.
Macro practice as responsive global engagement	Research agendas are developed in collaboration with local and global community members. Research questions emerge from shared problems with local and global community members (Tuhiwai-Smith, 1999).	Concepts denoting a pathway to responsive global engagement are a common discussion topic in curricula. Information about diversity, inclusion, multiculturalism, and multilingualism is part of the curriculum.	Practical activities requiring demonstration of the concepts of responsive global engagement are commonly utilized.	Clinical services are carried out in collaboration with local and global communities. Clinicians are able to make seamless transitions between local and global communities.

Source: Reprinted with permission from Hyter, Y. D. (2014). A framework for responsive global engagement in Communication Sciences and Disorders. *Topics in Language Disorders, 34*(2), 103–120.

Using a conceptual framework will facilitate your ability to provide culturally responsive services in any circumstances with any person from any cultural group. You will develop some principles to follow as you engage in culturally responsive practices. There are a number of conceptual frameworks and models for understanding cultural diversity, and that serve as support for culturally responsive practices, that have been discussed in the literature—WHO-ICF; World Report on Disability; The Meaning of Illness, Disease and Disability; the Iceberg Theory; Cultural Dimensions; as well as the VISION Model; a Pedagogical Framework; the Hierarchy of Cultural Knowledge Model; and a Conceptual Framework for Responsive Global Engagement

EXTENDED LEARNING

- Begin to identify, explain, and question one's own cultural values/beliefs.
- Begin to develop your own conceptual framework that will facilitate culturally responsive practices, and will guide the decisions you make as a SLP or audiologist. Some things to think about as you develop your own conceptual framework or philosophy of practice are to
  - □ Begin by identifying a social theory to guide your thinking.
  - □ Identify concepts consistent with the social theory (or theories) but that also are meaningful for your field.
  - □ Define the concepts.
  - □ Arrange them in a way that demonstrates their relationship one to another. (Reviewing the article by Hyter, 2014, will be helpful as a guide for developing your own conceptual framework or philosophy of practice.)
  - □ Students in Dr. Hyter's class also work for a semester on a conceptual framework for culturally and globally responsive practice. Examples of three of those frameworks are shown in Figures 3–5, 3–6, and 3–7.
- Engage in critical and dialectical thinking by journaling in response to prompts that are part of the PluralPlus companion website.
- Solve the case study presented on the PluralPlus companion website from the perspective of each of the social theories discussed in this chapter.

DISCUSSION QUESTIONS

1. How are the theoretical frameworks presented in this chapter similar? How are they different?
2. Which theoretical frameworks seem to overlap? Which ones seem to be 180 degrees different from each other?
3. Which theoretical framework(s) resonates with your current thinking? Why?

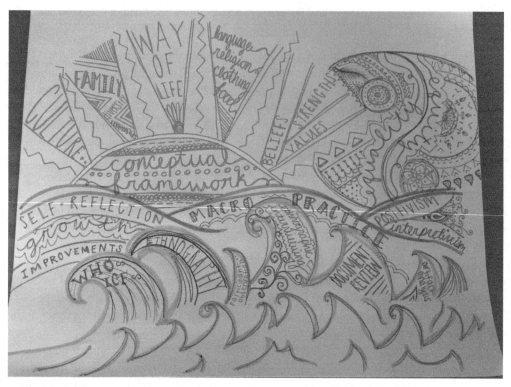

FIGURE 3–5. Conceptual framework example. Image courtesy of Lindsay Marie Hunt.

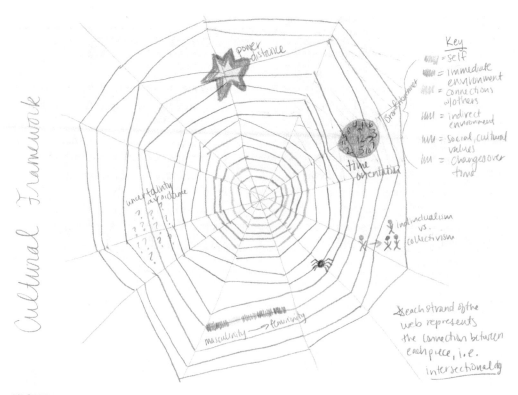

FIGURE 3–6. Conceptual framework example. Image courtesy of Jennifer Elise Otwell.

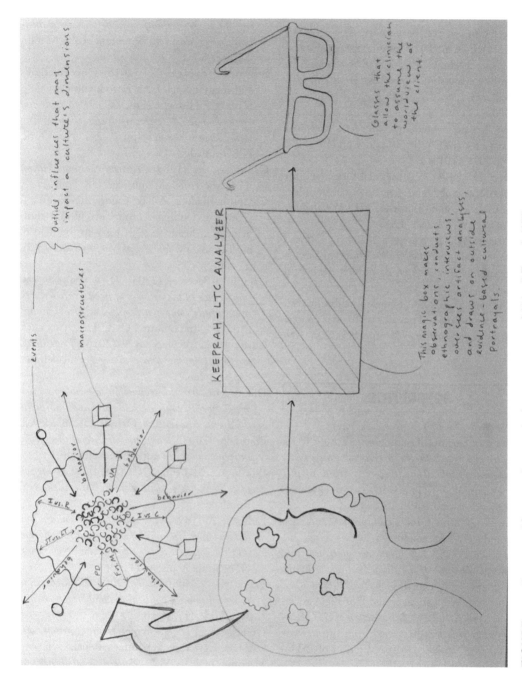

FIGURE 3–7. Conceptual framework example. Image courtesy of Abigail Francis Williams.

FURTHER READING

Bellon-Harn, M. L., & Garrett, T. T. (2008). VISION: A model of cultural responsiveness for speech-language pathologists working in family partnerships. *Communication Disorders Quarterly, 29*(3), 141–148.

Hofstede, G. (2011). Dimensionalizing cultures: The Hofstede model in context. *Psychology and Culture, 2*(1). http://dx.doi.org/10.9707/2307-0919.1014

Hyter, Y. D. (2014). A conceptual framework for responsive global engagement in communication sciences and disorders. *Topics in Language Disorders, 34*(2), 103–120.

Kalyanpur, M., & Harry, B. (2012). *Cultural reciprocity in special education: Building family-professional relationships.* Baltimore, MD: Paul H. Brookes.

McCormack, B. (2003). A conceptual framework for person-centered practice with older people. *International Journal of Nursing, 9*(3), 202–209.

REFERENCES

Academy of Doctors of Audiology (ADA). (2017). *ADA supports S.9, the over-the-counter hearing aid act of 2016.* Retrieved from http://www.audiologist.org/about/ada-news-archive/1707-ada-supports-s9

Agger, B. (2006). *Critical social theories* (2nd ed.). Boulder, CO: Paradigm.

Al-Haj, M. (1995). *Education, empowerment and control: The case of the Arabs in Israel.* Albany, NY: State University of New York Press.

American Speech, Language and Hearing Association (ASHA). (2016). *Introduction of OTC hearing aid legislation.* Retrieved from http://www.asha.org/News/2016/Introduction-of-OTC-Hearing-Aid-Legislation/

Baert, P. (1998). *Social theory in the twentieth century.* New York, NY: New York University Press.

Bellon-Harn, M. L., & Garrett, T. T. (2008). VISION: A model of cultural responsiveness for speech-language pathologists working in family partnerships. *Communication Disorders Quarterly, 29*(3), 141–148.

Brookfield, S. (2012). *Teaching for critical thinking: Tools and techniques to help students question their assumptions.* San Francisco, CA: John Wiley & Sons.

Browne, K., & Nash, C. J. (2016). Queer methods and methodologies: An introduction. In C. J. Nash & K. Browne (Eds.), *Queer methods and methodologies: Intersecting queer theories and social science research* (pp. 1–24). New York, NY: Routledge.

Callinicos, A. (1989). *Against postmodernism: A Marxist critique.* Cambridge, UK: Polity Press.

Campinha-Bacote, A., & Campinha-Bacote, J. (2009). Extending a model of cultural competence in health care delivery to the field of health care law. *Journal of Nursing Law, 13*(2), 36–44.

Campinha-Bacote, J. (2003). *The process of cultural competence in the delivery of health care services. A culturally competence model of care.* Cincinnati, OH: Transcultural C. A. R. E. Associates.

Chitty, K. K., & Black, B. P. (2010). *Professional nursing: Concepts and challenges.* Philadelphia, PA: Saunders.

Dillon, M. (2010). *Introduction to sociological theory: Theorists, concepts, and their applicability to the twenty first century.* Oxford, UK: Blackwell.

Elliott, A. (2009). *Contemporary social theory: An introduction.* New York, NY: Routledge.

Elliott, A., & Lemert, C. (2014). *Introduction to contemporary social theory.* New York, NY: Routledge.

Fadiman, A. (1997). *The spirit catches you and you fall down: A Hmong child, her American doctors and the collision of the two cultures.* New York, NY: Farrar, Straus, and Giroux.

Fraser, N., & Honneth, A. (2003). *Redistribution or recognition?: A political-philosophical exchange.* New York, NY: Verso.

Gramsci, A. (1971). *Selections from the prison notebooks.* New York, NY: International.

Harrington, A. (2005). *Modern social theory: An introduction.* Oxford, UK: Oxford University Press.

Herman, E. S., & Chomsky, N. (2002). *Manufacturing consent: The political economy of mass media.* New York, NY: Pantheon Books.

Hofstede, G. (1984). Cultural dimensions in management and planning. *Asia Pacific Journal of Management, 1*, 81–99.

Hofstede, G. (2010). The GLOBE debate: Back to relevance. *Journal of International Business Studies, 41*(8), 1339–1346.

Hofstede, G. (2011). Dimensionalizing cultures: The Hofstede model in context. *Psychology and Culture, 2*(1). http://dx.doi.org/10.9707/2307-0919.1014

Horton-Ikard, R., Munoz, M. L., Thomas-Tate, S., & Keller-Bell, Y. (2009). Establishing a pedagogical framework for the multicultural course in communication sciences and disorders. *American Journal of Speech-Language Pathology, 18*, 192–206.

Hyde, A. (2004). *Sociology for health professionals in Ireland.* Dublin, Ireland: Institute of Public Administration.

Hyter, Y. D. (2014). A conceptual framework for responsive global engagement in communication sciences and disorders. *Topics in Language Disorders, 34*(2), 103–120.

Jones, P., Bradbury, L., & Le Boutillier, S. (2011). *Introducing social theory* (2nd ed.). Cambridge, UK: Polity

Kalyanpur, M., & Harry, B. (2012). *Cultural reciprocity in special education: Building family-professional relationships.* Baltimore, MD: Brookes.

Kirst-Ashman, K. K. (2013). *Human behavior in the macro social environment: An empowerment approach to understanding communities, organizations, and groups* (3rd ed.). Belmont, CA: Wadsworth.

Kleinman, A. (1989). *The illness narratives: Suffering, healing, and the human condition.* New York, NY: Basic Books.

Kleinman, A., & Benson, P. (2006). Anthropology in the clinic: The problem of cultural competency and how to fix it. *PloS Medicine, 3*(10), 1673–1676.

Kuttner, P. (2016, October 29). The problem with that equity vs. equality graphic that you're using. *Cultural Organizing.* Retrieved from http://culturalorganizing.org

Leininger, M. M. (2004). *Culture care diversity and universality: A theory of nursing.* Sudbury, MA: Jones & Bartlett.

Marcuse, H. (2012). *One-dimensional man: Studies in the ideology of advanced industrial society.* Boston, MD: Beacon Press.

Monette, D. R., Sullivan, T. J., & DeJong, C. R. (2011). *Applied social research: A tool for the human services* (8th ed.). Australia: Brooks/Cole Cengage Learning.

Mukherji, P., & Albon, D. (2014). *Research methods in early childhood: An introductory guide* (2nd ed.). Thousand Oaks, CA: Sage.

Munoz, C. C., Conrad DoBroka, C., & Mohammad, S. (2009). Development of a multidisciplinary course in cultural competence for Nursing and Human Service professions. *Journal of Nursing Education, 48*(9), 495–503.

Neuman, W. L. (2003). *Social research methods: Qualitative and quantitative approaches* (5th ed.). Boston, MA: Allyn & Bacon.

Neuman, L. (2006). *Social research methods: Qualitative and quantitative approaches.* (6th ed.). New York, NY: Pearson Education.

Ortega, R. M., & Coulborn Faller, K. (2011). Training child welfare workers from an intersectional cultural humility perspective: A paradigm shift. *Child Welfare, 90*(5), 27–49.

Over-the-Counter Hearing Aid Act of 2016, S.9, 114th Cong. (2006).

Parsons, T. (1937). *The structure of social action.* New York, NY: McGraw-Hill.

Prasad, P. (2005). *Crafting qualitative research: Working in the postpositivist traditions.* London, UK: Routledge.

Purnell, L. 2002. The Purnell model for cultural competence. *Journal of Transcultural Nursing, 13*, 193–196.

Robinson, C. (1983). *Black Marxism: The making of the Black radical tradition.* London, UK: Zed Press.

Salas-Provance, M. B. (2010). Counseling in a multicultural society: Implications for the field of communication sciences and disorders. In L. Flasher & P. Fogel (Eds.), *Counseling skills for speech-language pathologists and audiologists* (pp. 159–189). Clifton Park, NY: Delmar.

Santiago-Valles, W. F. (1998). *Memories of the future: Maroon intellectuals from the Caribbean and the origins of their communication strategies, 1925–1940* (Unpublished doctoral dissertation). Simon Fraser University, Canada.

Santiago-Valles, W. F. (2005). Producing knowledge for social transformation: Precedents from the Diaspora for twenty-first century research and pedagogy. *The Black Scholar, 35*(2), 50–60.

Santiago-Valles, W. F. (2006). Resistance among those displaced to the Caribbean: Suggestions for future research. In R. Gowricharn (Ed). *Caribbean transnationalism: Migration, pluralization, and social cohesion* (pp. 59–78). Oxford, UK: Lexington Books.

Santiago-Valles, W. F. (2011, September). *Excluded intellectual traditions in Africa and the African Diaspora: Transdisciplinary research procedures, methodologies, bibliographies and allies.* Talk sponsored by the African Studies Center at Michigan State University, East Lansing, MI.

Scheper-Hughes, N., & Lock, M. M. (1987). The mindful body: A prolegomenon to future work in medical anthropology. *Medical Anthropology Quarterly, New Series, 1*(1), 6–41.

Sinclair, M. (2007). Editorial: A guide to understanding theoretical and conceptual frameworks. *Evidenced-Based Midwifery, 5*(2), 39.

Sivanandan, A. (2005). *Race & Class: The future. Race & Class, 46*(3), 1–6.

Stockman, I., Boult, J., & Robinson, G. (2004). Multicultural issues in academic and clinical education: A cultural mosaic. *ASHA Leader, 9*, 7 & 20.

Suh, E. (2004). The model of cultural competence through an evolutionary concept analysis. *Journal of Transcultural Nursing 15*(2), 93–102.

Tervalon, M., & Murray-Garcia, J. (1998). Cultural humility versus cultural competence: A critical distinction in defining physician training outcomes in multicultural education. *Journal of Health Care for the Poor and Underserved, 9*(2), 117–125.

Ting-Toomey, S. (1999). *Communicating across cultures.* New York, NY: The Guilford Press.

Ting-Toomey, S., & Chung, L. C. (2012). *Understanding intercultural communication.* Oxford, UK: Oxford University Press.

Tuhiwai-Smith, L. (1999). *Decolonizing methodologies: Research and indigenous peoples.* Dunedin, New Zealand: University of Otago Press.

United Nations New Centre. (2016). *News focus: Mali.* Retrieved from http://www.un.org/apps/news/infocusRel.asp?infocusID=150

Verschueren, J. (2012). *Ideology in language use: Pragmatic guidelines for empirical research.* Cambridge, UK: Cambridge University Press.

Vygotsky, L. (1978). *Mind in society: The development of higher psychological processes.* Cambridge, MA: Harvard University Press.

World Health Organization. (2011). World Report on Disability 2011. Geneva: World HealthOrganization.

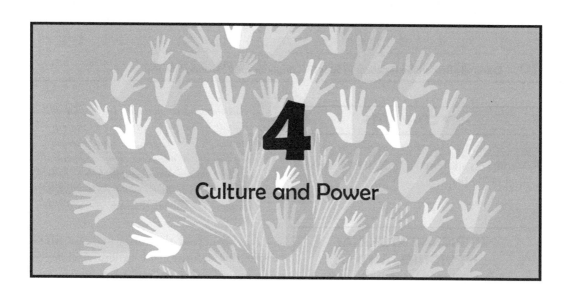

4

Culture and Power

Culture, as we mentioned in Chapter 2, is composed of the assumptions, values, and beliefs held by groups of people, which drive behaviors, ways of using language, and ways of organizing daily life (Hyter, 2014; Ting-Toomey & Chung, 2012). These assumptions, values, and beliefs are passed from one generation to the next and are based on the histories that groups of people have with solving shared problems.

In this chapter, you learn about the relationship between culture and power. The purpose of this chapter is to facilitate your knowledge of power in its various forms, and the ways that unequal relations of power affect cultural beliefs and behaviors, and could impact effective professional or clinical practices.

LEARNING OBJECTIVES

After reading, discussing and processing the information presented in this chapter, you will be able to demonstrate the following knowledge, skills, and attitudes:

1. Knowledge
    a. Define power and its various iterations.
    b. Discuss the relationship between culture and power.
    c. Explain the potential for increased power that a person in a caregiving role in a relationship has over the person in the care-receiving role.
2. Skills
    a. Recognize institutionalized (systemic) power and the ways that it has the potential to affect cultural beliefs and practices, and the provision of professional services.
    b. Work to reduce power inequities between those you serve.
    c. Recognizing your own power in your role as a service provider, and the influence you may have on the decisions and actions of the person you are serving.
3. Attitudes demonstrated through journaling
    a. Demonstrate the valuing of equity and justice.
    b. Demonstrate a willingness to gain additional information and knowledge about unequal power relations.
    c. Demonstrate the desire to minimize and eliminate unequal power relations between you and those you serve.

KEY CONCEPTS

Key concepts addressed in this chapter are presented in Table 4–1.

HURRICANE KATRINA, ITS VICTIMS, AND POWER IN THE FORM OF STRUCTURAL VIOLENCE

Dr. Paul Farmer defines structural violence in this way:

> Structural violence is one way of describing social arrangements that put individuals and populations in harm's way. The arrangements are structural because they are embedded in political and economic organization of our social world; they are violent because they cause injury to people (typically not those responsible for perpetuating such inequalities). (Farmer, 2004; Farmer, Nizeye, Stulac, & Keshavjee, 2006, p. 1686)

TABLE 4–1. Key Concepts

Power	Microaggressions
Structural violence	Linguistic profiling
Manufactured consent	Linguicism
	Intersectionality
Symbolic violence	Equity
Ideology	
Standard language ideology	
Equality	

> . . . neither culture nor pure individual will is at fault; rather historically given (and often economically driven) processes and forces conspire to constrain individual agency. Structural violence is visited upon all those whose social status denies them access to the fruits of scientific and social progress. (Farmer, 2001, p. 79)

As you read the following case, think about this definition of structural violence. As you read the chapter, think about the relationship between culture, structural violence, and power. Farmer and colleagues (2006) also state that clinicians (that would include speech-language pathologists and audiologists) do not usually receive education about structural violence and its social forces. Nevertheless, "interventions will fail if we are unable to understand the social determinants of disease" (p. 1687).

Box 4–1

Between August 23 and August 31, 2005, unequal relations of power were revealed up close and personal through the disaster of Hurricane Katrina, and its aftermath in New Orleans, Louisiana. Hurricane Katrina was one of the deadliest hurricanes that occurred in the United States (Knabb, Rhome, & Brown, 2005).[1] It started as a category 5 and then became a category 3 that hit cities along the Gulf coast but devastated New Orleans, producing 43 tornadoes around the Gulf states (Knabb et al., 2005). New Orleans had been perceived by many in the United States as a place for wonderful jazz music, exciting Mardi Gras parties, great food, and a place to

---

[1]After this book went to press, Hurricane Harvey was a category 4 and was followed by Hurricane Irma, which started as a category 5 and Hurricane Maria, which made landfall in Puerto Rico as a category 4. These hurricanes all occurred in September of 2017.

experience the mixture of Cajun and Creole cultures (Simmons & Casper, 2012). "The hurricane provoked tourists and consumers alike to see the city in a new and profoundly disturbing light" (p. 676). In the wake of Katrina, those who suffered the most were those who were impoverished and marginalized in the city. But among those individuals, the group that received the most media coverage was African American. The groups rendered practically invisible were the victims who were Latin@/Hispanic, Asian American, people with disabilities, as well as those who were elderly (Simmons & Casper, 2012).

It is important to start this chapter with a definition of power, which can be individual or social. It is the ability to "control our own destiny" (Newton, 2002, p. 227). More specifically, power is the capacity of groups of people to exert control of their lives in their own interest, even amid opposition from others (Hardcastle, Powers, & Wenocur, 2011; Weber, 1947). Power is usually thought about as primarily being in the hands of those who own and use natural, material, and financial resources to shape the world for their own benefit (Simmons & Casper, 2012). Groups with power can decide what topics get covered in the media or during political debates, or can determine what the rules of a process are, and then change them when it is in their own interest (Bachrach & Baratz, 1962). Groups with power can advance interpretations of those without power (Lukes, 2005), such as those that are marginalized in a society. Lukes (2005) states that "power is . . . most effective when least observable" (p. 64).

Power is dynamic in that who or which groups hold power can shift based on the context. For example, students (the group in schools usually thought to have little power)

negotiating with the administration for a better studying environment (e.g., removal of fluorescent lighting) can exercise power by staging a walkout if negotiations with the school administration stall.

Culture and power intersect within communicative interactions (Martin & Nakayama, 2000). When one of the authors (Dr. Hyter) traveled to Paris, France, for the first time, she was able to communicate using a little rudimentary French. When she and her husband went to a restaurant for breakfast, she went to the counter and ordered in English, "I would like to order eggs and a croissant, please." The waiter very politely said in French, we do not have eggs and a croissant. Dr. Hyter understood what he said, but realized that something else was going on because it was clear that they had a counter full of croissants, and she could see the chefs making eggs. From a cultural perspective, it is important to know that many French citizens would prefer for guests in their country to speak French, not English. Dr. Hyter realized her error and reordered breakfast in French, but by then, it was too late. The waiter refused to consider Dr. Hyter's order. The only way she could eat breakfast that morning was because her husband ordered it for her—in French. The waiter exercised individual power in this communicative interaction.

Power can be exerted using at least six different tools. One, structural violence, was defined and discussed at the beginning of the chapter. Following are other historical examples of the way power has been exerted in the world using: (1) physical violence, (2) symbolic violence, (3) manufactured consent, (4) the organization of work, and (5) the organization of leisure time.

Physical Violence

In 1963, the Southern Christian Leadership Conference (SCLC) organized a campaign in

Birmingham, Alabama, to end racial segregation practiced by businesses in this city. The methods used to protest racial segregation included sit-ins at lunch counters of stores like Woolworth's or Kresge's,[2] in churches that were open only to White people, as well as by marching throughout cities and towns. You can find pictures of Woolworth's store front and lunch counter at https://ephemeralnewyork.wordpress.com/tag/1960s-protests-in-new-york-city/ and https://www.washingtonpost.com/national/franklin-mccain-who-helped-inspire-sit-ins-for-civil-rights-as-part-of-greensboro-four-dies/2014/01/13/8c39840e-7c6e-11e3-9556-4a4bf7bcbd84_story.html?utm_term=.0d67b6173d24

These peaceful protests were met by physical violence, such that the protesters were beat with bully clubs, rocks, and fists (by police and White citizens who were against integration), assaulted by attack dogs, and hit with water from fire hoses turned up "high enough to remove bark from trees" (Isserman & Kazin, 2000, p. 89). This particular form of physical violence (i.e., use of water cannons or water hoses) was used again as "crowd control" in 2016 in North Dakota when groups of people, primarily composed of members of the Standing Rock Sioux Tribe and others, were peacefully protesting the construction of the Dakota Access Pipeline (Barajas, 2016). These acts of violence were (and still are in many cases) sanctioned and carried out by the arm of the law (e.g., police and the courts) and supported by the state government. Unfortunately, physical violence continues to occur even in professional settings such as between a boss and her or his employee, or between a service provider and her or his client. Each year, approximately 2 million workers in the United States report having experienced workplace violence (U.S. Department of Labor,

n.d.). Violence still occurs in the workplace and in professional settings, but it is now primarily symbolic rather than physical.

Symbolic Violence

Symbolic violence occurs because of the implicit (and often unnoticed) economic exploitation, political domination, and social exclusion of certain groups (Bourdieu, 2005). Economic exploitation is based on three criteria (Wright, 1997). First, benefits to one group depend on the disadvantage or deprivation of another group (Wright, 1997, p. 10). In other words, there is an inverse interdependence among those groups that have material resources and those that do not. Second, the first criterion for exploitation as stated above depends on the exclusion of groups from access to certain resources. This exclusion may be supported by laws, such as the housing policy of the United States between 1934 and 1968 (Hannah-Jones, 2012). Between 1934 and 1968 the Federal Housing Administration (FHA) denied mortgages to people of color. With this policy, the FHA legalized and institutionalized racism; that is, a division of the government implemented racist laws deliberately to exclude segments of U.S. society. Third, those who control access to resources, appropriate [*this is the verb, as in the intentional taking of something that belongs to someone else to present as if it were one's own*] the work efforts produced by those who are exploited (Buraway & Wright, 2006; Wright, 1997). In other words, the exploiters depend on the efforts of the exploited for their own welfare and benefit (Buraway & Wright, p. 471).

In this text we define politics as the ability to exercise power in one's own interest. Specifically, politics is " . . . the process

---

[2]Woolworth's and Kresge's were what would be considered "five and dime" stores that sold items (e.g., candy, clothing, toys, etc.) for little money. In the 1960s, these stores had lunch counters where they would serve lunch, sodas, and shakes.

of conflict (and conflict resolution) among private interests carried into the public arena" (Parenti, 2011, p. 2). Politics includes groups with competing interests and varying degrees of power working within the existing political and economic system. For example, some groups may be working to make the system more hospitable to diverse and marginalized groups, as well as to demolish the existing structures in favor of creating more equitable alternatives to it (Parenti, 2011). At the same time, other groups may be working to ensure multinational corporations and the people who run them have acquired more profits at the expense of diverse and marginalized groups and/or countries. An example of symbolic violence in the form of political domination is the closing of public schools that were primarily located in the neighborhoods of African American and Latin@/Hispanic children because of a movement designed to promote private, religious, and charter schools over public ones. Some research has shown that charter school outcomes are not better or worse than public school outcomes (U.S. Department of Education, 2010). Those with power have shaped schooling systems to be organized in the interests of their own ideas. This act of power can be "misrecognized" (Bourdieu, 2005, p. 60) by the public, meaning that it is not perceived as being an act that exploits, dominates, or excludes, but as a legitimate need for certain types of communities.

Language can be used in a variety of ways, including as an instrument of symbolic power (Ball & Alim, 2006; Baugh, 2003, 2007), and can contribute to exploitation, domination, or the exclusion of others (Lecercle, 1990). In this way, language and communication are not neutral endeavors (Fairclough, 2001; Lippi-Green, 1997, 2012; Schiffman, 1996). An example of language being used as an instrument of symbolic power is when one communication partner decides to not uphold his or her responsibility in the communica-

tive interaction. Let's explore this point a little more. There is a tacit agreement between speakers and listeners based on the principle of *mutual responsibility* (Clark & Wilkes-Gibbs, 1986). This agreement is not necessarily consciously thought about by communicative participants, but the basic assumption is that communicative partners collaborate during an interaction. When engaged in communicative activities with persons who are different than themselves, however, people often make decisions about whether or not they will "accept their responsibility in the act of communication" (Lippi-Green, 1997, p. 70). Those with more power in the communicative undertaking may decide to reject their responsibility within the communicative act.

Rejection of the principle of mutual responsibility is related to *language ideology* or *linguistic culture*. Language ideology (Ahearn, 2012) and linguistic culture (Schiffman, 1996) refer to the beliefs, values, and assumptions that people have about language (Ahearn, 2012; Irvine & Gal, 2000; Lippi-Green, 2012; Schiffman, 1996). If communication partner "A" believes that person "B" is speaking with an accent that is not comprehensible, it is less likely that speaker "A" will uphold his or her end of the communicative act. *Standard language ideology*, or better stated, the ideology of the standard language (Milroy, 2001, p. 530), is the unquestioned belief that there is a certain model of language that is "normal," the correct way to speak, or the standard against which other variations of a language should be measured (Irvine & Gal, 2000; Milroy, 2001). According to Milroy (2001), "English, French, and Spanish are believed by their speakers to exist in standardized forms, and this kind of belief affects the way in which speakers think about their own language and about 'language' in general" (p. 530).

Another example of symbolic violence in the form of social exclusion is the role played by microaggressions in creating exclusive rather than inclusive environments. Not taking part in a communicative act can be considered a microaggression. Microaggressions are the "brief and commonplace daily verbal, behavioral, and environmental indignities, whether intentional or unintentional, that communicate hostile, derogatory, or negative racial, gender, sexual-orientation, and religious slights and insults to the target person or group" (Pierce, Carew, Pierce-Gonzalez, & Willis, 1978; Sue, 2010, pp. 4–5). Microaggressions can go beyond race, gender, sexual, and religious categories to include groups with disabilities, psychological impairments, and those from low socioeconomic backgrounds (Capodilupo & Sue, 2013).

According to Sue (2010), there are three primary types of microaggressions: microinsults, microassaults, and microinvalidations. Microinsults are racialized, gendered, or sexualized demeaning comments and behaviors. An example is when an African American or Latin@/Hispanic person is waiting in line to make a purchase, and a White person arrives later but steps in front of the person already waiting in line, as if the African American or Latin@/Hispanic person was not visible. The insult is made worse when the store clerk proceeds to wait on the White person as if he or she arrived in line first.

Microassaults are what is called "old fashioned racism, sexism, or heterosexism" (Sue, 2010, p. 29) carried out by individuals. These are deliberate, overt or covert attitudes, beliefs, or behaviors against groups of people (e.g., First Nations, African Americans, Latin@s/Hispanics, Asians, or other marginalized groups such as members of the LGBTQIA[3] community, persons who are impoverished, or individuals with disabilities). A pretty public microassault was committed when a director of a government-funded nonprofit organization in a town in West Virginia insinuated

on her Facebook page that Mrs. Obama, the first African American first lady of the United States, was an "ape in heels." The mayor of that town then approved (liked) that Facebook message (see the series of articles about this topic printed in the *Washington Post* at https://www.washingtonpost.com/news/post-nation/wp/2016/11/14/ape-in-heels-w-va-officials-under-fire-after-comments-about-michelle-obama/?utm_term=.20081ec667ee) (Browning & Bever, 2016). These comments are considered racist because of the long history in the United States of African Americans and Black people as well as First Nations people having been compared to animals, and specifically for African Americans, referred to as monkeys, apes, and orangutans since the 1600s (DeMello, 2012; Feagin, 2013). These overtly racist comments—microassaults—are made worse when the perpetrators claim that they "are not racists" or their supporters suggest that they "didn't really mean it in a racist way" rather than condemning the statements and the sentiments behind them. Another public display of a microassault was committed in 2016 by then presidential candidate Donald Trump (who would go on to become president of the United States in 2016), when he "mocked" a reporter with a disability (see http://heavy.com/news/2016/09/donald-trump-mocks-disabled-reporter-serge-kovaleski-denies-mocking-reporter/).

Microinvalidations are the negation of the feelings, perceptions, and people who experience racist, sexist, gendered microinsults and microassaults. One common example is when a woman, for example, is explaining how her comments in a meeting are ignored, but when a man parrots what she just said the comments are highly valued by those participating in the meeting. Let's say this woman who experienced this event in a meeting was expressing concern about the sexist nature

---

[3]LGBTQIA stands for lesbian, gay, bisexual, transgender, queer, intersexual, and asexual.

of the meeting, as well as the sexist nature of professional meetings in general for groups of women, and the man she was talking to said, "but that could happen to anyone—it happened to me once, too." At that moment, the woman's concern was invalidated by the man to whom she was speaking.

A shocking event occurred in 2009 during a speech made early in the presidential term of President Barack Obama, the first African American president in the United States. While President Obama was giving a speech to the joint session of Congress, a Republican congressman, Joe Wilson Sr., representative of South Carolina's second congressional district, yelled "you lie," in the middle of the speech. Although there previously had been negative *collective* responses to a presidential address (e.g., head shaking, not standing, or not clapping), this particular event was the first time in the history of the United States that such a public show of disrespect for the presidency occurred. Since this elevated level of disrespect occurred during the term of the first Black president of the United States, this behavior was deemed racist by many, particularly because nothing of the sort ever occurred before with the White presidents. This outburst seemed to serve as an attempt to invalidate or negate the authority of the presidency. What makes this microinvalidation worse is that although Wilson received a formal "rebuke" by the House of Representatives, he did not lose his job when he ran for office in 2010, 2012, or again in 2014, suggesting that the public he represented agreed with this racist behavior.

Microaggressions are daily experiences for many groups in the United States. These negative experiences, although subtle and indirect, wreak havoc emotionally and psychologically for groups that are the target of these aggressions. Sue (2010) states that microaggressions "assail self-esteem of recipients, produce anger and frustration, deplete psychic energy, lower

feelings of subjective well-being and worthiness" (p. 6), which result in increased physical health problems and shortened life expectancy, as well as denying populations of color and those that are marginalized based on race, ethnicity, nationality, ability level, gender, and sexual orientation "equal access and opportunity in education, employment and health care" (Smith, Hung, & Franklin, 2011; Sue, 2010, p. 6).

Consider the examples of microaggressions in the following list. After reviewing the list, identify microaggressions that you experienced yourself, or that you noticed have been perpetrated by individuals or by a system (e.g., the way an educational system is organized) against others.

1. When a woman at John McCain's (a U.S. Senator who ran for president in 2008) town hall meeting said that she did not trust Obama (who became President Barack Obama serving for two presidential terms between 2008 and 2016) because he was an "Arab," McCain's response was, "No ma'am. He's a decent family man, a citizen that I just happen to have disagreements with. He's not!"

An underlying assumption of the statements made by John McCain and by the woman who made the statement is that there would be, in fact, something wrong if President Obama was an Arab. Although McCain corrected the woman's perception, his response also served to facilitate the myth that an Arab man is not necessarily a "decent family man, a citizen . . . " or should ever be president of the United States.

2. After a female faculty member from the Cherokee nation, and who has a PhD, makes a statement during a faculty meeting, a Caucasian male faculty

member with a PhD, says, "I don't understand anything you are saying." This event reoccurs during most faculty meetings.

This scenario illustrates one communication partner deciding to not sustain his end of the communicative contract. It is likely that the linguistic culture or language ideology of the male faculty member is that the discourses of First Nations women are not comprehensible.

3. A supervising audiologist makes the following statement to his or her students: "Cultural competence only means that it's important to treat everyone with respect. We all know how to do that." This statement made by the audiologist is similar to someone saying that they "do not see color; everyone is the same." What the audiologist is missing is that being treated with respect and treating others with respect mean different things to different groups of people.

Statement 3 above is a clear example of cultural blindness, which occurs when everyone is treated the same. If everyone is being treated the same (the meaning of equality), specific cultural perspectives or needs are being ignored, minimized, or marginalized. Implementing a policy of treating everyone the same can lead to: (1) developing and providing services that do not utilize cultural strengths; (2) attributing limited progress or external circumstances to the individuals or groups being served; and (3) placing limited value on facilitating cultural responsiveness among service providers, such as having limited resources dedicated to helping employees gain cultural awareness and knowledge (Cross et al., 1989; National Center for Cultural Competence [NCCC], n.d.). Cultural blindness is the third step, following cultural destructiveness and cultural incapacity, in the continuum of cultural competence from Cross et al., discussed in Chapter 2. This issue of cultural blindness and the problems with treating everyone the same raise the issue of the important differentiation between equality and equity.

Equality refers to treating everyone the same or making sure everyone has the same rights, resources, and opportunities. What is equally as important, if one truly understands being culturally and linguistically responsive, is equity. Equity means that everyone has what they need to make use of available resources, and opportunities. In other words, "people with unequal need require different or differential treatment to achieve identical results" (Srivastava, 2007, p. 68). What one person or group may need could be different than other persons or groups. Let's consider an example about the educational achievement gap that persists between children attending schools in high-income communities and those attending schools in low-income communities. An achievement gap happens when there is a disparity between academic performance on such measures as standardized test scores, retention rates, and grade point averages (NCES, 2015).

It is important to know School A is in a high-income tax bracket community. School B is in a low-income tax bracket community. Since in the United States the amount of resources available for schools is pegged to the income of the community surrounding the school, School A receives many more resources for educating students than does School B (Kuttner, 2016). Equality would be making sure that all schools in the United States had the same amount of resources for each student, whether the school was in a high-income, middle-income, or low-income community. This would require changing the U.S. schooling policy—an important goal. Equity, however, would be ensuring that all students had the resources needed to be successful; meaning that the low-income school would need more resources than the high-income school to eliminate the achievement gaps between the groups (Kuttner, 2016). There are several visual representations of equality versus equity circulating on the Internet. Figure 4–1 shows three people of different heights standing. The picture on the left shows *equality*—all of the people are standing on the same-size block trying to look over a wall. Although the people are standing on blocks of equal size, the shortest person is still at a disadvantage. The picture on the right is a representation of *equity*, in that none of the people are disadvantaged. They all have what they need, per se, to see over the wall.

4. An African American female faculty member receives an award after over 30 years of working in her field, and a European American part-time faculty member with a master's degree with less than 10 years of experience says to her, "Oh, you know so many people. I see

how you got that award. Now I know what I need to do to get one."

5. One student says to a classmate from an impoverished background, "How did YOU get an A on that test?" or "How did YOU get into this program?"

6. Rachel Jeantel, a friend of Trayvon Martin, a young man who was murdered while Rachel was on the telephone with him testified in the murder trial of the man accused of Martin's murder. During Jeantel's testimony, the defense lawyer opened by saying, "I know you grew up in a Haitian family so make sure that everybody can hear you—try to speak as clear . . . " (Bernie de la Rionda, Assistant Prosecutor). Then within an 8-minute time span during the first 15 minutes of Ms. Jeantel's testimony, there were 22 statements made by the prosecutor about her not being understandable.

Example 6 is another example of a communicative contract not being upheld by the speakers with power (the prosecutor or

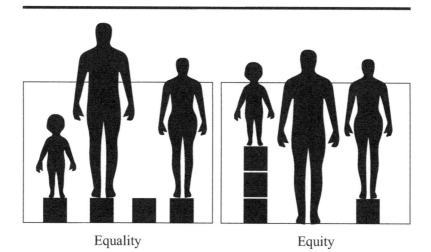

Equality   Equity

FIGURE 4–1. Equality versus equity. Illustrated by Severin Provance.

defense lawyer) when questioning a young woman who probably had very limited experience in the judicial system. Unfortunately, Ms. Jeantel's multilingualism (she speaks three languages) and her speech impairment were used to discredit her testimony.

We do not want to become distracted with thinking that racist, gendered, sexist acts are only between individuals. There are policies and structures embedded into the way society is organized (Farmer, 2001, 2004; Farmer et al., 2006), and these policies operate in a way that facilitates and maintains microaggressions, as well as unequal relations of power (Chomsky, 2016). Also, all of the "isms," such as racism, sexism, disability-ism, linguicism, class-ism, and gender-ism cannot be considered separate from each other but are intricately linked; we must consider their intersectionality (Cho, Crenshaw, & McCall, 2013; Collins, 2000; Crenshaw, 2005; hooks, 1994). Intersectionality, a concept coined by Kimberlé Crenshaw, emerged from the work of Black feminist writers such as Crenshaw, Patricia Hill Collins, and bell hooks. These writers wrote about the inequalities and power differences within society (Powell Sears, 2012). Intersectionality means that people have various and overlapping identities (i.e., social locations) that are experienced at the same time, including but not limited to gender, sexual orientation, economic class, age, nationality, disability, race, and language use. These varied "social locations interact to create distinct meanings in the lives of" people (Powell Sears, 2012, p. 546). Considering intersectionality in culturally responsive practice may help service providers more accurately understand the diversity that exists within cultural, racial, and ethnic groups, as well as be more effective in recognizing "the impact of intersecting social locations on" health, and communication outcomes (Powell Sears, 2012).

Manufactured Consent

Symbolic violence is a tool of manufactured consent (Herman & Chomsky, 2002). Manufactured consent is the ability to make people believe and act in ways that are in opposition to their own good (Lukes, 2005). It occurs when cultural tools, such as the media, churches, and schools, are used to convince the public to act in ways that are against their own interest (Herman & Chomsky, 2002). One example that we have had in recent history (between 2005 and 2016) is the discussion in the United States about universal health care. Discussions about universal health care have been happening in the United States since the early 1900s (Starr, 2013) and have been occurring in other countries[4] since the 1800s. Most recently, in 1993 First Lady Hillary Clinton proposed a Health Security Act that proposed to provide comprehensive and universal health care for every person in the United States. This was going to occur by requiring employers to provide health care for their employees. There was a great deal of opposition to this plan by organizations that had employees, as well as the health care industrial complex,[5] and the act never made it out of the Senate. Fast forward to 2010, President Obama's health care plan—the Patient Protection and Affordable Care Act—changed the way insurance was offered in that it expanded Medicaid to millions of people in the United States who oth-

---

[4]Other countries that have had some form of universal health care include Germany, Austria, Hungary, Norway, Britain, Russia, Netherlands, Sweden, Denmark, France, and Switzerland.

[5]*Industrial complex* was popularized by President Dwight D. Eisenhower in 1961. He used this phrase in a presidential address to the public when referring to the military. Industrial complex refers to entities that are interconnected (e.g., military, health insurance, prison industry) and that provide services or materials for profit.

erwise did not have health insurance, required insurance companies to insure those who had preexisting conditions, and allowed children under the age of 25 to stay on their parents' insurance plans. The plan also stipulated that all citizens in the United States were required to purchase health care. Although the plan was approved in the House and the Senate and signed into law in 2010, the Republican party continued with efforts to undermine and dismantle the law (some sources say that there were at least 60 or more attempts within an 8-year time span to dismantle the law). As of March 2016, the U.S. Department of Health and Human Services reported that 20 million more people in the United States now have health insurance, and that over 6 million youth between 19 and 25 years of age are now insured, resulting in a "46.5 percent drop in the number of uninsured" youth (HHS, 2016). Manufactured consent occurred when the media pundits and "politicians" consistently discussed how universal health care was not a good policy for the United States, resulting in many people who would or who do benefit from the health care policy actually being against health care for all.

Organization of Work

Power can be enacted through the way work is organized. The organization of work focuses on what work is done, and who does what work. Many organizations undergo changes in the way work is organized to help the worker be more efficient; however, the changes in the organization of work can also have the effect of increased stress for the worker. Such stress could result from workers being required to "do more with less," meaning less personnel, less resources, and sometimes, less autonomy. Work is organized in various ways including

the: (1) form of work (teaching versus supervising clinical practice, or providing assessments versus intervention); (2) caseload or the number of clients one is required to see per day (e.g., speech-language pathologists working in health care settings average productivity levels of 77% or 6 hours and 10 minutes per 8-hour day [ASHA, 2017]); and (3) workload (i.e., the total number of activities that one is engaged in to perform his or her duties). These factors affect the number of hours in a day someone might work, and one's responsibilities or division of labor. We probably all agree that working is necessary and can be a fulfilling activity; however, in many societies work is similar in that "(1) it always coincides with a particular set of hierarchical relations between individuals, social groups, and in certain periods of history, nations . . . and (2) it is always taken over, shaped, and reproduced by (and often for) the dominant social group (*the group with the most power*[6]), generally comprising those who own or control the primary means of production" (Magdoff, 2006). Additionally, in the United States, for much of the population, work is tied to ones' access to resources—this idea, of course, does not hold for people who have inherited wealth from family lines. There are ideologies that exist about the differences between manual and mental workers, the roles that women should have in the workplace, and the value of the work that is done by people of color. A critical examination of how work is organized can reveal implicit power structures.

Leisure Time

Because of the way work is organized, groups of people often have very little time for leisure. Power relations are displayed during leisure time—how it is defined, whether it is regulated

---

[6]Italicized phrase was added by the authors.

or considered valid leisure activity, and the space in which leisure activities occur (Van Krieken, Habibis, Smith, Hutchins, Martin, & Maton, 2013). Some forms of leisure traditionally engaged in by people who are working class or impoverished have been categorized as illegal, such as cock fights and dog fights. Some forms of leisure engaged in by people of higher socioeconomic status have been categorized as sport, such as racing horses and dogs. All of the aforementioned activities may potentially bring harm to animals, but only the animal sports likely to be engaged in by people who are impoverished or by people of color are considered illegal.

Power plays a role in every facet of our social lives (Delpit, 2006a). Although we have altered some of the language used by Delpit (2006b), in the following, we present a list of characteristics of power (pp. 24–25), which Delpit calls the "culture of power" (p. 24):

- First, power is an element in *all* contexts and interactions, including but not limited to such contexts as churches, schools, hospitals, and prisons, and to such interactions as those between parents and children, husbands and wives, teachers and students, doctors and patients, and clinicians and clients. There are no neutral spaces in which power relations do not exist.

There are power differences between clergy and parishioners, and even between clergy at different levels within the same church, such as between a bishop and a pastor or between the lead pastor and an associate pastor. There are also differences in power between teachers and students, men and women, doctors and other medical personnel, and service providers and their clients or patients. One way that service providers have more power than their clients is that they have specialized knowledge (Srivastava, 2007). Professionals in speech,

language, and hearing sciences attend university for 6 or 7 years before being able to practice in their field. This time span for gaining knowledge gives the professional a certain sense of authority. Power relations exist in all aspects of society and in every social and professional relationship.

- Power is usually not equally available across racial, class, gender, cultural, national, economic, or political lines.
- There are rules for ways to behave in the face of power.

One example of these rules can be exemplified in the ways people think and talk about language and its use. It is not uncommon to hear legitimate and rule governened language variations (e.g., African American English) being called "bad English," or "broken English." Also, individuals or groups of people who speak language variations, particularly ones who are stigmatized in the United States, are also delegitimized. Recall the earlier discussion about Rachel Jeantel who was a witness during a murder trial. She was castigated online because she: (1) spoke African American English, and (2) had a speech impediment, both of which broke the unstated rules of power in a U.S. courtroom.

- The "rules" of power are in the interest of those who have power.

How success and effectiveness in social institutions are determined is based on "the culture of those who are in power" (Delpit, 2006, p. 24). Power comes from the way social institutions are organized. If the witness mentioned above spoke general American English dialect, presented with speech production skills that were not impaired, and used the pragmatic behaviors of middle-class Euro-Americans, it is unlikely that her character would have been so heavily criticized in public, and her testimony would have been treated as having some level of validity.

- There is an inverse correspondence between power and recognition of power. In other words, those with the most power are least willing to recognize power differences between people and groups, and least willing to acknowledge that they hold power over others. People with the least power, however, are most aware of unequal power relations.

It is imperative for service providers to be aware of the relationship between culture and power. Ideology plays a large part in maintaining unequal relations of power, because people often personify assumptions that validate existing power relations. Recognizing power dynamics within professional relationships is important for being an effective service provider (Formosa, 2015). When professionals are aware of power imbalances between them and their constituents, they can deliberately make efforts to balance power relations (Srivastava, 2007).

CHAPTER SUMMARY

Power is dynamic rather than static, and it plays a role in every facet of life. Power can be exerted through structural violence, physical violence, symbolic violence, manufactured consent, the organization of work, and the organization of leisure time, but it is typically unequal across race, class, gender, sexual orientation, cultures, nationalities, and economic and political lines. The rules of power are designed in the interest of those who have the most power in society; yet, those with the most power usually do not recognize that they have power. Rather, those with the least power are most aware of unequal power relations. To be effective service providers, we need to under-stand and acknowledge unequal relations of power, and strive to balance power relations between ourselves and those we serve.

EXTENDED LEARNING

- Engage in a quick writing task by writing one paragraph identifying and explaining the ways that you have been privileged and disadvantaged by unequal power relations. Then write a second paragraph identifying how you could have changed that power dynamic.
- Develop your own visual model differentiating equality and equity.
- Form a group with three others and discuss the intersectionality of the various identities among you.

DISCUSSION QUESTIONS

1. Identify and explain how professionals in your field and their corresponding practices may create or maintain unequal power relations.
2. What are some of the ways that you have observed power being exerted? Give examples of each.
3. What are some of the ways that you have benefited from structural or symbolic violence?

FURTHER READING

Delpit, L. (2006b). The silenced dialogue. In L. Delpit (Ed.), *Other people's children* (pp. 21–47). New York, NY: W.W. Norton.

Farmer, P. (2003). *Pathologies of power: Health, human rights, and the new war on the poor*. Berkeley, CA: University of California Press.

Freire, P. (1985). *The politics of education: Culture, power and liberation.* Westport, CT: Bergin and Garvey.

Hodgson, D. L. (2015). *The gender, culture and power reader.* Oxford, UK: Oxford University Press.

Johnson, A. (2005). *Privilege, power and difference* (2nd ed.). New York, NY: McGraw-Hill.

REFERENCES

Ahearn, L. M. (2012). *Living language: An introduction to linguistic anthropology.* Chichester, UK: Wiley-Blackwell.

American Speech-Language-Hearing Association (ASHA). (2017). *Caseload and workload: Practice portal.* Retrieved from http://www.asha.org/PRPSpecificTopic.aspx?folderid=8589934681&section=Overview

Bachrach, P., & Baratz, M. (1962). Two faces of power. *American Political Science Review, 56*(4), 947–952.

Ball, A., & Alim, H. (2006). Preparation, pedagogy, policy and power: Brown, the King case, and the struggle for equal language rights. *National Society for the Study of Education, 105*(2), 104–124.

Barajas, J. (2016, November 21). *Standing Rock protest: Police deploy water hoses, tear gas against Standing Rock protesters.* Available from PBS News Hour at http://www.pbs.org/newshour/rundown/police-deploy-water-hoses-tear-gas-against-standing-rock-protesters/

Baugh, J. (2003). Linguistic profiling. In S. Makoni, G. Smitherman, A. Ball, & A. Spears (Eds.), *Black linguistics: Language, society and politics in Africa and the Americas* (pp. 155–168). New York, NY: Routledge.

Baugh, J. (2007). Attitudes toward variation and earwitness testimony. In R. Bayley & C. Lucas (Eds.), *Sociolinguistic variation: Theories, methods, and applications* (pp. 338–348). Cambridge, UK: Cambridge University Press.

Bourdieu, P. (2005). *Language and symbolic power.* Malden, MA: Polity Press.

Browning, L., & Bever, L. (2016, November 16). "Ape in heels": W. Va. Mayor resigns amid controversy over racist comments about Michelle Obama. *The Washington Post.*

Buraway, M., & Wright, E. O. (2006). Sociological Marxism. In J. H. Turner (Ed.), *Handbook of sociological theory* (pp. 459–486). New York, NY: Springer.

Capodilupo, C. M., & Sue, D. W. (2013). Microaggressions in counseling and psychotherapy. In D. W. Sue & D. Sue (Eds.), *Counseling the culturally diverse: Theory and practice* (pp. 147–174). Hoboken, NJ: John Wiley & Sons.

Cho, S., Crenshaw, K. W., & McCall, L. (2013). Toward a field of intersectionality studies: Theory, applications and praxis. *Intersectionality: Theorizing Power, Empowering Theory, 38*(4), 785–810.

Chomsky, A. (2016, May 23). Will the millennial movement rebuild the ivory tower or be crushed by it? *Truthdig* report. Retrieved from http://www.truthdig.com/report/page3/will_the_millennial_movement_rebuild_the_ivory_20160523

Clark, H. H., & Wilkes-Gibbs, D. (1986). Referring as a collaborative process. *Cognition, 22*(1), 1–39.

Collins, P. H. (2000). *Black feminist thought: Knowledge, consciousness and the politics of empowerment.* New York, NY: Routledge.

Crenshaw, K. (2005). Mapping the margins: Intersectionality, identity politics, and violence against women of color. In R. K. Bergen, J. L. Edleson, & C. M. Renzetti (Eds.), *Violence against women: Classic papers* (pp. 282–313). Auckland, NZ: Pearson Education.

Cross, T., Bazron, B., Dennis, K., & Isaacs, M. (1989*). Towards a culturally competent system of care* (Vol. 1). Washington, DC: CASSP Technical Assistance Center, Center for Child Health and Mental Health Policy, Georgetown University Child Development Center.

Delpit, L. (2006a). *Other people's children.* New York, NY: W.W. Norton.

Delpit, L. (2006b). The silenced dialogue. In L. Delpit (Ed.), *Other people's children* (pp. 21–47). New York, NY: W. W. Norton.

DeMello, M. (2012). *Animals and society: An introduction to human-animal studies.* New York, NY: Columbia University Press.

Fairclough, N. (2001). *Language and power*. New York, NY: Routledge.

Farmer, P. (2001). *Infections and inequalities: The modern plagues*. Berkeley, CA: University of California Press.

Farmer, P. (2004). An anthropology of structural violence. *Current Anthropology 45*, 305–326.

Farmer, P. E., Nizeye, B., Stulac, S., & Keshavjee, S. (2006). Structural violence and clinical medicine. Policy Forum. *PLOS Medicine*, *3*(10), 1686–1691.e449.

Feagin, J. R. (2013). *The White racial frame: Centuries of racial framing and counter-framing* (2nd ed.). New York, NY: Routledge.

Formosa, C. (2015). Understanding power and communication relationships in health settings. *British Journal of Healthcare Management*, *21*(9), 420–425.

Hannah-Jones, N. (2012). *Living apart: How the government betrayed a landmark civil rights law*. New York, NY: Open Road Media.

Hardcastle, D. A., Powers, P. R., & Wenocur, S. (2011). *Community practice: Theories and skills for social workers* (3rd ed.). Oxford, UK: Oxford University Press.

Herman, E. S., & Chomsky, N. (2002). *Manufacturing consent: The political economy of the mass media*. New York, NY: Pantheon Books.

hooks, b. (1994). *Teaching to transgress: Education as the practice of freedom*. New York, NY: Routledge.

Hyter, Y. D. (2014). A conceptual framework for responsive global engagement in communication sciences and disorders. *Topics in Language Disorders*, *34*(2), 103–120.

Irvine, J. T., & Gal, S. (2000). Language ideology and linguistic differentiation. In P. Kroskrity (Ed.), *Regimes of language: Ideologies, polities, and identities* (pp. 35–84). Santa Fe, NM: School of American Research Press.

Isserman, M., & Kazin, M. (2000). *America divided: The civil war of the 1960s*. Oxford, UK: Oxford University Press.

Knabb, R. D., Rhome, J. R., & Brown, D. P. (2005, December 20). *Tropical cyclone report: Hurricane Katrina, 23–30 August 2005*. National Hurricane Center. Retrieved from http://www.nhc.noaa.gov/data/tcr/AL122005_Katrina.pdf

Kuttner, P. (2016, October 29). The problem with that equity vs. equality graphic that you're using. *Cultural Organizing*. Retrieved from http://culturalorganizing.org

Lippi-Green, R. (1997). *English with an accent: Language, ideology and discrimination in the United States*. New York, NY: Routledge.

Lippi-Green, R. (2012). *English with an accent: Language, ideology and discrimination in the United States* (2nd ed.). New York, NY: Routledge.

Lucercle, J. J. (1990). *The violence of language*. London, UK: Routledge.

Lukes, S. (2005). *Power: A radical view* (2nd ed.). New York, NY: Palgrave: MacMillan.

Magdoff, H. (2006, October). The meaning of work: A Marxist perspective. *Monthly Review: An Independent Socialist Magazine*, *58*(5). Retrieved from http://monthlyreview.org/2006/10/01/the-meaning-of-work-a-marxist-perspective/

Martin, J. N., & Nakayama, T. K. (2000). *Intercultural communication in contexts* (2nd ed.). London, UK: Mayfield.

Milroy, J. (2001). Language ideologies and the consequences of standardization. *Journal of Sociolinguistics*, *5/4*, 530–555.

National Center for Cultural Competence. (n.d.). *Cultural competence continuum: Cultural and linguistic competence in health promotion training*. Retrieved from https://nccc.georgetown.edu/projects/sids/dvd/continuum.pdf

Newton, H. P. (2002). Black capitalism reanalyzed I: June 5, 1971. In D. Hilliard & D. Weiss (Eds.), *The Huey P. Newton reader* (pp. 227–233). New York, NY: Seven Stories Press.

Parenti, M. (2011). *Democracy for the few* (9th ed.). Boston, MA: Wadsworth, Cengage Learning.

Pierce, C., Carew, J., Pierce-Gonzalez, D., & Willis, D. (1978). An experiment in racism: TV commercials. In C. Pierce (Ed.), *Television and education* (pp. 62–88). Beverly Hills, CA: Sage.

Powell Sears, K. (2012). Improving intercultural competence education: The utility of an intersectional framework. *Medical Education*, *46*, 545–551.

Schiffman, H. P. (1996). *Linguistic culture and language policy*. New York, NY: Routledge.

Simmons, W. P., & Casper, M. J. (2012). Culpability, social triage, and structural violence in the aftermath of Katrina. *Perspectives in Politics, 10*(3), 675–686.

Smith, W. A., Hung, M., & Franklin, J. D. (2011). Racial battle fatigue and the "mis" education of black men: Racial microaggressions, societal problems, and environmental stress. *Journal of Negro Education, 80*(1), 63–82.

Srivastava, R. H. (2007). *The healthcare professional's guide to clinical cultural competence.* Toronto, ON, Canada: Elsevier Canada.

Starr, P. (2013). *Remedy and reaction: The peculiar American struggle over health care reform* (Rev. ed.). New Haven, CT: Yale University Press.

Sue, D. W. (2010). *Microaggressions in everyday life: Race, gender and sexual orientation.* Hoboken, NJ: John Wiley & Sons.

Ting-Toomey, S., & Chung, L. C. (2012). *Understanding intercultural communication* (2nd ed.). Oxford, UK: Oxford University Press.

U.S. Department of Education. (2010). *The evaluation of charter school impacts: Executive summary.* Washington, DC: Author.

U.S. Department of Health and Human Services. (2016, March 3). *20 million people have gained health coverage because of the Affordable Care Act, new estimates show.* Retrieved from https://www.hhs.gov/about/news/2016/03/03/20-million-people-have-gained-health-insurance-coverage-because-affordable-care-act-new-estimates

U.S. Department of Labor Occupational Safety and Health Administration. (n.d.). *Workplace violence.* Retrieved from http://www.pbs.org/newshour/rundown/police-deploy-water-hoses-tear-gas-against-standing-rock-protesters/

Van Krieken, R., Habibis, D., Smith, P., Hutchins, B., Martin, G., & Maton, K. (2013). *Sociology* (5th ed.). Francis Forest, NSW: Pearson Australia.

Weber, M. (1947). *The theory of social and economic organization.* Translated by A. M. Henderson & Talcott Parsons. New York, NY: Free Press.

Wright, E. O. (1997). *Class counts: Comparative studies in class analysis.* Cambridge, UK: Cambridge University Press.

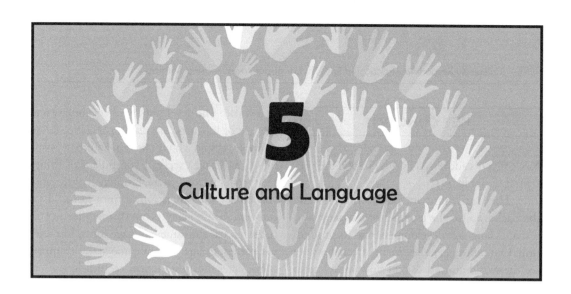

5

Culture and Language

The influence of culture on the development of language is well established, and language occurs within a sociocultural context (Barrueco, Lopez, Ong, & Lozano, 2012; Imai, Kanero, & Masuda, 2016; Otto, 2014). Language is part of culture, as it reflects culture and is influenced by culture (Kidd, Kemp, Kashima, & Quinn, 2016). Language is a symbolic system, in which language forms (words, morphemes) and uses, have meaning. Culture also is symbolic in that it represents historical memory and experiences and "ways of living and thinking" (Wenying, 2000, p. 328). One way to learn about culture and increase cultural responsiveness is by learning a language. For example, one can learn a great deal about cultural assumptions of some groups in the United States by understanding the concept of "independence." Similarly, one can understand life in Senegal by learning the concept of the Wolof word, "Teranga." Although there is not a direct translation into English, Teranga includes the values of hospitality, courtesy, politeness, and gratitude (Dr. Souleymane Faye, Linguist, personal communication, May 30, 2017). In this chapter, we review definitions of communication and language and their relationship to culture, and then discuss spoken and written language variations, variations in nonverbal communication, and linguistic politics.

KEY CONCEPTS

Key concepts addressed in this chapter are presented in Table 5–1.

The family unit and the community are the backdrop for the learning of language and it shapes language development and its production. Our cultural environment affects how we see the world around us and how we relate to that world. The development of vocabulary and the use of language are culture specific. As an example, a child who is raised in an urban apartment may have excellent vocabulary of things seen in a city like a *metro*, but may have limited vocabulary for things found on a farm, like a *combine*. Additionally, people from different cultures can use the same language form, but refer to different things. Review some of the examples of the ways these differences occur below.

Box 5–1

- *College* in the United States refers to the educational institution one attends after high school. In France, however, it refers to the level of education that occurs *before* high school, which is middle school or junior high school.
- *Breakfast* in Puerto Rico will likely include a hot cereal, such as *harina de avena* (oatmeal) or *crema de maiz* (cornmeal cereal). In Mexico, however, it more than likely refers to *huevos rancheros* (corn tortillas topped with fried eggs, cheese, and salsa with a side of refried beans), and in Senegal, it will refer to a baguette of French bread, Nutella, and a cup of tea or coffee.
- *Market* in the United States usually refers to a place where you can purchase fresh fruits and vegetables, but in Senegal it refers to an open air "Mall" where you can purchase fruits and vegetables, and also clothing, shoes, electronics, office supplies, and so on.

Can you think of other ways that the same concepts have very different meanings in other countries or among cultural groups different than your own?

TABLE 5–1. Key Concepts

Language variation	Innatist theory
Multilingualism	Bilingualism
Paralinguistic	Nonverbal communication
Proxemics	Kinesics
Linguistic human rights	Language policies
Simultaneous bilingual	Sequential bilingual
Dual language learning	Second language learning
English as an additional language	Conceptual scoring
	Assimilation
Acculturation	

LINGUISTIC RELATIVITY

One of the most prominent theories on the relationship between language and culture is linguistic relativity—the theory associated with Franz Boas, Edward Sapir, and Benjamin Lee Whorf (Leavitt, 2015). The theory of linguistic relativity is that the characteristics of language affect one's worldview (Lucy, 1997). Linguistic relativity has come under significant criticism over the years, particularly due to the limited empirical research available to support it (Lucy, 1997). Leavitt (2011) contends, however, that Boas, Sapir, and Whorf did not believe that language determined or limited one's worldview, but that language characteristics tended to guide the way ideas were conceptualized. We agree with this idea, and that there is a mutual effect between language and culture. Language guides the way ideas are conceptualized and culture influences language. In addition to language, communication conventions vary across cultures.

COMMUNICATION AND LANGUAGE

Communication is the ability to engage in an exchange of ideas with another or several other people. Communication can be fraught with unequal power relations, particularly when it occurs between cultural, linguistic, or racial groups (see Chapter 4 for more detailed discussion on Culture and Power). A person is successful at communicating when he or she is able to get her point across to the person or persons with whom she is interacting, but this interaction can be verbal or nonverbal.

Communication includes linguistics as well as paralanguage or paralinguistics (Ottenheimer, 2013; Trager, 1958), kinesics (Birdwhistell, 1952), and proxemics (Hall, 1963,

1966). Also all languages have systematic rule-governed ways where sounds are combined into words, and words are combined into sentences, and sentences are combined into discourse. For example, all languages around the world have diverse phonotatic rules. The sounds /mb/ can only occur at the end of words in English, but can occur at the beginning of words in Wolof (i.e., *lamb* in English or *mbokk* in Wolof).

Paralinguistics refers to anything that occurs alongside of language, and has been referred to as voice cues because it can provide cues about someone's intentions (Ottenheimer, 2013; Trager, 1958). A term that is used to describe paralinguistic features is *prosody*. Paralinguistic cues are the variations in pitch, loudness, vocal quality, tone of voice, and duration of speech, as well as characteristics used during writing. For example, a smiley face following a statement in an e-mail may indicate that the writer is intending to convey happiness with something (e.g., "I think the quilt was perfect. ☺"). Capitalized letters in the body of an e-mail (e.g., "Please ARRIVE at NOON") could indicate someone being emphatic. Speaking with a whisper could intend secrecy (Ottenheimer, 2013).

Kinesics (Birdwhistell, 1952, 1970) refers to gestures and body movements and postures, and facial expressions that are used in communication. These aspects of communication can occur along with spoken language, but can also be used independent of spoken language in meaningful ways. McNeill (1992) describes a continuum of body movements from those that are used while speaking to those that are not necessarily used while speaking: gesticulations, language-like gestures, pantomimes, emblems, and sign language. Gesticulations refer to movements of extremities that accompany speech. For example, a person who says, "He threw the ball," may accompany this statement with the physical gesture of throwing while making the statement. Language-like gestures take the place of words in a sentence, for example, "she then [gesture]." Both gesticulations and language-like gestures occur with language being produced (Hyter, 1994). Pantomimes are similar to gesticulations but do not require any accompanying language. Emblems are gestures that are culturally specific, such as the thumbs up or a fist bump. Figures 5–1 and 5–2 are examples of emblematic gestures. Sign languages are full linguistic systems and do not require accompanying speech, although some Deaf signers do incorporate speech and other paralinguistic forms (see Chapter 6).

Paralinguistics and kinesics can vary across cultural and linguistic groups. In the oral narratives of adolescents who were African American English (AAE) speakers, Hyter (1994) found that they used gesticulations in the form of deictic points in a specific plane of space to mark the introduction of new characters into a scene 44% of the time; this characteristic of gesture use is not unique to AAE speakers. These data also showed, however, that the AAE speakers participating in this study used vowel elongation 18% of the time when introducing new characters using a pronoun (e.g., "he:"). In some cultures, bidding someone to approach using your index finger is an insult. In others bidding someone to approach is done with the palm pointed outward, and then simultaneously moving the four fingers up and down. In the United States that gesture would be the same as waving "goodbye" or "hello." For years, Dr. Hyter confused these gestures, misinterpreting a bid for her to follow or come to someone with a wave goodbye. In addition to unique uses of paralinguistics to convey new information in narratives, some speakers of AAE also use gesticulations in creative ways. Table 5–2 includes descriptions of some of the kinesic aspects of AAE.

Hall (1963) developed the theory of proxemics, which is how a person "unconsciously

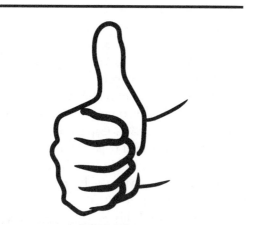

FIGURE 5–1. Example of emblematic gesture. Illustrated by Severin Provance.

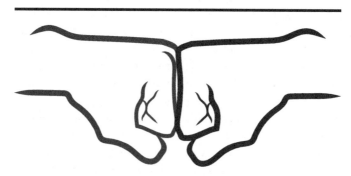

FIGURE 5–2. Example of emblematic gesture. Illustrated by Severin Provance.

TABLE 5–2. Some Kinesic Aspects of AAE

Name of the Speech Act Produced as a Gesticulation	Meaning	Description	Source
Suck teeth	Disgust, disbelief	Sound made by pressing the tongue against the front teeth and then making an implosive by sucking in and releasing the tongue	Green, 2002; Rickford & Rickford, 1976; Smitherman, 2000; DeJarnette, Rivers, & Hyter, 2015
Cut eye	Disbelief, distrust	A gesture made by looking at a person from the side of one's eye rather than directly	Green, 2002; Rickford & Rickford, 2000; Smitherman, 2000
Neck-roll	Usually made when making a point, telling someone off, giving a person a piece of their mind	Neck rolls side to front to side without moving shoulders or turning the head	Green, 2002; Rickford & Rickford, 2000; Rivers, Hyter, & DeJarnette, 2012; Smitherman, 2000
Givin' skin/givin' five*	Solidarity, affirmation	Hold your hand out and the person you are interacting with will tap your hand with his or her hand or will place his or her palm on yours and slide it off	Alim & Smitherman, 2012

Note. *This gesture has been largely co-opted by other groups as of 2017.

Sources: Adapted from Hyter (1994) and DeJarnette et al. (2015).

structures space" (p. 1003). Hall (1966) identified four distances, but how these distances are interpreted varies among cultural groups. In Hall's schema the distances are intimate, personal, social, and public. Intimate distance (6–18 inches apart) indicates an intimate or close relationship with the person to whom one is speaking. Personal distances 1.5 to 4 feet apart occur among family members and close friends. Social distances (4–12 feet apart) are used by people who are colleagues, between professors and students, or people who are seen regularly but with whom you do not have a personal relationship, such as a bank teller or postal worker. Public distance (12–25 feet) is typically used during public speaking engagements or classroom teaching. These distances will vary depending on how members of cultural groups conceptualize space. In Western cultures (e.g., North American, European) people are more likely to interact with each other at great distances; also, touching in one cultural context may be appropriate and not in another (Hall, 1968). When in Puerto Rico, Dr. Hyter greets friends and family members, particularly if they are older than her, with a kiss on both cheeks. While in Senegal, Dr. Hyter is typically greeted by her female friends with three kisses—alternating cheeks.

HIGH- AND LOW-CONTEXT CULTURES

Ed T. Hall (1976) describes high- and low-context cultures as a way to differentiate cultural groups by how much context is taken into consideration during communication exchanges. These cultures, as described by Hall, can be thought about along a continuum with high-context communication on one end of the continuum, and low-context communication on the other end. Hall was able to plot certain cultural groups on one end of the continuum or the other, but it is probably accurate to think that most cultural groups will not necessarily fall *only* on one end of the continuum or the other. Rather people's positions on the continuum will shift based on the circumstances. For high-context cultures, meaning is conveyed through nonverbal means, including gestures, and indirect ways of speaking. These ways of speaking include "code words, nuances, and forms of etiquette that express a persons' emotions or intent sometimes in indirect ways that are difficult to perceive by those who are unfamiliar with the culture and its norms for communicating meaning" (Ingraham, 2006, p. 111). Low-context cultures, on the other hand, use the linguistic code to convey meaning in messages; that is, to make sense of the information being communicated, one does not need to know or understand the cultural context as all of the content is carried in the linguistic code. Hall categorized cultures in Japan and China as high-context cultures, and Sweden, Germany, and the United States to low-context cultures (Ingraham, 2006). Of course, we need to be careful not to generalize, because cultural groups are not homogeneous. Dr. Hyter, who identifies as Black and was born in the United States, consistently looks to the context and unspoken signals (paralinguistics, facial expressions, gestures, and body postures) to comprehend what someone is saying. It is an automatic response, and these are the strategies she uses to understand the full picture. If there is inconsistency between the words spoken and the paralinguistic and nonlinguistic contextual cues, she questions (not always out loud) the veracity of what the person is saying. There are other variations in communication and language use, which are discussed below.

LANGUAGE VARIATION

Variations in languages have always existed, and these variations can occur within the same language. Bailey (2004) has said that "We all speak English but not two of us speak it in the same way" (p. 6). Rather than using the term "English," it may be more appropriate to call it "Englishes." This idea can be extended to all languages, as all languages have variations. Many languages contributed to English including African, Dutch, Spanish, and German (Bailey, 2004). For example, *vigilante, mosquito, tobacco,* among others are borrowed from Spanish (Durkin, 2014). Arabic has contributed to Spanish, such as *alfombra* (rug), *azul* (blue), *azúcar* (sugar), *arroz* (rice), and *aciete* (oil) (Dworkin, 2012). We use the concept "language variation" rather than "dialect." Dialect means language variation (Wolfram & Schilling-Estes, 2006) but can be perceived negatively by those who do not study languages and linguistics. In this case, we are defining language variation as a variety of talking/language that is associated with a socially defined group. Language variations differ with respect to pronunciation, vocabulary, grammar, and use. Language variations include bilingualism and multilingualism. Bilingualism is the ability to communicate with and comprehend two languages. Multilingualism means that you have proficiency in more than two languages. Language variations can be regional, such as southern or eastern variations, or social, such as with Spanish-influenced English or AAE.

There are many reasons for language variations. Historically, language variations occurred as a result of language contact—a common occurrence for the majority of people in the world. Language contact often occurs under circumstances of unequal power relations such as during war, trade, colonization, enslavement, or immigration. With language contact, there are increasing tensions between languages that were valued (those usually associated with the groups that had more economic and political power), and other languages becoming marginalized, resulting in social inequality or the increased regulation of language use. For example, in 1980 the Refugee Act (PL 96-212) served as an amendment to earlier acts focused on immigration and refugees (i.e., Immigration and Nationality Act and Migration and Refugee Assistance Act). This act was designed to provide a procedure for admitting refugees to the United States based on humanitarian concerns. In 1981, English Only legislation began being introduced across the U.S. (Schmid, 2001). Note that there have been efforts to make English the "official" language of the United States since the 1700s. Most of the efforts have coincided with a major fissure in society with respect to immigrants and/or refugees. In addition to historical/social reasons for language variations, there are linguistic reasons, too. For example, phonological variations occur when there are alterations made to words borrowed from one language and used in another, such as *déjà vu*. Features of one language are imported into another language (Treffers-Daller, 2010). Lexical borrowing will also lead to language variations, such as the borrowing of words from one language to another as mentioned earlier in this chapter. There are also institutions that facilitate the maintenance of language variations—social networks and communities of practice.

Social Networks

A social network is composed of a "web of ties" among individuals that happen to be connected to each other through various contexts that can include settings such as work, schooling, neighborhood, or church (Milroy & Llamas, 2013, p. 411). Social networks help people solve problems of daily life (Milroy & Llamas, 2013). A social network of the first order is one where individuals have direct contact and interact regularly (Figure 5–3). For example, Dr. Hyter and Dr. Salas-Provance, and let's say, two other people (represented in Figure 5–3 as the four dots within the innermost circle) were part of a social network through the American Speech-Language-Hearing Association's (ASHA) SIG 17, Global Issues in Communication Sciences and Related Disorders. These four people represent a social network of the first order, as they are all connected with each other and working together. They met when Dr. Hyter joined the group in 2008, the first year that Dr. Salas-Provance chaired the organization. A social network of the second order refers to people who are connected to at least one person in the first-order network (as indicated on the figure). A third-order social network (represented by the outermost circle) includes individuals connected to people in the second order, but not the first order.

Communities of Practice

Communities of practice make up a group of people who deliberately come together to solve a common problem (Eckert & Wenger, 1992). As the group is working to solve this common problem, "practices emerge" or a "way of

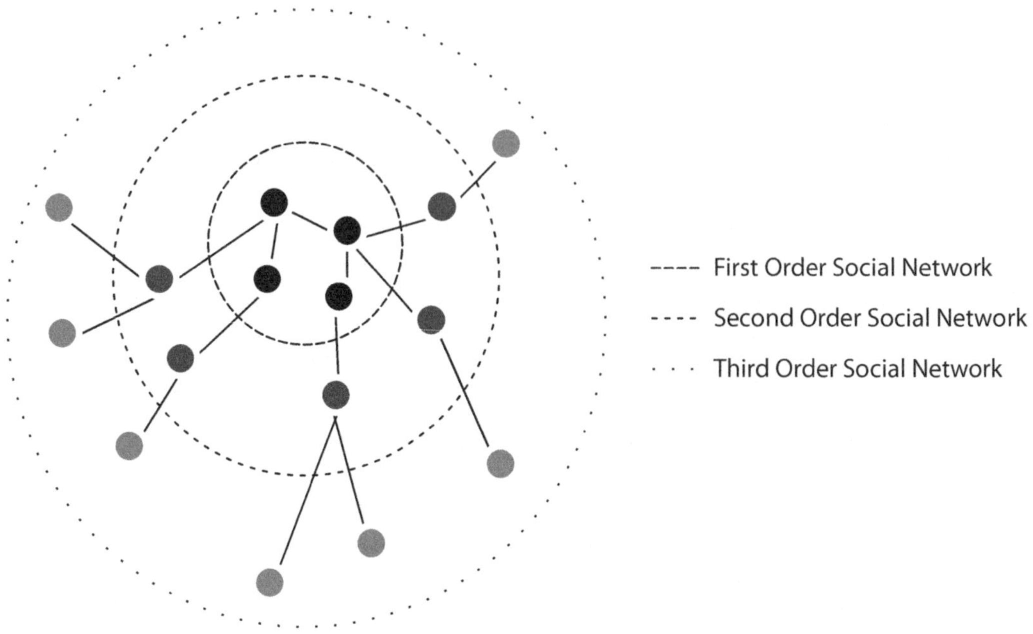

FIGURE 5–3. Social network map showing web of ties among individuals across first-, second-, and third-order networks. Illustrated by Severin Provance.

doing things" (Myerhoff & Strycharz, 2013, p. 429). There are three criteria for being a community of practice. First, there needs to be mutual engagement among members of the community; that is, the members get together to participate in their shared practice. This getting together can be in person, over the phone, or through electronic media, for example (Myerhoff & Strycharz, 2013). Second, the members of the community of practice share a "jointly negotiated enterprise" (Myerhoff & Strycharz, 2013, p. 430). Third, members have shared resources. For example, Dr. Hyter is a member of a community of practice that includes persons from various ethnicities, economic standings, genders, and generations that focus on making decisions about social justice projects taking place in a Midwestern city using direct democracy processes. This is a group of people who have come together specifically to develop and implement a direct democracy event (called Urban Democracy Feast © http://www.urbandemocracyfeast.org), meet twice per month in person and over e-mail. During the meetings, members of this community of practice negotiate what processes and activities will take place during the planned event, and they all have access to the same resources for engaging in the planning and in the event. In addition to the macro level issues with respect to language variation, next we focus on specific types of language variation—bilingualism and African American English.

Bilingual Language Development

The number of children in the United States who are being raised in a home where they hear languages other than English has grown exponentially over the past 10 years. A robust wave of immigration from Mexico over the past 15 years of nearly 3 million people and the arrival of over 10.3 million immigrants from around the world between 2000 and 2007 (the highest 7-year period of immigration in American history) contributed to this growth (NCES, 2011). The subsequent births to immigrant parents will enssure that those numbers will grow further. In fact, many speech-language pathologists around the country will find that these children are the majority in their schools. Children who are receiving dual language input and developing English as a second language present the clinician with opportunities and challenges. Some children develop a second language from birth through a simultaneous language acquisition process (dual language acquisition). Others develop the second language at a later point and are called *sequential bilinguals* (or second language learners) (Genesee, 2008; Kohnert, 2008a, 2012).

Therefore, consideration of the information from a cultural perspective is imperative. It is important to note that beyond cultural variation, the grammatical development of a bilingual child lags behind that of the child's monolingual peers, and a bilingual-monolingual difference in vocabulary size is present when the two languages in the bilingual child are measured separately. When the vocabulary is summed (i.e., conceptual scoring), the vocabulary development is similar (Bedore, Peña, Garcia, & Cortex, 2005; Kester & Peña, 2002; Pearson & Fernandez, 1994).

Many bilingual children or those learning English as an additional language (i.e., "English as an additional language learners" is used to refer to people who may be learning English as a third or fourth or even seventh language rather than a second language) live in an environment where two or more languages are spoken at home, and those languages may be different than the language spoken at school (Whiteside, Gooch, & Norbury, 2016). Additionally, when bilingual or multilingual people live in a context where their language is not the dominant language in the area (e.g., the United States), they are affected by acculturation or assimilation. Acculturation occurs when members of cultural groups decide to maintain cultural values, beliefs, worldviews, traditions, and language(s) but are able to incorporate some of the dominant culture into their way of life, resulting in a "blended cultural or linguistic patterns" (Ovando, 2008a, p. 9). Assimilation is when members of a cultural group give up their cultural values, beliefs, worldviews, traditions, and language to "take on the traits of another culture," adopting that other culture as a way of life (Ovando, 2008b, p. 43). Read the story of Lina Chavez presented in Box 5–2, as an example of the issues that her family must navigate with regard to acculturation or assimilation, and their perceptions of how their decisions may affect Lina's language development.

Box 5–2

Lina Chavez is 4 years old, the youngest of five children, with ages that range from 4 to 15 years. Lina has been brought to a clinic by her parents because she is not speaking like the other four children in the family were at the same age. The family came to the United States 5 years ago from El Salvador, and Lina was born in the United States. She attends preschool two days a week. The other children are in school, have been learning English at school, and have been placed in the bilingual immersion program at school. The mother was educated in her country as a social worker and works as a certified nurse assistant (CNA) in the United States. The father is a truck driver who is gone from home for long periods of time. Lina and the other children are cared for at home by their grandparents, who live with the family, while the parents are at work.

The use of Spanish in the family is strong. It is their native language and there do not appear to be any family members who have speech, language, hearing, or other communication problems in Spanish. Lina was born in the United States, so it is likely that she has been exposed to both English and Spanish her entire life; therefore, she may be a bilingual. The fact that she has heard English on TV daily is not a strong predicting factor for English language development, however. The grandparents have not learned English, and their cultural experiences have remained limited to their Spanish-speaking friends at church and the surrounding block of immigrants from South American countries. They have remained in a restricted ethnic enclave of Spanish-language use. It has been found that groups who remain isolated in this manner have a more difficult time acculturating to the new language and new culture (Borjas, 2006). Lina's parents have both been working long hours; thus, her major language experiences at home have been influenced by her grandparents. Her brothers and sisters have been learning English in school for the past 5 years, and some of them have done well, while others are struggling. It is important to know the level of language mixing to which Lina is exposed and their proficiency in English. Research has shown that language use in the home is a positive predictor of language development if the language user has a high degree of proficiency in the home language (Hoff & Core, 2013). We know that her oldest brother was 10 when he came to the United States as a fluent Spanish speaker. He may have established

excellent English skills from the base of solid Spanish language skills, but yet, he was older when he began learning a second language. However, each member of Lina's family may have a different level of proficiency in English, making it difficult to establish a solid linguistic foundation in English. If the children are having a difficult time learning English, there may be fewer opportunities for Lina to hear English at home, but we are sure that she is receiving significant English input in school. Lina's mother spoke "some" English in El Salvador and has improved her English significantly in her time in the United States and while working as a CNA (Certified Nursing Assistant). The father is most comfortable in Spanish but can get by with little English as a truck driver.

Lina's mother is educated, and maternal education is a predictor of the literacy and language development of children (Lyon, 1996) in both monolingual and bilingual children. This may be an advantage for Lina and her expected language development. However, Mrs. Garcia-Lopez was told by her mother, Mrs. Valles-Garcia, that they should not speak to Lina in English, because she can see that the other children have been losing their Spanish over the past 5 years. The grandparent's level of acculturation is more limited as compared to the family, and she wants to hold on to their native language and the cultural connotations of that language. A nurse at work has told Mrs. Lopez the opposite of the grandparent's advice in terms of the use of language at home; that they should only speak in English to Lina so she would not get confused. The nurse is speaking from a framework of assimilation to her environment and wants the same for Lina. It has been well reported in the literature that a child raised in a simultaneous bilingual language environment can learn the two languages well, and the parents should not be advised to give up their first language in order for a child to learn English. It is important to preserve the heritage language (Cummins, 2001; Paradis, Genesee, & Crago, 2010).

The first language in this case, Spanish, provides many advantages to the child in terms of maintaining the child's cultural identity. The family shares their values and traditions through the first language. It allows the children to continue participating in family and community events where the language is used, and to continue relationships with older family members (e.g., grandparents) who may not speak English. When parents or older family members do not speak English and the teenagers in the family do not speak the native language well, this can set up a pattern of low intimacy communication with high conflict communication (Cohen & Wickens, 2015). Neither party can express themselves fully. This adds to the conflict and challenge for the family members who remain dominant in the native language. Research has shown that the continued use of L1, the home language, maintains the richness of the culture and does not take away from L2 development (Hoff & Core, 2013). The home language is the language with special sayings that are integral to the family connection that may not translate well into English. The saying "*ven mi hita*"/vɛn mi jita/, come my little girl, does not translate well into English as it loses the intonation, gentleness, or cariño /karinjo/ and smoothness evoked in Spanish. Spanish, in this case, is the language most developed linguistically and provides the best foundation for language learning. The child can

speak this language with confidence. To stop the Spanish language exposure would be to leave Lina with a weak language foundation in English and a language loss in Spanish. The negative effects of this can easily be foreseen, whereby language, literacy, and educational success can be compromised. Lina is in an environment where she is receiving L1 support and the L2 can be added (additive bilingualism) in a natural manner (Fillmore, 1991). Families should be provided with the correct advice and information about the advantages of developing two languages simultaneously (Hoff & Core, 2013; Mahendra & Namzi, 2014). Parents should be informed that children will not acquire both languages at the same pace and they may appear delayed in their overall language development compared to their peers, which is within the norm for bilingual children. There is no benefit to speaking English only and avoiding the heritage language.

Another positive aspect for Lina's potential to establish a second language well is that Mrs. Lopez and her husband had a high-level command of the Spanish language in their country, providing Lina with a strong Spanish foundation. They are adding to this strong foundation a second language. Lina's parents are supportive of the use of English in order for the entire family to continue their educational and professional success. She is satisfied with the bilingual program her children have been part of in the schools. There is a pull toward maintaining the Spanish language use at home as it represents the language of her childhood, her parents in the United States, and her extended family in El Salvador. Culturally, there are many difficult decisions to make for acculturation, while maintaining ethnic roots. Language use is but one of many

> aspects. Hammer and Rodriquez (2012) speak more broadly to these parameters that are important in the socialization process of the child learning a second language. We revisit Lina's case in the PluralPlus companion website.

Theories About Second Language

There are many theories used to describe the process of acquiring a second language. There is the "innatist theory," which postulates that a second language is acquired unconsciously, similar to the acquisition of a first language (Krashen, 1985). There is the one-way communication theory where clear input is required, and the two-way communication theory where conversations must occur during meaningful activities (Krashen, 1994; Lightbown & Spada, 1999; Pica, 1996). Second language acquisition can be a five-stage process (Tabors, 2008). Stage one, the Preproduction Stage, is also called the silent period. This can be a confusing time, but an appropriate assessment can explain if the child is experiencing language delay, selective mutism, social anxiety, a speech and language impairment, or is in the first stage of acquiring a second language (Preston, 2014). There is no agreement in the literature about how long the silent period

may last. It can last less than a month or up to 6 months. During this time the child listens but does not speak. In the Early Production stage, the child may use one to two word statements for a period, which could be last 1 year. The Speech Emergence stage can take up to 3 years, and the child is using words more often, longer phrases, and more words overall. A child can remain in Stage 4, the Intermediate Fluency stage, for 3 to 5 years. The child is now engaging in social language communication. Finally, the Advanced Fluency stage can occur over a 5- to 7-year period, and the child is fluent in the second language in all contexts (Table 5–3).

Beyond English, the language most commonly used in the United States is Spanish (American Community Survey, 2016). Study of the acquisition of language by Spanish speaking children is extensive (Goldstein, 2012; Kohnert & Goldstein, 2005; Marchman, Martínez-Sussmann, & Dale, 2004; Wallner, 2016). However, it is likely that in

TABLE 5–3. Typical First Language and Second Language Acquisition

Typical First Language Acquisition		Typical Second Language Acquisition			
6–8 months	Babbling	Stage One	Preproduction	0–6 months	Silent period
9–18 months	Single words	Stage Two	Early Production	6 months–1 year	Short words
24 months	Two words	Stage Three	Speech Emergence	1–3 years	More and longer words
24–30 months	Early multiword stage	Stage Four	Intermediate Fluency	3–5 years	Social language communication
Beyond 30 months	Late multiword stage	Stage Five	Advanced Fluency	5–7 years	Fluent in all contexts

your practice or caseload today, you will have students and patients who speak a variety of languages, such as Arabic, Mandarin, Thai, Turkish, Slovenian, Samoan, Portuguese, or Vietnamese, among others. Approximately 20% of English language learning children in the United States do not have Spanish as their first language (Paradis, 2014), yet there are few resources to learn the language acquisition patterns of languages beyond Spanish and English (McLeod, 2007).

There also is a large body of literature on language and cognition in bilingual adults and bilingual adults with aphasia (Kohnert, 2008a). For example, it has been found that language experiences can influence disease progression in the age of onset of dementia (Craik, Bialystok, & Freedman, 2010), memories may be preserved in the language in which the original experience occurred, and the adult with a dual language system may lose control of this system as he or she gets older. It is especially important to know the level of function in each language prior to the neurological event in order to standardize the assessment and have a complete understanding of the current abilities of the patient or client.

We next discuss language variation. We focus on AAE, but the additional reading list in the PluralPlus student companion website, includes suggested readings about other language variations.

African American English[1]

AAE is a variation of English and is a rule-governed language system (ASHA, 2003). Yet, at the same time that research in fields of linguistics, speech-language pathology, psychology, and anthropology confirm the richness and importance of this language variation (Chun, 2001; Harris, & Moran, 2006; Labov, Cohen, Robins, & Lewis, 1968; Pearson, Velleman, Bryant, & Charko, 2009; Pollock & Meredith 2001; Rickford, et. al., 2015; Van Hofwegen &Wolfram, 2010; Wolfram & Fasold, 1974) the use of AAE is also negatively stigmatized (Lippi-Green, 2012; Hanming & Loury, 2005). AAE is spoken by many individuals in African American communities, but not all African Americans speak AAE, and not all people who speak AAE are African American. Some of the factors that may influence the use of AAE are age, gender, socioeconomic status, education, and geographic location (Washington & Craig, 1998). In many instances, the use of AAE is part of cultural identity formation (Craig & Grogger, 2012).

Green (2002) and Lanehart (2015) provide an extensive overview of AAE in books that include discussions on the historical perspective for AAE, child language acquisition, and AAE topic discussions in childhood and adolescence with a final overview of the language and identity connection. These sources provide current and relevant information for your work with children and adults who use African American English.

Seymour and Seymour (1977) provided a theoretical framework, wherein the use of this linguistic system is a part of "normal communication behavior" (p. 247). They refer to AAE as a conglomerate of language variations similar to Southern American English. There are three basic theories about the origins of AAE. One theory is the substratist hypothesis, which asserts that AAE is influenced by Niger Congo African languages (Green, 2002; DeBose & Faraclas, 1993). The second theory is the Creolist hypothesis that states that AAE was a creole (Edwards & Winford, 1991;

---

[1]African American English (AAE) has been called several names since the 1960s, such as Negro dialect, Black English, African American vernacular English, Black Linguistics, and Ebonics (Green, 2002; Makoni, Smitherman, Ball, & Spears, 2003; Williams, 1975, 1997).

Green, 2002; Rickford, 1998; Rickford & Rickford, 2000). A third way of talking about the origins of AAE is the dialectologist view, indicating that features of AAE are found in other language dialects or varieties of English, "especially in Southern varieties or earlier stages of English" (Green, 2002, p. 9). In the text that follows, we review some of the morphological, semantic, syntactic, and pragmatic aspects of AAE.

Morphosyntactic Features of AAE

There are some morphemes used in general American English (GAE) that are optional in AAE. Such morphemes include plural /s/, possessive /'s/, regular past tense marker /ed/, main verb (copula), and zero copula (Bland-Stewart, 2005; Green, 2002). Table 5–4 lists some of the morphosyntactic features of AAE.

Lexicon of AAE

AAE has specific creative uses of words that are used across age groups (Green, 2002). A lexicon refers to the words and phrases of a language. Green (2002) defines lexicon as an "abstract dictionary in which meanings and other information such as pronunciations of words can be found." (p. 12) Smitherman (1998) states that the AAE lexicon "is the commonality that takes us across boundaries. Regardless of job or social position, most African Americans experience some degree of participation in the life of the community." (p. 221) The AAE lexicon includes words and phrases, some of which are listed in Table 5–5. There are three types of question forms in AAE: (1) subject auxiliary inversion, (2) noninversion, and (3) questions without auxiliaries (Green & Sistrunk, 2015). See Table 5–6 for examples of these question forms.

Pragmatic Characteristics of AAE

AAE features are included in all aspects of language, including pragmatic language. We are referring to pragmatics using a holistic definition, and it includes linguistic, nonlinguistic, and cognitive aspects of communication that occur within macrolevel contexts, which influence communicative behaviors (Hyter,

TABLE 5–4. Some Morphological Features of AAE

Pluralization	Nouns that refer quantity (e.g., two, age) do not require a plural marker in AAE. For example, two dogs may be produced like "two dog" as the plurality is marked already with the word "two."
Possession	Word order usually marks possession in AAE, such as in "the lady car."
Regular past tense marker	The /ed/ is not required, resulting in "Last week he cook dinner."
Negation	Multiple negatives are acceptable, "I hope it don't be no leak."
Zero copula	The form of be is not required in contractible forms. The verb is included in uncontractible forms, e.g., "He running" is acceptable; whereas, "Yes, he" is not.
Irregular verb form usage	Use of a past tense verb form rather than a past participle or vice versa, e.g., "She seen him" or "She knowed him."

Source: Based on Bland-Stewart (2005) and Green (2002, pp. 76–105).

TABLE 5–5. Some Common Aspects of the AAE Lexicon

Word/Phrase	Definition	Example of Use
Get over (verb)	This verb is constructed with a verb and a preposition or particle. To take advantage of.	He tried to get over on the principle
Call-self (verb)	A person is making a poor attempt at something in the eyes of someone else. In this verb, any preposition can be attached to -self.	She call herself dressing up. They call they-self cooking.
Come (semi auxiliary)	This semi auxiliary comes before a main verb that ends in -ing. It is used to express resentment, anger, offense.	They come walking in here like they owned the place.
Own (adjective)	This adjective is used to intensify a reflexive pronoun.	Listen, I can do it myownself.
Stay (verb)	To reside at a place or to be at a particular place often for long periods of time.	She stay on Pembrook Street. He stay in that room.
be (verbal markers)	This verbal marker indicates the repetition of some event or activity	They be walking too fast. (i.e., they usually walk too fast).
BIN (verbal marker)	Indicates that some event or activity occurred in the remote past.	They BIN walking too fast (i.e., they have been walking too fast for a long time)
be dən (verbal marker)	Indicates some event or activity that ended some point in the future.	They be dən finished when I get there
BIN dən (verbal marker)	Indicates an event or activity that ended at some point in the distant past	The parents BIN dən left (i.e., The parents left a long time ago).

Source: Adapted from Green, L. (2002). *African American English: A linguistic introduction* (pp. 12–33). Oxford, UK: Oxford University Press.

TABLE 5–6. AAE Question Forms

Question Type	Example
Subject auxiliary inversion	Do you want to read my book? What did you say?
Noninversion auxiliary	You can see my book? How she was doing when you saw her?
Zero auxiliary	You saw my book? (i.e., Did you see my book?) What he said? (i.e., What did he say?)

Source: Adapted with permission from Green, L. J., & White-Sustaita, J. (2015). Development of variation in child African American English. In S. Lanehart (Ed.), *The Oxford Handbook of African American English* (pp. 475–491). Oxford, UK: Oxford University Press.

2007; Hyter, Rivers, & DeJarnette, 2015, p. 9). Pragmatics includes the following components: speech acts, discourse management and production, and the ability to recognize listener's needs during an interaction, which requires social cognitive skills. Research on African American pragmatics is very limited (as of 2017), and what does exist focuses on narrative assessment and intervention. In a systematic synthesis of the literature, Hyter et al. (2015) identified only 55 refereed published articles and dissertations that included at least 30% of the subjects who were African American. The reviewed studies were conducted over a 45-year period. Of these 55 articles, 73% focused on discourse (primarily narrative discourse), 11% on speech acts, and 16% on presupposition (Hyter et al., 2015). Table 5–7 shows some information about African American pragmatics.

Written Language Variation

Language variation does not only occur orally. It can also occur in writing. There is not much data in the literature on the expository writing of African American children and adolescents. In a systematic synthesis of the literature on the pragmatic language skills of African American children and adolescents, Hyter, Rivers, and DeJarnette (2015) found that of the 55 published articles that met their inclusion criteria, 40 focused on discourse. Of these 40, only two (5%) addressed expository discourse produced by AAE speakers. Ball (1992, 1996) found that adolescents creating expository discourse incorporate culturally influenced discourse strategies. Koonce (2015) found that children who speak AAE perform similarly to their Euro American peers in expository discourse when their texts were examined for *t*-units,

TABLE 5–7. A Sample of Pragmatic Language Skills of Child Speakers of African American English (AAE)

Pragmatic Component	Characteristics Identified in AAE Speakers
Speech acts	• AAE children use diverse speech acts, but what is needed are the mainstreamed uses of emic taxonomies during assessment and intervention of pragmatic language in the area of speech acts.
	• Basic speech acts develop at 2 years of age and are used in conversational discourse by 3–4 years.
	• Early language functions reflect a cultural style of communication.
Narrative discourse	• Speakers of AAE and general American English exhibit similar narrative skills.
	• Narrative structures (referential cohesion, mental state expression) do not seem to be dialect dense.
	• Children who learn to dialect shift will do better on literacy activities than their peers who do not learn to dialect shift.
Presupposition skills	• Social cognitive skills guide communicative interactions and facilitate dialect-shifting.
	• AAE speakers are more likely to have false belief activities, and AAE speakers who passed false belief activities told better stories.

Source: Based on Hyter, Rivers, and DeJarnette (2015) and Stockman (2010).

mean length of *t*-unit, clausal density, topic maintenance, informativeness, and fluency.

Additionally, Kersting, Anderson, Newkirk-Turner, and Nelson (2015) found that African American students used more features from the African American oral tradition, although these features showed up in the written narratives of both African American and Euro American students. When story length was controlled, they found that African American students produced significantly more AAE discourse features in their written stories compared to their Euro American counterparts. The two features that occurred statistically more in AAE speakers than in the writings of GAE speakers are parallelism ("It can be red; it can be white; it can be any color, really.") and the use of cultural references (e.g., AAE lexicon such as, "He got the ball back and *took it to the hole.*" (Kersting et al., p. 97). See the more extensive list of AAE discourse forms in the Kersting et al. (2015) article and in Champion (2003).

LANGUAGE POLITICS

One thing is constant and that is that language is always changing. *The Canterbury Tales*, written by poet Geoffrey Chaucer, is a good example for exploring which words were used, and how they were spelled in the 14th century (1300s). These tales were about people migrating to Canterbury England in the late 1300s and early 1400s, which serves as an example of society in the 14th century (Rigby, 2014, p. 1). The prologue to *The Cook's Tale* included words spelled like, Londoun, spak, thoughte, and hadde. Today, in the 21st century, these same words would be spelled differently—London, spoke, thought, and had. Other words that are used in these tales were words such as Reve (i.e., Reeve), millere

(i.e., miller), and harbergage. A Reeve was an elected official; the miller was the person who ran or managed the grain mill; and harbergage refers to refuge.

Word meanings, spellings, and sentence structures have changed over time. For example, the word *language* was spelled, "langage" in the 1400s and 1500s. By the 1640s it was spelled the way we spell it today (Lippi-Green, 2012). There have always been efforts to stop or alter language change through language legislation and linguistic human rights. Language is a living organism and has a lifespan like any other living organism. Languages are born, live, and then eventually die. A language dies when there are no more speakers of the language (Crystal, 2000). On one hand, language death is a natural event. On the other hand, languages are dying at "epidemic proportions" (Wolfram, 2004, p. 764). In other words, languages are dying much faster than they should be. Some languages die suddenly because the speakers are killed off or die, such as Tasmanian. Language can die a radical death when there is an abrupt end to speakers using the language because they change to another language due to life or death circumstances. For example, in 1930 there were uprisings by indigenous people living in El Salvador. When the uprisings were over, those who looked like they were indigenous or spoke the indigenous languages were killed. Speakers decided to stop speaking the language to preserve their lives. Some First Nations languages, for example, were victims of sudden death. Most languages die gradually over time. Some of the causes of gradual language death are natural, and others result from structural processes. When groups of people are displaced (forcefully or otherwise) from their home countries, typically the first generation acculturates but holds on to their language and culture. The second generation may understand their heritage language but may not become fluent in it, and the third generation likely will not speak the heritage language at all (McWhorter, 2004). Other causes of gradual language death may be associated with economic development (Harbert, 2011), and to the imperialism of English (Skutnabb-Kangas, 2000).

There are characteristics of language death that show up on language form, content, and use. With regard to morphology, when a language is dying, the speakers omit prefixes and suffixes. If we use Spanish as an example, to refer to the future one would begin to produce *hablar* (to talk) rather than *hablare* (will talk). With a dying language, there tends to be a reduction in the use of complex syntax; that is, there is a decrease in the use of subordinate and relative clauses. Some words are no longer used when a language is dying, and there is a narrowing of language registers.

Death of languages has consequences for our ability to maintain cultural heritage, and has implications in our relationship with ecology (Nettle & Romaine, 2000). Simons and Fennig (2017) report that there are currently 7,099 languages in the world, one-third of which are at risk of disappearing because they have less than 1,000 speakers. Only 23 languages are spoken by more than half of the world's populations (Simons & Fennig, 2017). Loss of a language means that you lose a way of thinking—cultural traditions (Woodruff & Brown, 2015), since language is the primary way these traditions are passed from one generation to the next. Language loss also has implications for biodiversity (Nettle & Romaine, 2000). Studies have shown that 70% of the world's languages are located in the "planet's biodiversity hotspots" (Kivner, 2012). As these areas become degraded, the cultures and languages in the area are also being lost (Kivner, 2012), which means losing a way of thinking and cultural traditions. Although languages die gradually anyway, politics, economics, and attitudes, such as linguistic culture, can play a role in ushering in the death of a language more rapidly.

Linguistic Culture and Language Policy

Linguistic culture and language policy are intricately linked. Linguistic culture refers to the beliefs, values, and assumptions that people have about the languages that they speak and that others speak (Schiffman, 1996). Language policies—that is, making decisions about language regarding whether multiple languages being spoken in a society, for example, are an asset (a resource) or a problem (Kontra, Phillipson, Skutnabb-Kangas, & Varady, 1999) or whether certain languages should be used as the language of instruction or the news (Brock-Utne, 2014; Brock-Utne & Hopson, 2005)—are very much linked with linguistic culture. Language policies can be top-down or official governmental policies, or bottom-up resulting from the general attitudes, assumptions about languages, and their value in a society (Schiffman, 1996). Linguistic culture is maintained by ideologies—unquestioned assumptions—of the existence of standard and correct ways to speak and use languages. This assumption of an idealized standard or correct way to use language is called standard language ideology (Milroy, 2001). Linguistic culture also includes attitudes, beliefs, and values about language codification (being able to be written)—whose language should be codified and justified through the existing power structures in a society.

There have been long-standing struggles against language variation and change in the United States. A little bit of the history of these struggles over language is presented in Table 5–8. As you read this part of the chapter, work with two or three others to make a contextualized timeline of your field (speech-

TABLE 5–8. Contextualized History of Language Legislation

Decade	Events	Context
1700s	**Naturalization Act of 1790** indicated that to be naturalized to a citizen, a person had to be a "white free person." This act left out indentured servants, those who were enslaved, free Blacks, Asian Americans, and those in the First Nations.	1700s—The slave trade was occurring. 1700s—Germans were migrating to the United States. 1787—The United States Constitution was being written. **Andrew Hamilton, Ben Franklin,** and **John Adams** all wrote about the problem of Dutch and German speakers in the United States. **John Adams** proposed an English Language Academy to serve as a standard. **Noah Webster** promoted a book on language standardization as a way to prescribe English Language use. **Robert Lowth** and **Lindley Murray** both wrote documents defining "good" English (McWhorter, 2003; Schmid, 2001).
1800s	**Civilization Act of 1819**—The goal was to "civilize" First Nations groups. **Indian Removal Act**—Signed into law by Andrew Jackson in 1830, it required the removal of First Nations to west of the Mississippi River.	**Thomas Jefferson** wanted to settle 30,000 Americans in Louisiana, which was an acquired territory, in order to stop the use of French. Increased immigration from Europe. Immigrants created their own schools, and bilingual education was common. The Elocution movement was ongoing. Psychological testing of immigrants was taking place, and there were brain studies being completed (McWhorter, 2003; Schmid, 2001).

language pathology or audiology), by identifying the following:

1. What was happening within social structures (economic, political, sociocultural, and state violence [military])?
2. What struggles over language variation and what advances were made in your field during a particular 50-year period between 1600s and the current year?

An empty chart for completing this assignment is located in Appendix 5–1. In addition, Table 5–9 shows several language legislations that were acted on in the United States since the 1600s.

CHAPTER SUMMARY

This chapter introduced you to the relationship between culture and language. You learned that the family and community are foundations for language development and production. We reviewed the differences between communication and language and discussed different linguistic and paralinguistic

TABLE 5–9. History of Language Legislation in the United States Since 1600

Year	Legislation
1600s	Bilingualism was common for members of working classes, particularly in New York, Pennsylvania, New Jersey, and Delaware.
1770–1820	Non-English speakers became "problematic."
1830–1840s	Bilingual instruction was common. It was mandated in Ohio (English/German) in 1839 and in Louisiana (French/English) in 1847. There were German language schools in Baltimore, Cincinnati, Cleveland, Indianapolis, Milwaukee, and St. Louis.
1903–1949	Policy of "Americanization" in the schools in Puerto Rico focused on making the Spanish speakers, English speakers, and at the same time, this policy included "patriotic activities," for example, flag raising, saluting, and singing the national anthem (Schmid, 2001,[a] p. 26).
1919–1920	Twenty-three states implemented restrictive language legislation.
1923	*Meyer v. Nebraska*—banned teaching a foreign language.
1968	The Bilingual Education Act addressed the linguistic needs of students speaking limited English.
1973	*Diana v. State Board of Education*—Diana was a Spanish speaker who was put in a class with children who had cognitive impairments. The rule resulted in a requirement to test in a person's native language.
1974	*Lau v. Nichols*—1800 Chinese students who did not speak English were at the center of this case. The court rules that not having supplemental language instruction for students with limited English proficiency was a violation of their civil rights.
1979	*MLK Jr. Elementary School children v. Ann Arbor*—The ruling that came out of *Lau v. Nichols* was used to protect the rights of children who speak a language variation; that is, educational agencies are required to take appropriate action to overcome language barriers that impede students' learning (20 U. S. C. §1703[f]).
	Larry P. v. Riles—Classified students as learning disabled based on race. The court ruled that testing should not discriminate based on race.
1980s	English Only—In 31 states as of 2014 (*Washington Post*, 2014[b]).
1990	Proposition 227—Essentially this proposition ended formalized bilingual education in California for the 1.4 million students who spoke English as a second or additional language (California State Government, 1998). Parents can sign a waiver to get bilingual education for their children.
	Native American Language Act (PL 101-477) states that Native Americans are entitled to use their own languages.

TABLE 5–9. *continued*

Year	Legislation
2002	George W. Bush, Republican president of the United States in 2002, repealed the Bilingual Education Act.[c]
2010	Plain Writing Act, signed into law by Democratic President Barak Obama, required federal agencies/organizations to use language and communication that the public can understand and use. It requires the government to "ensure that regulations are accessible, consistent, written in plain language, and easy to understand" (PL 111-274).

Notes. [a]Schmid, C. (2001). *The politics of language: Conflict, identity and cultural pluralism in comparative perspective.* Oxford, UK: Oxford University Press. [b]Schwarz, H. (2014, August 12). States where English is the official language. *The Washington Post.* Retrieved from https://www.washingtonpost.com/blogs/govbeat/wp/2014/08/12/states-where-english-is-the-official-language/?utm_term=.02cf458737b9 [c]Crawford, J. (2008). *The Bilingual Education Act, 1968–2002: An obituary.* Retrieved from http://www.languagepolicy.net/books/AEL/Crawford_BEA_Obituary.pdf

aspects of communication, including kinesics and proxemics. We also discussed Hall's High-Low Context Cultures. Included in this chapter was a discussion on language variation, including bilingualism, multilingualism, and AAE. Social networks and communities of practice are two ways that groups of people interact with each other, and typically, they help to maintain ways of communicating—language variations. We ended the chapter with a discussion on how language variations have been legislated throughout the history of the United States.

EXTENDED LEARNING

The following activities are designed to extend your learning about the topic of culture and language:

1. Conduct a literature search for articles that document the characteristics of language variations in the United States.
2. Conduct a literature search and write an annotated bibliography on the benefits of bilingualism.

3. Write a case study that includes a client or patient who is bilingual or who speaks a language variation, and whose daily life has been affected by economic, political, and cultural social structures.

FURTHER READING

Champion, T. B. (2003). *Understanding storytelling among African American children: A journey from Africa to America.* New York, NY: Routledge.

Hyter, Y. D., Rivers, K. O., & DeJarnette, G. (2015). Pragmatic language of African American children and adolescents: A systematic synthesis of the literature. *Topics in Language Disorders, 35*(1), 8–45.

Kersting, J., Anderson, M. A., Newkirk-Turner, B., & Nelson, N. W. (2015). Pragmatic features in original narratives written by African American students at three grade levels. *Topics in Language Disorders, 35*(1), 90–108.

Lippi-Green, R. (2012). *English with an accent: Language, ideology and discrimination in the United States* (2nd ed.). New York, NY: Routledge.

Schiffman, H. (1996). *Linguistic culture and language policy.* New York, NY: Routledge.

Shin, S. J. (2012). *Bilingualism in schools and society: Language, identity and policy.* New York, NY: Routledge.

Stockman, I. (2010). A review of developmental and applied language research on African American children: From a deficit perspective on dialect differences. *Language, Speech and Hearing Services in Schools, 41*(1), 23–38.

REFERENCES

Alba, R., Logan, J., Lutz, A., & Stults, B. (2002). Only English by the third generation? Loss and preservation of the mother tongue among the grandchildren of contemporary immigrants. *Demography, 39*(3), 467–484.

Alim, S., & Smitherman, G. (2012). *Articulate while Black: Barack Obama, language and race in the U.S.* Oxford, UK: Oxford University Press.

American Community Survey 5-Year Estimates. Language spoken at home by ability to speak English for the population 5 years and over. (2016). Retrieved from https://factfinder.census.gov/faces/tableservices/jsf/pages/productview.xhtml?pid=ACS_15_5YR_B16001&prodType=table

Bailey, R. W. (2004). American English: Its origins and history. In E. Finegan & J. R. Rickford (Eds.), *Language in the USA: Themes for the twenty-first century* (pp. 3–17). Cambridge, UK: Cambridge University Press.

Ball, A. F. (1992). Cultural preference and the expository writing of African American adolescents. *Written Communication, 9*, 501–532.

Ball, A. F. (1996). Expository writing patterns of African American students. *The English Journal, 85*(1), 27–36.

Barrueco, S., Lopez, M., Ong, C., & Lozano, P. (2012). *Assessing Spanish-English bilingual preschoolers: A guide to best approaches and measures.* Baltimore, MD: Brookes.

Bates, E. (1976). *Language and context: The acquisition of pragmatics.* New York, NY: Academic Press.

Bedore, L., & Peña, E. D. (2008). Assessment of bilingual children for identification of language impairment: Current findings and implications for practice. *International Journal of Bilingual Education and Bilingualism, 11*, 1–29.

Bedore, L. M., Peña, E. D., García, M., & Cortez, C. (2005). Conceptual versus monolingual scoring: When does it make a difference? *Language, Speech, and Hearing Services in Schools, 36*, 188–200

Birdwhistell, R. L. (1952). *Introduction to kinesics: An annotation system for analysis of body motion and gesture.* Washington, DC: Department of State, Foreign Service Institute.

Birdwhistell, R. L. (1970). *Kinesics and context: Essays on body motion communication.* Philadelphia, PA: University of Pennsylvania Press.

Bland-Stewart, L. M. (2005). Difference or deficit in speakers of African American English: What every clinician should know . . . and do. *ASHA Leader, 10*, 6–7, 30–31.

Bloom, L., & Lahey, M. (1978). *Language development and language disorders.* New York, NY: McMillan.

Borjas, G. J. (2006). Making it in America: Social mobility in the immigrant population. *The Future of Children, 16*(2), 55–71.

Brock-Utne, B. (2014). Language of instruction in Africa—The most important and least appreciated issue. *International Journal of Education and Development in Africa,* 14–18.

Brock-Utne, B. & Hopson, K. (2005). *Languages of instruction for African Emancipation: Focus on postcolonial contexts and considerations.* Dar Es Salaam, Tanzania: Mkuki n Nyota.

Brown, R. (1973). *A first language: The early stages.* London, UK: George Allen & Unwin.

California State Government. (1998). *Proposition 227 Education. Public Schools. English as required language of instruction. Initiative statute.* Retrieved from http://www.lao.ca.gov/ballot/1998/227_06_1998.htm

Champion, T. B. (2003). *Understanding storytelling among African American children: A journey from Africa to America.* New York, NY: Routledge.

Chomsky, N. (1957). *Syntactic structures* (2nd ed.). Berlin, Germany: Mouton de Gruyter.

Chun, E. (2001). The construction of white, black, and Korean American identities through African American vernacular English. *Journal of Linguistic Anthropology 11*, 52–64.

Cohen, J., & Wickens, C. M. (2015). Speaking English and the loss of heritage language. *TESL-EJ, 18*(4). Retrieved from http://www.tesl-ej.org/wordpress/issues/volume18/ej72/ej72a7/

Craig, H. K., & Grogger, J. T. (2012). Influences of social and style variables on adult usage of African American English features. *Journal of Speech, Language, and Hearing Research, 55,* 1274–1288

Craik, F. I. M., Bialystok, E., & Freedman, M. (2010). Delaying the onset of Alzheimer disease: Bilingualism as a form of cognitive reserve. *Neurology, 75,* 1717–1725.

Crystal, D. (2000). *Language death.* Cambridge, UK: Cambridge University Press

Cummins, J. (2001). *Negotiating identities: Education for empowerment in a diverse society* (2nd ed.). Los Angeles, CA: California Association for Bilingual Education.

Cummins, J. (2002). Bilingual children's mother tongue: Why is it important for education? *Sprog Forum, 7*(19), 15–20.

Debose, C., & Faraclas, N. (1993). An Africanist approach to the linguistic study of Black English: Getting to the African roots of the tense/aspect/modality and copula systems in Afro-American. In S. Mufwene (Ed.), *Africanisms in Afro-American language varieties,* pp. 364–387. Athens, GA: University of Georgia Press.

DeJarnette, G., Rivers, K. O., & Hyter, Y. D. (2015). Ways of examining speech acts in young African American children: Considering inside-out and outside-in approaches. *Topics in Language Disorders, 35*(1), 61–75.

Durkin, P. (2014). *Borrowed words: A history of loanwords in English.* Oxford, UK: Oxford University Press.

Dworkin, S. N. (2012). *A history of the Spanish lexicon: A linguistic perspective.* Oxford, UK: Oxford University Press.

Eckert, P., & Wenger, É. (2005). Communities of practice in sociolinguistics. *Journal of Sociolinguistics, 9*(4), 582–589.

Edwards, W., & Winford, D. (eds.) (1991). *Verb phrase patterns in Black English and creole.* Detroit, MI: Wayne State University Press.

Fenson, L., Dale, P. S., Reznick, J. S., Bates, E., Thal, D., Pethick, S. J., . . . Stiles, J. (1994). Variability in early communicative develop-ment. *Monographs of the Society for Research in Child Development, 59*(5) i, iii–v, 1–85.

Fillmore, L.W. (1991). When learning a second language means losing the first. *Early Childhood Research Quarterly, 6,* 323–346.

Genesee, F. (2008), What do we know About bilingual education for majority-language students? *The Handbook of Bilingualism.* 547–576.

Goldstein, B. (2000). *Cultural and linguistic diversity resource guide for speech-language pathologists.* San Diego, CA: Singular.

Goldstein, B. (2012). *Bilingual language development and disorders in Spanish-English speakers* (2nd ed.). Baltimore, MD: Brookes.

Green, L. (2002). *African American English: A linguistic introduction.* Cambridge, U.K: Cambridge University Press.

Green, L., & Sistrunk, W. (2015). Syntax and semantics in African American English. In S. Lanehart, (Ed.), *The Oxford handbook of African American language* (pp. 355–370). Oxford, UK: Oxford University Press.

Gutierrez-Clellan, V., Simon-Cereijdo, G., & Sweet, M. (2012). Predictors of second language acquisition in Latino children with specific language impairment. *American Journal of Speech-Language Pathology, 21*(1), 64–77.

Hall, E. T. (1963). A system for the notation of proxemics behavior. *American Anthropologist, 65,* 1003–1025.

Hall, E. T. (1966). *The hidden dimension.* New York, NY: Anchor Books.

Hall, E. T. (1968). *An essay on language.* Philadelphia, PA: Chilton Books Education Division.

Hall, E. T. (1976). *Beyond culture.* New York, NY: Anchor Books.

Hammer, C., & Rodriquez, B. (2012). Bilingual language acquisition and the child socialization process. In B. Goldstein (Ed.), *Bilingual language development and disorders in Spanish-English speakers* (pp. 3–30). Baltimore, MD: Brookes.

Hanming, F. & Loury. G. C. (2005). "Dysfunctional identities" can be rational. *American Economic Review, 95*(2), 104–111.

Harbert, W. (2011). Endangered languages. In P. K. Austin & J. Sallabank (Eds.), *The Cambridge handbook of endangered languages* (pp. 403–422). Cambridge, UK: Cambridge University Press.

Harris, K. L., & Moran, M. J. (2006). Phonological features exhibited by children speaking African American English at three grade levels. *Communication Disorders Quarterly, 27*, (4), 195–205.

Harrison, G. (2007). Language as a problem, a right or a resource? A study of how bilingual practitioners see language policy being enacted in social work. *Journal of Social Work, 7*(1), 71–92.

Hoff, E., & Core, C. (2013). Input and language development in bilingually developing children. *Seminars in Speech and Language, 34*(4), 215–226.

Holman, E. W., Wichmann, S., Brown, C. H., & Eff, C. A. (2015). Diffusion and inheritance of language and culture: A comparative perspective. *Social Evolution & History, 14*, 49–64.

Hyter, Y. D. (1994). *A cross-channel description of reference in the narratives of African-American vernacular English speakers* (Unpublished doctoral dissertation). Temple University, Philadelphia, PA.

Hyter, Y. D. (2007). Pragmatic language assessment: A pragmatics-as-social practice model. *Topics in Language Disorders, 27*(2), 128–145.

Hyter, Y. D., Rivers, K. O., & DeJarnette, G. (2015). Pragmatic language of African American children and adolescents: A systematic synthesis of the literature. *Topics in Language Disorders, 35*(1), 8–45.

Imai, M., Kanero, J., & Masuda, T. (2016). The relation between language, culture, and thought. *Current Opinion in Psychology, 8*, 70–77.

Ingraham, C. L. (2006). Context communication. In Y. Jackson (Ed.), *Encyclopedia of multicultural psychology* (pp. 110–111). Thousand Oaks, CA: Sage.

Kersting, J., Anderson, M. A., Newkirk-Turner, B., & Nelson, N. W. (2015). Pragmatic features in original narratives written by African American students at three grade levels. *Topics in Language Disorders, 35*(1), 90–108.

Kester, E. S., & Pena, E. D. (2002). *Limitations of current language testing: practices for bilinguals.* College Park, MD: ERIC Clearinghouse on Assessment and Evaluation. (ERIC Document Reproduction Service No. ED470203)

Kidd, E., Kemp, N., Kashima, E. S., & Quinn, S. (2016). Language, culture and group membership: An investigation into the social effects of colloquial Australian English. *Journal of Cross-Cultural Psychology, 47*(5), 713–733.

Kivner, M. (2012, May 13). Study links biodiversity and language loss. *BBC News.* Retrieved from http://www.bbc.com/news/science-environment-18020636

Kohnert, K. (2008a). *Language disorders in bilingual children and adults.* San Diego, CA: Plural.

Kohnert, K. (2008b). Primary language impairments in bilingual children and adults. In J. Altarriba & R. Heredia (Eds.), *An introduction to bilingualism: Principles and processes.* New York, NY: Taylor and Francis.

Kohnert, K. (2012). Processing skills in early sequential bilinguals. In B. Goldstein (Ed.), *Bilingual language development and disorders in Spanish-English speakers* (2nd ed., pp. 95–112). Baltimore, MD: Brookes.

Kohnert, K., & Goldstein, B. (2005). Speech, language, and hearing in developing bilingual children: From practice to research. *Language, Speech, and Hearing Services in Schools, 36*(3), 169–171.

Kontra, M., Phillipson, R., Skutnabb-Kangas, T., & Varady, T. (1999). Conceptualising and implementing linguistic human rights. In M. Kontra, R. Phillipson, T. Skutnabb-Kangas & T. Varady (Eds.), *Language: A right and a resource: Approaching linguistic human rights* (pp. 1–24). Budapest, Hungary: Central European University Press.

Koonce, N. (2015). When it comes to explaining: A preliminary investigation of the expository language skills of African American school-age children. *Topics in Language Disorders, 35*(1), 76–89.

Krashen, S. (1985). *The input hypothesis.* Beverly Hills, CA: Laredo.

Krashen, S. (1994). The input hypothesis and its rivals. In N. Ellis (Ed.), *Implicit and explicit learning of languages* (pp. 45–77). London, UK: Academic Press.

Labov, W., Cohen, P., Robins, C., & Lewis. J. (1968). *A study of the non-standard English of Negro and Puerto Rican speakers in New York city.* Final Report, Cooperative Research Project 3288, 2 Vols. (Philadelphia, PA: U.S. Regional Survey, 204 N. 35th St Philadelphia 19104).

Lanehart, S. (Ed.). (2015). *The Oxford handbook of African American language*. Oxford, UK: Oxford University Press

Leavitt, J. (2015). Linguistic relativity: Precursors and transformations. In F. Sharifian (Ed.), *The Routledge handbook of language and culture* (pp. 18–30). New York, NY: Routledge.

Lightbown, P. M., & Spada, N. (1999). *How languages are learned*. Oxford, UK: Oxford University Press.

Lippi-Green, R. (2012). *English with an accent: Language, ideology and discrimination in the United States* (2nd ed.). New York, NY: Routledge.

Loury, G. C. (2005). Racial stigma and its consequences. *FOCUS, 24*(1), 1–6.

Lucy, J. (1997). Linguistic relativity. *Annual Review of Anthropology, 26*, 291–312.

Lyon, J. (1996). *Becoming bilingual: Language acquisition in a bilingual community*. Clevedon, UK: Multilingual Matters.

Mahendra, N., & Namzi, M. (2014). Becoming bilingual. *ASHA Leader. 19*, 40–44.

Makoni, S., Smitherman, G, Ball, A. F., & Spears, A. K. (2003). Introduction: Toward Black linguistics. In S. Makoni, G. Smitherman, A. F. Ball, & A. K. Spears (Eds.), *Black l inguistics: Language, society, and politics in Africa and the Americas* (pp. 1–18). London, UK: Routledge.

Marchman, V. A., Martínez-Sussmann, C., & Dale, P. (2004). The language-specific nature of grammatical development: Evidence from bilingual language learners, *Developmental Science, 7*(2), 212–224.

McLeod, S. (Ed.). (2007). *The international guide to speech acquisition*. Clifton Park, NY: Thomson Delmar Learning.

McNeill, D. (1992). *Hand and mind: What gestures reveal about thought*. Chicago, IL: University of Chicago Press.

McWhorter, J. (2003). *The power of Babel: A natural history of language*. New York, NY: Perennial.

McWhorter, J. (2004). *The story of human language* [Audio CD]. Chantilly, VA: The Great Courses.

Milroy, J. (2001). Language ideology and the consequences of standardization. *Journal of Sociolinguistics, 5*(4), 530–555.

Milroy, L., & Llamas, C. (2013). Social networks. In J. K. Chambers & N. Schilling-Estes (Eds.), *The handbook of language variation and change* (2nd ed., pp. 409–427). Oxford, UK: Wiley-Blackwell.

Myerhoff, M., & Strycharz, A. (2013). Communities of practice. In J. K. Chambers & N. Schilling (Eds.), *The handbook of language variation and change* (2nd ed., pp. 428–447). Oxford, UK: Wiley-Blackwell.

National Center for Education Statistics (NCES), Institute of Education Sciences, U.S. Department of Education. (2011). *The condition of education 2011*. Washington, DC: U.S. Government Printing Office.

Nettle, D., & Romaine, S. (2000). *Vanishing voices: The extinction of the world's languages* Oxford, UK: Oxford University Press.

Ottenheimer, H. J. (2013). *The anthropology of language: An introduction to linguistic anthropology* (3rd ed.). Belmont, CA: Wadsworth.

Otto, B. (2014). *Language development in early childhood education* (4th ed.). Upper Saddle River, NJ: Pearson Education.

Ovando, C. J. (2008a). Acculturation. In J. M. Gonzalez (Ed.), *Encyclopedia of bilingual education* (pp. 9–10). Thousand Oaks, CA: Sage.

Ovando, C. J. (2008b). Assimilation. In J. M. Gonzalez (Ed.), *Encyclopedia of bilingual education* (pp. 43–45). Thousand Oaks, CA: Sage.

Paradis, J., Genesee, F., & Crago, M. B. (2010). *Dual language development and disorders*. Baltimore, MD: Paul H Brookes.

Paradis, J. (2014). Discriminating children with SLI among English language learners. *CREd Library*. Retrieved from http://cred.pubs.asha.org/article.aspx?articleid=2442989

Pearson, B. Z., & Fernández, S. C. (1994). Patterns of interaction in the lexical growth in two languages of bilingual infants and toddlers. *Language Learning, 44*, 617–653.

Pearson, B. Z., Velleman, S. L., Bryant, T. J. & Charko, T. (2009). Phonological milestones for African American English-speaking children learning mainstream American English as a second dialect. *Language, Speech, and Hearing Services in Schools, 40*, 1–16.

Pica, T. (1996). Second language learning through interaction: Multiple perspectives. *Working Papers in Educational Linguistics, 12*(1), 1–22.

Pollock, K. E., & Meredith, L. H. (2001). Phonetic transcription of African American vernacular

English. *Communication Disorders Quarterly, 23*, 47–53.

Preston, K. (2014, November). When a child goes silent. *ASHA Leader, 19*, 34–38.

Rickford, J. R. (1998). The Creole origins of African American vernacular English: Evidence from copula absence. In S. Mufwene, J. Rickford, G. Bailey, & J. Baugh (Eds.), *The structure of African American English* (pp. 154–200). London, UK: Routledge.

Rickford, J. R., Duncan, G. J., Gennetian, L. A., Gou, R. Y., Greene, R., Katz, L. F., . . . Ludwig J. (2015). Neighborhood effects on use of African-American vernacular English. *Proceedings of the National Academy of Sciences, 112*(38), 11817–11822.

Rickford, J., & Rickford, A. (1976). Cut eye and suck teeth: Africa words and gestures in New World guise. *Journal of American Folklore, 89*(353), 194–309.

Rickford, J.R., & Rickford, R.J. (2000). *Spoken soul: The story of Black English.* New York, NY: Wiley and Sons.

Rigby, S. H. (2014). Reading Chaucer: Literature, history and ideology. In S. H. Rigby (Ed.), *Historians on Chaucer: The "general prologue" to the Canterbury Tales* (pp. 1–23). Oxford, UK: Oxford University Press.

Rivers, K. O., Hyter, Y. D., & DeJarnette, G. (2012). Parsing pragmatics. *ASHA Leader, 17*, 14–17.

Schiffman, H. (1996). *Linguistic culture and language policy.* New York, NY: Routledge.

Schmid, Carol L. (2001). *The politics of language: Conflict, identity, and cultural pluralism in comparative perspective.* Oxford, UK: Oxford University Press.

Schmitt, M. B., Logan, J. A. R., Tambyraja, S. R., Farquharson, K., & Justice, L. M. (2017). Establishing language benchmarks for children with typically developing language and children with language impairment, *Journal of Speech, Language, and Hearing Research, 60*, 364–378.

Seymour, H. N., & Seymour, C. M. (1977). A therapeutic model for communication disorders among children who speak Black English vernacular. *Journal of Speech and Hearing Disorders, 42*, 247–256.

Simons, G. F. & Fennig, C. D. (Eds.). (2017). *Ethnologue: Languages of the world, Twentieth edition.* Dallas, TX: SIL International, Online version: http://www.ethnologue.com

Skutnabb-Kangas, T. (2000). *Linguistic genocide in education or worldwide diversity and human rights?* Mahwah, NJ: Erlbaum.

Smitherman, G. (1998). The lexicon of AAVE. In S. S. Mufwene, J. R. Rickford, G. Bailey, & J. Baugh (Eds.), *African-American English: Structure, history and use* (pp. 203–225). London, UK: Routledge.

Smitherman, G. (2000). *Talkin that talk.* New York, NY: Routledge.

Tabors, P. O. (2008). *One child, two languages: A guide for preschool educators of children learning English as a second language* (2nd ed.). Baltimore, MD: Brookes.

Trager, G. L. (1958). Paralanguage: A first approximation. *Studies in Linguistics, 13*, 1–12.

Treffers-Daller, (2010). Borrowing. In M. Fried, M. Ostman, & J. Verschueren (Eds.), *Variation and change: Pragmatic perspectives* (pp. 17–25). Amsterdam, The Netherlands: Benjamins.

Van Hofwegen, J., & Wolfram, W. (2010). Coming of age in African American English: A longitudinal study. *Journal of Sociolinguistics, 14*, 427–455.

Van Hofwegen, J., & Wolfram, W. (2016). On the utility of composite indices in longitudinal language study. In S. E. Wagner & I. Buchstaller (Eds.), *Using panel data in the sociolinguistic study of variation and change.* Routledge Studies in Language Change Series. London, UK: Routledge.

Wallner, K. (2016). The effects of bilingualism on language development of children. *Communication Sciences and Disorders: Student Scholarship & Creative Works.* Retrieved from http://digitalcommons.augustana.edu/csdstudent/5

Washington, J. A., & Craig, H. K. (1998). Socioeconomic status and gender influences on children's dialectal variations. *Journal of Speech, Language, and Hearing Research, 41*, 618–626.

Wenying, J. (2000). The relationship between culture and language. *ELT Journal, 54*(4), 328–334.

Whiteside, K. E., Gooch, D., & Norbury, C. F. (2016). English language proficiency and early school attainment among children learning English as an additional language. *Child Development, 88*, 812–827.

Williams, R. L. (1975). *Ebonics: The true language of Black folks*. St. Louis, MO: Institute for Black Studies.

Williams, R. L. (1997). The Ebonics controversy. *Journal of Black Psychology*, *23*(3), 208–214.

Wolfram, W. (2004). Language death and dying. In J. K. Chambers, P. Trudgill, & N. Schilling-Estes (Eds). *The handbook of language variation and change* (pp. 764–787). Oxford, UK: Oxford University Press.

Wolfram, W., & Fasold, R. (1974). *The study of social dialects in American English*. New York, NY: Prentice Hall.

Wolfram, W., & Schilling-Estes, N. (2006). *American English: Dialects and variation* (2nd ed.). Cambridge/Oxford, UK: Basil Blackwell.

Woodruff, J., & Brown, J. (2015, January 27). *What does the world lose when a language dies?* Interview with Gwyneth Lewis, National Poet of Wales & Bob Holman, Host of *Language Matters, PBS Newshour*. Oxford, UK: Oxford University Press.

Appendix 5–1

Contextualized Timeline Chart

Work with two to three others to complete this chart for one 50-year period between 1600s and today.

Decade	Cultural Events	Political Events	Economic Events	State-Sanctioned Violence Events (Military)	Events in Speech, Language, and Hearing Sciences
Early 1600s (1600–1649)					
Late 1600s (1650–1699)					
Early 1700s (1700–1749)					
Late 1700s (1750–1799)					
Early 1800s (1800–1849)					
Late 1800s (1849–1899)					
Early 1900s (1900–1949)					

Decade	Cultural Events	Political Events	Economic Events	State-Sanctioned Violence Events (Military)	Events in Speech, Language, and Hearing Sciences
Late 1900s (1950–1999)					
Early 2000s (2000–2049)					
Late 2000s (2050–2099)					

1. Summarize the events that happened during the 50-year period that you investigated.

2. Discuss if there were cultural, political, economic, or military events that occurred in the 50-year period that you investigated that may have affected the developments in speech, language, and hearing sciences.

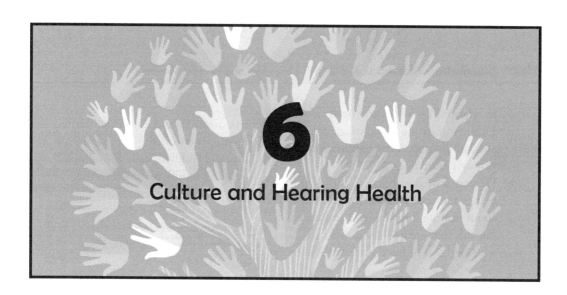

6

Culture and Hearing Health

The loss of hearing can have a significant impact on child development, the development of language, and educational outcomes. Hearing loss occurs in every region of the world but is unevenly distributed, where some regions have a much higher prevalence rate (i.e., those with lower income levels) than others (WHO, 2012). This chapter focuses on the relationship between culture and hearing health care, including considerations for assessment and rehabilitation or intervention with persons who have a hearing loss and who may have a cultural background different from your own, or who may speak a language (or languages) other than English. Also covered in this chapter is information on Deaf culture, and the difficulty that those who are Deaf or hard of hearing may have with due process in the judicial system.

LEARNING OBJECTIVES

After reading, discussing, and processing the information presented in this chapter, you will be able to demonstrate the following knowledge, skills, and attitudes:

1. Knowledge
   a. Discuss the prevalence of hearing loss and Deafness in the United States and the world.
   b. Explain the relationship among hearing health and cultural health beliefs.
   c. Discuss the importance of understanding the effects of culture and linguistic diversity on providing effective services to those who are Deaf and hard of hearing.
2. Skills
   a. Identify ways to modify assessment and rehabilitation practices to be more culturally and linguistically responsive.
   b. Demonstrate through journaling and assignments the ability to incorporate suggested considerations for assessing and providing rehabilitation to persons with hearing loss, particularly those for whom English is not their first language.
3. Attitudes demonstrated through journaling
   a. Demonstrate the ability to consider cultural and linguistic diversity

in relationship to hearing health, Deafness, hearing loss, assessment, and habilitation and rehabilitation through journaling.

b. Demonstrate the ability to value the beliefs and concerns, and stigmas about hearing, hearing loss, and hearing aids that are held by individuals who are Deaf or have a hearing loss.

KEY CONCEPTS

Key concepts addressed in this chapter are presented in Table 6–1.

> **Box 6–1**
> **Michael, audiologist; Jennifer, speech language pathologist; and Fatimatou**
>
> Michael and Jennifer, two clinicians, were faced with difficult decisions regarding the intervention recommendations of a child. Fatimatou is a 19-month-old child with multiple conditions. At birth, she was diagnosed with congenital cytomegalovirus (CMV), a leading cause of "birth defects and hearing loss globally" (Mwaanza et al., 2014, p. 728), which was the cause of her moderate to severe hearing loss,
>
> seizure disorder, and cognitive deficits. Fatimatou is enrolled in a program for infants and toddlers with disabilities. Fatimatou's family migrated to the United States after being forcefully displaced from Malawi due to the severe drought and flooding that caused hundreds of thousands of families to leave their homes and country. This long-standing drought and the accompanying floods practically wiped out Malawi's food production abilities (Lamble, 2016). Her family's faith/religious practices did not allow for her to eat foods that were not produced on their own land from their own crops, livestock, or water well, meaning that food from other sources was not allowed. Additionally, Fatimatou's parents were suspicious of Westernized health care; their trust of formalized medical treatments and doctor visits was low resulting in limited follow-through on recommendations for them to seek medical intervention for Fatimatou's seizures, hearing difficulties, and other medical issues.

There are several factors going on with Fatimatou. Identify the issues that will challenge ways that speech, language, and audiology services could be offered to (and accepted by) Fatimatou and her family:

1. _____

2. _____

3. _____

4. _____

5. _____ [1]

TABLE 6–1. Key Concepts

Hearing health	Sign language
Deaf	Hard of hearing
Hearing loss	Stigma
Dual language learner	Second language learner

---

[1]A list of items that should be considered is provided on the PluralPlus companion website.

Fatimatou was born with CMV, which is one of the leading causes of hearing loss in the world, and can be acquired from maternal infections during pregnancy (Mocarski, Shenk, & Pass, 2007; Mwaanza et al., 2014). CMV can cause serious defects in a fetus, although it might not cause disease in a healthy adult carrying the fetus (CDC, 2016a). As of 2011, it was reported that "0.7% of all births worldwide" are born with CMV, and 15% to 20% of babies infected with CMV have "permanent disability, including hearing loss, visual impairment, and cognitive deficit" (Dollard, Staras, Amin, Schmnid, & Cannon, 2011, p. 1895). CMV occurs all over the world; some report that in sub-Saharan Africa it is an infection of AIDS progression in children. A higher prevalence of CMV has been found in children infected with HIV when compared to those not infected with HIV (Mwaanza et al., 2014). One outcome of CMV infection is hearing loss, and for our purposes in this chapter, we focus on that issue with Fatimatou.

As we discuss in this text, the demographics of the United States and other countries are changing, largely due to global processes that compel groups of people to move from their home countries to another country. Some are forced out by civil unrest and wars, or like Fatimatou's family, environmental disasters; yet others choose to leave in search of opportunities to improve their lives and those of their family members. In the United States, there is a high rate of immigration from countries where hearing loss is more prevalent. The prevalence of hearing loss in people 65 years old and older is highest in South Asia, Asia Pacific, and sub-Saharan Africa (McPherson & Swart, 1997; Stevens, Flaxman, Brunskill, Mascarenhas, Mathers, & Finucane, 2011;

WHO, 2017). Audiologists, hearing educators, and SLPs have increased opportunities to provide services to children with hearing loss who come from a cultural, ethnic, and/or linguistic background different from one's own (Rhoades, Price, & Perigoe, 2004). Although audiologists, like speech-language pathologists (SLPs), are experiencing increases in racial, ethnic, cultural, and linguistic diversity on their caseloads, publications in audiology (i.e., peer-reviewed journals, dissertations, books, and news articles) about culturally and linguistically responsive service delivery approaches seem to lag those produced in speech-language pathology.[2] To meet the needs of the current and future changing demographics, audiologists and hearing educators (as well as SLPs) need to be prepared to face these challenges and to be responsive to cultural and linguistic diversity.

HEARING LOSS, HARD OF HEARING, AND DEAFNESS

The American Speech-Language-Hearing Association (ASHA) defines hearing loss as resulting from "impaired auditory sensitivity and/or diminished speech intelligibility of the physiological auditory system" (ASHA, 2017e). There are different types of hearing loss as well as different degrees of hearing loss. Sensorineural hearing loss is caused by a disruption to or dysfunction of the sensory hair cells or auditory nerve in the inner ear. This is a type of hearing loss that is permanent, meaning that it usually cannot be eliminated (ASHA, 2017g). A conductive hearing loss results when sound waves are not able to travel

---

[2]In March 2017, a simple literature search using a university's library holdings of peer-reviewed journals, dissertation abstracts, books, and news articles between the years of 1990 and 2017, revealed that the concepts *"cultural competence"* + *audiology NOT Deaf* produced 261 publications; whereas, *"cultural competence"* + *"speech-language pathology" NOT Deaf* revealed 470 publications.

through to the inner ear; the obstruction of sound waves may occur at the outer ear canal, tympanic membrane, and/or middle ear ossicles. This type of hearing loss is often responsive to medical treatment such as removal of cerumen or surgery (ASHA, 2017c). A mixed hearing loss is one where there is both a problem with conducting sounds through the ear canal and tympanic membrane, as well as some damage to the nerves of the inner ear (ASHA, 2017f). In addition to *types* of hearing loss, there are differing *degrees* of hearing loss.

Hearing loss ranges from a mild to a profound loss, which is based on decibels hearing level (dB HL)—a measurement of sound intensity (i.e., the amount of energy in sound waves), which we hear as loudness (Trefil

& Hazen, 2004). By reviewing Figure 6–1, you can see that normal hearing threshold is between –10 and +20 dB HL. Being able to only hear sounds at levels greater than +20 dB HL is considered a mild to profound hearing loss depending on the intensity at which one's hearing threshold is measured. (Hearing threshold is the lowest [softest] sound a person can detect.) Hearing loss can occur in one ear (unilateral) or in both (bilateral). Depending on its severity, a hearing loss may affect an individual's ability to hear conversational speech as well as environmental sounds. Let's look at Figure 6–1 again for the degrees of hearing loss presented in an audiogram.

Mild hearing loss occurs between +25 and +40 dB HL. Moderate loss is +41 to +55

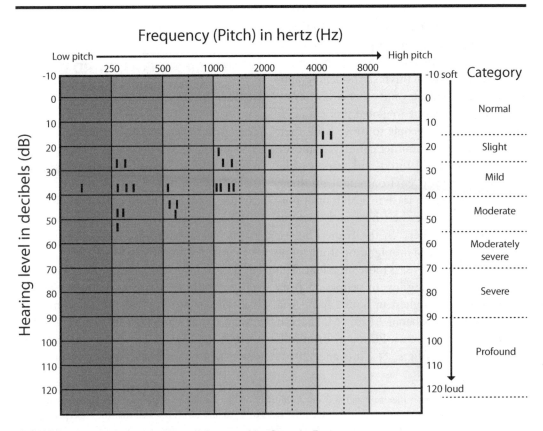

FIGURE 6–1. Hearing Thresholds. Illustrated by Severin Provance.

dB HL, severe is +70 to +90 dB HL, and profound loss is more than +90 dB HL (ASHA, 2017e). Typically, "hard of hearing" is used to refer to people who have a hearing loss in the mild to severe range. Those who are hard of hearing can often benefit from habilitation and rehabilitation, along with technology. Habilitation, facilitating the development of a skill, for children may include training in auditory perception (increasing awareness of sounds, sound discrimination, and connecting meanings to different sounds) and learning to use visual cues, as well as supporting speech and language development (ASHA, 2017b; Duncan, Rhoades, & Fitzpatrick, 2014). Rehabilitation, the restoration of skills, for adults may include such skills as learning to listen, using assistive listening devices, and using visual cues (ASHA, 2017a; Duncan, Rhoades, & Fitzpatrick, 2014). Technology that can be employed with those with hearing loss may include such items as hearing aids, FM systems, telephone amplifying devices, and cochlear implants. Individuals who are Deaf (or deaf) are those with hearing loss in the profound range, meaning that they have very little, if any, hearing acuity, and are likely to use sign language to communicate (WHO, 2017).

Prevalence of Hearing Loss

Both prevalence and incidence refer to the rate that a condition (hearing loss) occurs within a population (Peat, Barton, & Elliott, 2008). Prevalence refers to the number of people who are alive at a given time that have a condition; incidence refers to the number of new cases of a condition that occur within a certain timeframe. Both can be referred to as a percentage of the population (90% of children with hearing loss are born to hearing parents) or as the rate of a population (2–3 children out of

every 1,000 children in the United States have some level of hearing loss) (National Institute on Deafness and Other Communication Disorders [NIDCD], 2016b).

The World Health Organization (WHO, 2017[3]) reports that 360 million people in the world (about 5% of the world's population, and a number that is higher than the current U.S. population) have a disabling hearing loss—that is, a loss that exceeds 40 dB HL. Nearly 9% of this 360 million (i.e., 32 million) are children (WHO, 2017). In a systematic review of epidemiology of childhood hearing loss, Nicholson et al. (2015) reported a 3.1% prevalence rate of unilateral or bilateral childhood hearing loss when defined as >20 dB HL, and the prevalence rate was higher for Latin@/Hispanic children.

About 15% of the adult population in the world has hearing loss to some degree (WHO, 2011), and the prevalence of hearing loss decreases as income of the country increases. Hearing loss is one of the most prevalent disabilities in the United States and in the world (Nicholson, Martin, & Munoz, 2015; WHO & World Bank, 2011). In the United States, incidence of hearing loss among children is about 2/1,000 live births. For adults in the United States, about 15% (over 48 million) report having difficulty hearing. Of that 15%, a little more than half could benefit from hearing aids (NIDCD, 2016a).

Hearing loss can be caused by congenital diseases (present from birth), preventable causes, as well as complications that may occur during birth. Table 6–2 shows some of the causes of hearing impairment.

Hearing impairment can affect communication development and social functioning, and can be associated with anxiety and social isolation (Mick, Kawachi, & Lin, 2014), as well as contribute to accelerated cognitive decline in older adults (Lin et al., 2013).

---

[3]The World Health Organization (WHO) defines a disabling hearing loss as one that is more than a 40 dB HL loss.

TABLE 6–2. Some Causes of Hearing Impairment

Preventable causes	• Chronic ear infections
	• Fluid in the middle ear due to upper respiratory infections
	• Ototoxic medicines
	• Impacted cerumen
	• Noise exposure (ear buds and explosions during times of war)
Perinatal (occurs during birth)	• Birth hypoxia, ischemia
Congenital diseases (present at birth)	• Maternal infections (e.g., rubella)
Postnatal (occurs after birth or later in life)	• Childhood infections (e.g., mumps or measles)
	• Low birth rates
	• Age related, such as presbycusis

CULTURAL AND ETHNIC DIFFERENCES AND HEARING

Some studies have found that Blacks (people of African descent) have lower numbers of hearing loss compared with people who identify as White. In a study by Lin, Thorpe, Gordon-Salant, and Ferrucci (2011) of hearing loss in 717 older adults, a relationship between hearing loss and race was identified. Specifically, people of African descent (i.e., Black or African American) showed a prevalence of hearing loss that was significantly lower (43.3%) than their White counterparts (64.4%) in the study. Similar findings have been reported elsewhere (Agrawal, Platz, & Niparko, 2009; Helzner et al., 2005). Other studies have found that there may be a higher prevalence of hearing loss among individuals who are Latin@ or Hispanic in the United States. In a recent study on prevalence of hearing impairment in Latin@/Hispanic populations, it was found that Puerto Rican participants had a higher prevalence of hearing impairment than Mexican participants (Cruickshanks et al., 2015).

Researchers who conducted the Hispanic Health and Nutrition Examination Survey found that Hispanics and Latin@s showed a lower rate of hearing impairment than Non-Hispanic Whites, but that study primarily included Hispanics of Mexican backgrounds (Cruickshanks et al., 2015). Hearing impairment among Hispanic and Latin@s in the Cruickshanks et al. (2015) study was associated with environmental and personal factors such as socioeconomic status (SES) (lower income levels), noise exposure (occupational and recreational), less education, and diabetes (Cruickshanks et al., 2015, p. 645).

Disparities exist in health care in general, but also in relationship to hearing health (Manchaiah et al., 2015; Nieman, Marrone, Szanton, Thorpe, & Lin, 2016). These disparities, and research about hearing health within communities of color, however, have not typically been a focus of audiological research in the United States (Nash et al., 2013; Nieman et al., 2016; Shi, 2014). Understanding differences in race, ethnicity, and socioeconomic status is much needed in hearing health and hearing loss research. The limited quantity of research studies of this type make it difficult to determine *why* there may be racial/ethnic differences in the outcome of hearing assessments as well as hearing aid use. These racial/ethnic differences could confound research results if they are not systematically examined (Nieman et al., 2016).

Nieman and colleagues (2016) found that there are different rates of hearing aid use among African Americans, Whites, and Mexicans with hearing loss in the United States. African American older adults were more likely than Whites to report recent hearing testing; yet, interestingly, African American older adults were *less* likely to use hearing aids than their White counterparts with hearing loss. Specifically, African American older adults were 58% less likely, and Mexican older adults were 78% less likely than White older adults to report hearing aid use. Bainbridge and Ramachandran (2014) reported similar outcomes with respect to hearing aid use by 1,636 adults older than 70 years who participated in their study. Of these adults, over 86% of Whites reported wearing hearing aids, whereas only 12.7% of the participants who identified as "Non-Hispanic Blacks, Hispanics/Latinos, other race or multiracial" (p. 291) reported use of hearing aids. The authors speculate that the increase in hearing assessments by African American older adults could be due to their having Medicare coverage, which typically provides coverage for audiometric diagnostic testing under section 1861(s)(3) or 1861(s)(2)(C) if the testing is provided by an audiologist and ordered by a physician or medical practitioner (Centers for Medicare and Medicaid, 2016). Further speculation about the differences in hearing aid use was related to the possible limited access to insurance coverage for hearing aids. Medicare does not cover the cost of hearing aids (Centers for Medicare and Medicaid, 2016; Knudsen, Oberg, Nielsen, Naylor, & Kramer, 2010); a person would need to have

supplemental insurance to assist with acquiring them, and some supplemental insurance policies cover only a minimum of the cost of a hearing aid. For example, the cost of bilateral hearing aids could be as high as $4,500, but a person's supplemental insurance may only cover a fraction of that cost, such as $1,700. Additionally, contextual factors, as described in the WHO ICF (2001), could also be a barrier to hearing aid use. Such a contextual factor could be the stigma of wearing hearing aids (Bainbridge & Ramachandran, 2014; Diala et al., 2001; Givens, Katz, Bellamy, & Holmes, 2007; Manchaiah et al., 2015; Nieman et al., 2016; Wallhagen, 2010).

Manchaiah et al. (2015) used social representation theory to determine how members of a society perceive hearing loss. Social representation theory comes from the field of psychology, and through this theory "social psychological phenomena and processes can only be properly understood if they are seen as being embedded in historical, cultural, and macrosocial conditions" (Wagner et al., 1999, p. 96). Social representation theory explains how groups of people (a community or groups of people who identify as being part of the same cultural group) come to collectively understand, perceive, represent, communicate about, and behave in their world (Moscovici, 1963). The point we are making here is that social representation theory can be a tool for figuring out how groups of people share identities, marginalize or exclude others, and stigmatize illnesses or disorders (Howarth, 2001).

Not everyone with a hearing loss will utilize interventions for their hearing loss, with less than 20% of those with a hearing impairment using a hearing aid (Manchaiah et al., 2015). Hearing health, assessment, and interventions should be approached from "multidimensional," "multiprofessional," and "interdisciplinary" perspectives (Manchaiah et al., 2015, p. 1858). Several factors should be considered when providing hearing services to individuals and families from cultural and linguistic backgrounds that differ from one's own. These considerations are: (a) environmental and personal factors, as discussed in the WHO ICF framework (Manchaiah et al., 2015; Rhoades et al., 2004); (b) beliefs about, and attitudes and stigmas toward, hearing loss (Harris, Fleming, & Harris, 2012; Knudsen, Oberg, Nielsen, Naylor, & Kramer, 2010; Manchaiah et al., 2015); (c) health literacy (Hasseikus & Moxley, 2009); (d) language variations among users of sign language (Lucas, Bayley, McCaskill, & Hill, 2015); and (e) culturally and linguistically responsive practices to use during hearing assessment and intervention (Douglas, 2011a, 2011b; Kohnert & Derr, 2004; Lonka, Hasan, & Komulainen, 2011; Rhoades, Perusse, Douglas, & Zarate, 2008; Shi, 2014; Soman, Kan, & Tharpe, 2012; Wallhagen, 2010; Woods, Peña, & Martin, 2004).

Hearing loss can be defined in numerical terms, as we just did earlier in this chapter, and those numerical terms are based on how different a person's hearing is from those without a hearing loss. Hearing can also be defined differently, as it is in the Deaf culture communities. In the next section, we turn our attention to Deaf culture.

Deaf Culture

Deafness, according to the British Deaf Association (BDA, 2017), is "a state of being: it defines a group of people who share a perception of the world through an emphasis on visual and kinaesthetic input. This description of deafness is used most commonly for people who are deaf at birth or in very early childhood." In this way, deafness is different than having a physiological or audiological impairment (Knoors & Marschark, 2014). It refers to the underlying beliefs, values, and assumptions that groups of people have about their

way of life; it refers to a culture. Deaf communities have existed for centuries. The earliest recorded knowledge of Deaf communities was in the 1790s when schools were established for Deaf persons (Holcomb, 2013).

Deaf communities and Deaf culture have similar characteristics as other cultural groups; that is, they are diverse (not homogeneous) (Pray & Jordan, 2010), exist all over the world, and have a "link to a special heritage" (Knoors & Marshark, 2014, p. 26). In the field of Deaf studies, when deafness is used to refer to a cultural group, the "D" is capitalized, as in Deaf. When it is used to refer to someone with a profound hearing loss who is not associated with the Deaf culture or community, the lowercase "d" is used—deaf. Those who identify as being part of the Deaf culture or community see themselves as a cultural-linguistic group, are proud of their history, and do not consider their hearing status to be disabling (Holcomb, 2013). The language of Deaf communities is usually sign language (Holcomb, 2013; Woll & Ladd, 2011), but not only sign language as there are variations in how members of the Deaf community prefer to communicate (Fernandes & Myers, 2010).

Sign language in Deaf communities in the United States includes American Sign Language (ASL). The signed languages used by the members of Deaf communities could be thought about as existing on a continuum, with ASL on one end, finger spelling on the other, and a range of other signed languages that mix ASL and English in the middle (Pidgin Sign English, Signed English [SEE]) (Holcomb, 2013, p. 127). Within Deaf communities there is linguistic variation.

Language Variations Among Sign Language Users

As with spoken language, there are variations among sign languages (Lucas et al., 2015).

These variations exist for many reasons, including regional, age, gender, socioeconomic, racial, cultural, and familial differences, as well as due to the language policies implemented in deaf education (Lucas et al., 2015). Deaf education in the United States, for example, is primarily regulated by the Individuals with Disabilities Education Improvement Act (IDEA 2004) and the Regulations of the Offices of the Department of Education, Title 34 (Hult & Compton, 2012). Based on these laws, an annual Individualized Education Plan (IEP) is required for each student, and the IEP child study team (usually composed of teachers and parents or caregivers) determines the educational context in which the student who is Deaf or hard of hearing will be placed, including general education classrooms, self-contained classrooms, or schools for the Deaf (Hult & Compton, 2012).

Lucas and colleagues (2015) have identified the presence of African American English lexical items in sign language produced by African American persons who are Deaf or hard of hearing. African American lexicon contains words or phrases with "specialized or unique meaning" (Green, 2002, p. 12). For example, Lucas et al. (2015) report such phrases as "Stop trippin'!" "My bad," and "Girl, please" in the sign language of African American sign language users (Lucas et al., 2015, p. 156). These unique lexical items demonstrate that African American ASL users have contact with AAE speakers who are hearing (Lucas, 2015). African American users of ASL have also reported that they recognize that there are differences in the way Blacks sign and from the way Whites sign. Some of the differences include the unique lexical items mentioned before, as well as the use of a larger plane of space for signing, the incorporation of AAE gestures. Figure 6–2 shows a side-by-side comparison of a White person and a Black person making the same sign. You will see that the African American signer is using a larger space than the White signer to communicate the same idea.

Another feature of sign language that has been found to differ between White and Black signers is voiceless mouthing. Voiceless mouthing as it occurs in White signers has been studied a great deal (Lucas et al., 2015), and it usually accompanies nouns, verbs, predicates, adjectives, and adverbs, in that order. Voiceless mouthing can include mouth gestures that are related to English (mouthing "f-sh" while signing "finish"). They can also be part of the sign language without having any relationship to spoken English (mouthing "pah" while signing "at last") (Lucas et al., 2015, p. 159). Blacks do use voiceless mouthing, but it occurs intermittently. Also, older African Americans will engage in voiceless mouthing less often than younger African American signers (Lucas et al., 2015; Tabak, 2006).

ENVIRONMENTAL AND PERSONAL FACTORS

In Chapter 2, you learned that the WHO-ICF (2001), the framework for describing functioning, disability, and health internationally, includes contextual factors that interact with and can influence health, disability, and/or participation outcomes (Howe, 2008). Contextual factors "represent the complete background of an individual's life and living" (WHO, 2001, p. 16). Environmental factors include the "physical, social and attitudinal environment" of living that are outside of a person's life, but that may affect his or her ability to participate in daily life (WHO, 2001). For example, environmental factors could include an individual's home or school context, or access to services (Howe, 2008). Personal factors, on the other hand, include characteristics of the person that are not part

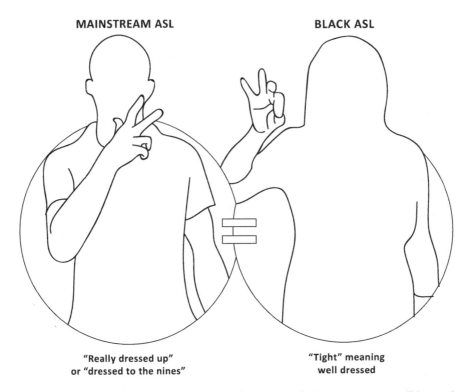

MAINSTREAM ASL   **BLACK ASL**

"Really dressed up"
or "dressed to the nines"

"Tight" meaning
well dressed

FIGURE 6–2. Comparison of White and Black sign of the same concept ("dressed up," signed by the man, and "tight," meaning well-dressed signed by the woman). Adapted from https://www.washingtonpost.com/national/health-science/whats-that-you-say/2012/09/17/95dc9ef6-010e-11e2-b260-32f4a8db9b7e_graphic.html?utm_term=.05cb966a3037. Illustrated by Severin Provance.

of the person's health condition (gender, age, cultural beliefs) (WHO, 2001, p. 17).

One contextual factor to consider when providing culturally responsive care is the changing structure of the family (Rhoades et al., 2008). When a family has a member that has a disability, the needs of that person affect the entire family (Rhoades et al., 2008). The family structure can change in various ways, such as: (a) higher rates of divorce; (b) working parents, which leads to changes in how child care happens and who is involved in raising children; and (c) diverse family structures (Rhoades et al., 2008). Another issue to consider is that increased impoverishment in the United States and other parts of the world can

make families more at-risk for health issues, including hearing loss, and limits their access to quality health care (Rhoades et al., 2008), as there are higher rates of recurrent serous otitis media in children who are impoverished (Auinger, Lanphear, Kalkwarf, & Mansour 2003). A personal factor to consider when being culturally responsive is the diverse nature of beliefs and attitudes about hearing loss, and stigmas toward hearing loss.

Cultural Beliefs and Stigmas

Folk beliefs are common in all cultural groups regardless of where they are in the world

(Harris, Fleming, & Harris, 2012; Kleinman, 1978; Salas-Provance, Good Erickson, & Reed, 2002). Kleinman (1978), through his theory of explanatory models, proposes that there are a wide range of ideas about health and disease among and within groups. It is not possible to separate these ideas about health or health beliefs from cultural beliefs because they are learned as people are socialized into their culture (Harris et al., 2012; Kleinman, 1978; Kleinman & Benson, 2006). Disparate health beliefs will expand as populations become more diverse (Shrestha & Heisler, 2011). For this reason, it is imperative for health professionals, including SLPs and audiologists, to understand the health beliefs of their clients. Being able to identify health beliefs and how those beliefs impact a person's response to his or her communication impairment (utilization of services, help seeking, compliance with recommendations) is an important step in being able to provide effective and culturally responsive services (Harris et al., 2012). There are models of practice that take health beliefs into consideration: explanatory models (Kleinman, 1978; Kleinman, Eisenberg, & Good, 2006), Biopsychosocial Model (Engel, 1980), and Health Beliefs Model (Champion, & Skinner, 2006).

Explanatory Models

Arthur Kleinman (1978), a psychiatrist and anthropologist, and colleagues (Kleinman et al., 2006) created a protocol for gaining access to how a person or group might perceive their own condition, illness, disease, or disorder. Perceptions of one's disorder are based on how one explains it. Kleinman identified eight questions that can be used to access a person's explanatory model about his or her illness or disorder. In Table 6–3, we included Klienman's questions and our revision of them based on how they could be formulated for Fatimatou's family.

If we were going to apply this model to Fatimatou, the clinicians working with her and her family would do well to ask these questions of Fatimatou's parents or family members to understand their experiences, concerns, and knowledge related to Fatimatou's hearing loss, as well as access to resources.

Biopsychosocial Model

This model incorporates biological, psychological, and social dimensions of illness and disease as essential components of a person's experiences (Borrell-Carrió, Suchman, & Epstein, 2004; Engel, 1980). In this way, the Biopsychosocial Model can be used to understand and address contextual factors facilitating or hindering a person's participation in daily life. This model also facilitates service providers' examination of the effects that socioeconomic factors can have on health outcomes by considering one's ability to access health care, and by acknowledging and working toward eliminating health disparities (Engel, 1980; Harris et al., 2012, p. 42).

Let's think about Fatimatou using the Biopsychosocial Model. Using this model, Michael and Jennifer (the clinicians working with Fatimatou and her family) would recognize that although Fatimatou's hearing loss was caused by biological factors, the family's response to Westernized medicine and Westernized clinical practices result from psychological and social factors. For example, the lack of trust in Westernized medicine could be due to previous experiences the family has had in the Westernized medical system. The family could be anxious (psychological) about Fatimatou's hearing loss but perceive that the service providers are not taking their family practices into consideration (sociocultural), resulting in their limited compliance with the intervention program. The service providers, then, would need to address each of these areas of concern (the biological—hearing loss; the

TABLE 6–3. Kleinman's Questions to Elicit Explanatory Models and Examples for Fatimatou's Family

Kleinman's Questions Kleinman et al., 2006, p. 147	Formulated for Fatimatou's Family by Hyter and Salas-Provance
What do you think caused your problem?	What do you think caused Fatimatou's hearing loss?
Why do you think it started when it did?	Why do you think Fatimatou lost her hearing when she did?
What do you think your sickness does to you? How does it work?	What do you think Fatimatou's hearing loss does to her? How does it affect her? How does it affect your family?
How severe is your sickness? Will it have a short or long course?	How severe is her hearing loss? Will it last a long time?
What kind of treatment do you think you should receive?	What type of treatment do you think Fatimatou should receive? What type of treatment would you like for her to receive?
According to Kleinman et al. (2006), the following questions will elicit a person's cultural meaning of his or her illness	
What are the most important results you hope to receive from this treatment?	What are you hoping will come out of the treatment?
What are the chief problems your sickness has caused for you?	What are the main problems that Fatimatou's hearing loss has caused for her? What problems has it caused for the family?
What do you fear most about your sickness?	What are your primary concerns about Fatimatou's hearing loss?

Source: Adapted from Kleinman et al., 2006.

psychological—lack of trust based on past experiences; the sociocultural—familial practices) to effectively treat Fatimatou's hearing loss.

Health Beliefs Model

The Health Beliefs Model (Glanz, Rimer, & Lewis, 2002) can be used to "either predict or explain a health-related action" (Harris et al., 2012, p. 43). In other words, it can be used to help determine what a person knows about his or her communication disorder, the person's beliefs and attitudes about or toward the com-

munication disorder, and what factors may influence one's decisions about accessing and utilizing services (Harris et al., 2012). There are several concepts that can be used to predict why those who are ill or have a disorder or condition will act to address it—that is, to go for an assessment or participate in intervention. These concepts include "susceptibility, seriousness, benefits and barriers to a behavior, cues to action, and self-efficacy" (Glanz et al., p. 46). If a person believes that he or she is susceptible to a disorder, that there could be consequences to having that disorder, and that there may be some therapy or intervention that will mitigate the consequences, he or she will be more likely to address the disorder. Champion, & Skinner (2006, pp. 47–49) define the concepts in the following ways:

- Perceived susceptibility—refers to beliefs about one's likelihood of contracting a disease or experiencing a disorder, such as a communication disorder.
- Perceived severity—refers to a person's beliefs about how serious an untreated disease or disorder might be, and the impact that the consequences (medical, social, educational, etc.) would have on their life.
- Perceived benefits and barriers—a person's belief about how the benefits of addressing a disease or disorder will influence his or her decision to address the issue. Similarly, the perceived barriers to acting to address a disease or disorder could prevent the person from addressing it. The person experiencing the disorder engages in a cost (i.e., susceptibility and severity) to benefit (i.e., benefits and barriers) analysis of sorts (Champion, & Skinner, 2006).
- Cues to action—one will be more prepared to act, if he or she has cues to act. Such cues could include, "bodily events (difficulty hearing) or environmental events (seeing an advertisement on the television about hearing loss)" (p. 49).
- Self-efficacy—the ability to successfully engage in behaviors to bring about certain outcomes (Bandura, 1997; Champion, & Skinner, 2006).

Let's think again about the case of Fatimatou, introduced in the beginning of this chapter, as we apply the Health Belief Model. Using the Health Belief Model, Fatimatou's parents are likely to already understand that Fatimatou was susceptible to a hearing loss. They will be more likely to seek help for her hearing loss if they: (a) believe that her hearing loss is a sufficiently severe condition; (b) perceive the benefits of hearing assessment and rehabilitation as being higher than the perceived barriers; (c) acknowledge and understand the cue to action (i.e., Fatimatou's difficulty hearing); and (d) have self-efficacy for navigating the audiological services available to Fatimatou and her family.

Stigma

A stigma refers to some sort of characteristic or behavior that is considered undesirable, "deeply discrediting" (Goffman, 1963, p. 3), or disgraceful, or that spoils one's reputation in a community or society (Goffman, 1963). The concept of a stigma can be considered from two points of view: (a) whether the person with the stigma thinks his or her "differentness" is already known by others, or (b) whether the person with the stigma thinks his or her differentness is not known or perceivable by others (Goffman, 1963, p. 4). Three types of stigma have been identified in the literature:

1. those that deal with the body—physical maladies;
2. those that refer to character traits (weak, rigid, or racist); and
3. those that are about races, nationalities, and religion (Goffman, 1963, p. 4).

Stigma, whether about hearing loss, the wearing of hearing aids, or the use of hearing devices, affects a person's coping behavior, acceptance of a hearing loss, and help-seeking behaviors for hearing habilitation or rehabilitation (Knudsen et al., 2010; Wallhagen, 2010). A person who believes that wearing a hearing aid is stigmatizing may be less likely to seek help with a hearing loss. If this person does seek help with a hearing loss, and was fitted for a hearing aid, he or she may not wear the hearing aid at all times, and may be more likely to wear the hearing aids less often if he or she thinks that others may be able to see the aids. Sometimes there are interactions among the types of stigma described earlier. For example, a person may believe that a physical stigma could be perceived by others as being related to a character trait, a hearing loss could signal a weakness.

HEALTH LITERACY

Health literacy is the ability to understand and process health information in a way that facilitates the ability to make informed decisions about one's own care, and to accurately follow instructions for intervention or treatment (U.S. Department of Health and Human Services, 2010; Hasseikus & Moxley, 2009). Low levels of health literacy result in higher incidences of health problems, including increased problems with mental disorders (Hardie, Kyanko, Busch, Losasso, & Levin, 2011; Wolf, Gazmararian, & Baker 2005).

Health literacy is related to culturally responsive care in that SLPs and audiologists not only need to understand cultural beliefs of clients, but also whether they have the capacity to process information about their hearing loss (or other communication disorder) and make decisions about their care that are in their best interest (Hasseikus & Moxley, 2009). Health literacy is not only focused on one's ability to read the literature provided by service providers, but also includes cultural beliefs (as discussed earlier), how information is communicated, the language in which information is communicated, and the format

of materials (materials that are densely written without whitespace and illustrations may be more difficult to process) (CDC, 2016b).

DEAF, HARD OF HEARING, SIGN LANGUAGE, AND DUE PROCESS

As we discussed in Chapter 5, Culture and Language, sometimes those who use languages in the United States other than general American English may not always receive due process during legal proceedings (Miller & Vernon, 2001). There are multiple factors that affect some sign language users' ability to understand and fully participate in legal proceedings, and to receive fair treatment within the judicial system. Some would argue that having an interpreter involved in the legal proceedings should facilitate sign language users' ability to have due process. In a document titled, "*An interpreter isn't enough: Deafness, language and due process*," LaVigne and Vernon (2003) discuss two legal cases where an interpreter was present, clearly indicated to the court that the client was not comprehending the proceedings, yet these concerns were ignored. Consider the excerpt from this paper of Jesse R who was Deaf and presented with "minimal brain dysfunction." He used a mix of various sign languages to communicate; these languages included ALS, English, signs that he learned and used only at home, and "street signs" (p. 844):

THE DEFENDANT [Jesse]: I want to enter no contest.

THE COURT: What does "no contest" mean to you?

THE DEFENDANT: I have a hard time explaining it, I think it means like, I'm not going to compete for anything. I'm not—that's what it means.

THE DEFENDANT: I don't want to have a jury or a trial.

THE COURT: I understand that you do not want to have a trial. However, if there was a trial, do you understand that you would have the rights that we're talking about?

THE DEFENDANT: I still don't want a jury or a trial?

THE COURT: Tell me why you don't want a jury, Mr. [R.].

THE DEFENDANT: I don't know.

THE COURT: Let me ask you again Mr. [R]. You have told me several times that you do not want a trial. Tell me why you do not want a trial.

THE DEFENDANT: Because I don't like to have a jury, trial or court. I just don't like it. I don't want it.

THE COURT: Have you ever had trial before?

THE DEFENDANT: No. Never.

THE COURT: So why have you decided that you don't like them?

THE INTERPRETER: No word response . . .

. . . .

THE COURT: I'm therefore satisfied the defendant based upon the record before this court today has knowingly and intelligently waived his right to trial in these matters, has entered a plea of no contest as to count two of the information knowingly and intelligently (LaVigne & Vernon, 2003, pp. 883–884).

In this case, there were linguistic and communication issues that affected adjudicative competence—that is, the ability of the defendant to understand and participate in the trial (LaVigne & Vernon, 2003). There are similar concerns, of course, for individuals who are hard of hearing (and for those who speak variations of English, as you read in Chapter 5). Even with hearing assistance technology, the speech perception of individuals who are hard of hearing may be compromised with the acoustics and dynamics of a courtroom (personal communication, Mary Peterson, AuD, March 20, 2017).

Another important factor that can influence due process in a trial is the level of cultural responsiveness enacted by the judicial officials (lawyers, judges, court recorders) and the interpreters. The courts undoubtedly believe that the presence of sign language interpretation provided Jesse an opportunity for due process. As we can see, however, with Jesse's case, even if there was an interpreter, that did not guarantee due process. This is particularly so if the defendant is speaking a language other than general American English.

CONSIDERATIONS FOR ASSESSMENT, HABILITATION, AND REHABILITATION

How to evaluate the hearing and speech perception of individuals who speak languages other than English or who are bilingual has "not been a priority in audiologists' research agendas" (Shi, 2014, p. 243). In this section, we summarize some of the existing literature on ways that hearing assessments can be conducted to be more culturally and linguistically responsive.

A common audiological assessment process is speech audiometry, which should be customized for individuals who speak language variations, including languages other than English (Shi, 2014). Speech recognition testing (SRT) is a routine assessment to measure the ability to hear speech. It is used to confirm pure-tone results (Dr. Mary Peterson, personal communication, March 22, 2017), recording the softest speech that can be heard 50% of the time (ASHA, 2017e). Although practically any material can be used for SRT testing, words composed of two syllables with equal stress on each syllable (spondees) are "preferred because they have the highest homogeneity of audibility" (Ramkissoon, Proctor, Lansing, & Bilger, 2002, p. 23). Some of the spondees may be unfamiliar to individuals who speak languages other than English. SRTs have been reported to be modified for individuals who speak languages other than English. Such modifications include reducing the number of words on the SRT list, which might provide false information indicating that the person's ability to recognize speech is better than it might be (Ramkissoon et al., 2002); developing a word list from the client's own language, which is problematic because most audiologists in the United States are monolingual (i.e., only 6% of audiologists and 6.6% of SLPs in the United States can provide services in a language other than English [ASHA, 2017d]); or using pairs of numbers (digits) for stimuli (Ramkissoon et al., 2002, pp. 23–24). Utilization of pairs of digits is a promising alternative to spondee words because numbers are familiar to most speakers around the world, whether they speak English or other languages. Ramkissoon et al. (2002) found that for bilingual (Spanish–English) speakers, SRTs obtained using digits were more like the pure-tone averages than were English spondee words (Shi, 2014). When there are discrepancies between language and speech perception scores among speakers of languages other than English, this discrepancy should be considered a reflection of the person's exposure to the second language (English) rather than an ability to learn the second language (Douglas, 2011a).

A test to determine the presence of an auditory processing disorder (SCAN-C; Keith, 2000) was examined for potential bias (Woods, Peña, & Martin, 2004). The SCAN-C requires repetition of stimuli (i.e., words and sentences). One concern with this measure is that there is potential for the repetitions produced by those who speak a dialectal variation of English or with accented English to be misinterpreted as an error (Goldstein & Iglesias, 2001; Woods et al., 2004). White and Latin@/Hispanic 8-year-old children from low and middle socioeconomic backgrounds were administered the SCAN-C. Findings of this study showed that there were no significant differences between the groups of participants based on ethnicity or socioeconomic status. The researchers did find that more Latin@/Hispanic participants than White participants were borderline to the disordered category based on SCAN-C scores (Woods et al., 2004). The researchers rescored the assessments using dialectal scoring; that is, a list of common Latin@/Hispanic American English phonological variations to the words in the SCAN-C was used to score the participants' productions. Table 6–4 shows the dialectal scoring that could be appropriate for using with the SCAN-C, particularly if the Latin@/Hispanic children being assessed fall into the borderline disordered category (Woods et al., 2004). The dialectal rescoring resulted in the Latin@/Hispanic children's performance becoming more closely matched to the performance of the White children on the SCAN-C (Woods et al., 2004).

It is appropriate to consider assessing individuals with hearing loss who speak variations of English, as well as languages other than English, by implementing the same practices that would be employed when assessing the spoken language of individuals speaking languages other than English (Douglas, 2011a, 2011b; Shi, 2014).

TABLE 6–4. Dialect Scoring

Filtered Words Subtest

Item	Target	Latino American English Acceptable Dialectal Variations
1	had	/hæ/, /hæt/
2	did	/dɪ/, /dɪt/, /di/, /dit/
3	need	/ni/, /nit/
5	leave	/lib/
6	you	/dzu/
9	find	/fain/, /faint/
10	if	/ɪ/
11	yes	/dzɛs/
12	while	/huail/
13	most	/moəst/
14	bad	/bæ/, /bæt/
17	ship	/tʃɪp /, /tʃɪ/, /tʃip/, /tʃi/
19	them	/dɛm/, /dɛ/
20	wait	/huɛit/, /huɛi/, /wɛi/
21	those	/doz/, /dos/, /ðos/
24	mouth	/mous/, /mout/, /mouʃ/
26	great	/grɛɪ/
27	such	/səʃ/
28	hot	/ha/
29	wide	/huaid/, /huai/, /wai/
30	duck	/dəg/
31	card	/gard/, /gar/, /kar/
32	way	/huɛɪ/
33	put	/pə/
36	ride	/rai/, /rait/
37	hit	/hit/, /hi/, /hɪ/
38	is	/is/, /iz/, /ɪs/
39	sing	/sin/

continues

TABLE 6-4. *continued*

Auditory Figure–Ground Subtest

Item	Target	Latino American English Acceptable Dialectal Variations
2	back	/bæ/, /bæg/
3	end	/ɛn/, /ɛnt/
4	take	/tɛɪ/, /tɛɪg/
5	coat	/goʊt/, /goʊ/, /koʊ/
8	case	/gɛɪs/
9	thick	/tɪk/, /sɪk/, /tɪg/, /sɪg/, /tɪ/, /sɪ/, /tik/, /sik/, /tig/, /sig/, /ti/, /si/, /θig/, /θi/, /θɪg/, /θɪ/
11	next	/nɛkəst/
12	got	/ga/
13	path	/pæt/, /pæs/, /pæʃ/
14	bag	/bæ/, /bæk/
16	feet	/fi/
19	waste	/huɛɪ/, /huɛɪəst/, /wɛɪəst/
21	sheep	/tʃip/, /tʃi/, /ʃi/
22	loud	/lou/, /lout/
23	hurt	/hɚ/
26	drop	/dra/
27	quick	/gwɪk/, /gwɪg/, /gwɪ/, /kwɪg/, /kwɪ/
28	nest	/nɛəst/
29	thank	/tɛɪnk/, /sɛɪnk/, /tɛɪŋ/, /sɛɪŋ/, /θɛɪŋ/
30	sled	/əslɛd/, /əslɛ/, /əslɛt/, /slɛ/, /slɛt/
31	frog	/fra/, /frak/
32	park	/par/, /parg/
33	neck	/nɛ/, /nɛg/
35	shop	/tʃap/, /tʃa/, /ʃa/
36	key	/gi/
37	fat	/fæ/
38	shoe	/tʃu/
40	feed	/fi/, /fit/

TABLE 6–4. *continued*

Competing Words Subtest

Item	Target	Right Ear Dialectal Variations	Target	Left Ear Dialectal Variations
1	waste	/huɛɪst/, /huɛɪəst/, /wɛɪəst/	cage	/gɛɪg/, /gɛɪʃ/, /kɛɪʃ/
2	need	/ni/, /nit/	case	/gɛɪs/
3			them	/dɛm/, /dɛ/, /ðɛ/
4	feed	/fi/, /fit/	path	/pæt/, /pæs/, /pæʃ/
5	large	/larʃ/	find	/fain/, /faint/
6	feet	/fi/	thank	/tɛɪnk/, /sɛɪnk/, /tɛɪŋ/, /sɛɪŋ/, /θɛɪŋ/
7	dog	/da/, /dak/	thick	/tɪk/, /sɪk/, /tik/, /sik/, /tɪ/, /sɪ/, /ti/, /si/, /tɪg/, /sɪg/, /tig/, /sig/, /θɪg/, /θig/, /θɪ/, /θi/
8	dark	/dar/, /darg/	hot	/ha/
9	show	/tʃou/	clown	/gloun/
10			home	/hoʊ/
11	bag	/bæ/, /bæk/		
13	white	/huait/, /huai/, /wai/	get	/gɛ/
14	dad	/dæ/, /dæt/		
15			cow	/gou/
16	most	/moʊəst/		
17			seed	/si/, /sit/
18			card	/gard/, /gar/, /gart/, /kar/, /kart/
19	laugh	/læ/		
21	ride	/rai/, /rait/		
22			you	/dzu/
23	name	/nɛɪ/	bank	/bɛɪn/, /bɛɪŋ/
24	hide	/hai/, /hait/		
25	shake	/tʃɛɪk/, /tʃɛɪg/, /tʃɛɪ/, /ʃɛɪg/, /ʃɛɪ/	car	/gar/
26	wide	/huaid/, /huai/, /wai/	use	/dzuz/, /dzus/, /jus/
27	yes	/dzɛs/	as	/æs/
28	mouth	/mous/, /mout/, /mouʃ/		
29			camp	/gæmp/, /gæm/, /kæm/
30	duck	/dəg/, /də/	ship	/tʃɪp/, /tʃɪ/, /ʃɪ/

continues

TABLE 6–4. *continued*

Competing Sentences Subtest

Item	Target	Latino American English Acceptable Dialectal Variations
1	The park is near the road.	/ðə (də) park (par/pard) ɪz (iz, ɪs, is) nir ðə (də) roʊd (roʊ, roʊt)/
2	The dinner plate is hot.	/ðə (də) dɪnɛr (dinɛr) plɛɪt (plɛɪ) ɪz (iz, ɪs, is) hat (ha)/
3	The floor looked clean.	/ðə (də) flor lukt (luk) klin (glin)/
4	People are going home.	/pipəl ar goʊɪŋ (goʊin) hom (ho)/
5	The washing machine broke.	/ðə (də) waʃɪŋ (huaʃɪŋ, huasɪŋ, huatʃɪŋ, wasɪŋ, watʃɪŋ, huaʃɪn, huasɪn, huatʃɪn, wasɪn) məʃin (məsin, mətʃin) brok (bro, brog)/
6	The ground was very hard.	/ðə (də) ground (groun, grount) wəz (huəz, huəs, wəs) vɛri (bɛri) hard (har, hart)/
7	They washed in cold water.	/ðɛɪ (dɛɪ) waʃt (huaʃt, huast, huatʃt, wast, watʃt, huas, was, huasʃ) ɪn (in) kold (gold, gol, golt, kol, kolt) wadɛr (huadɛr, huaθɛr)/
8	The room is getting cold.	/ðə (də) rum (ru) ɪz (iz, ɪs, is) gɪdɪŋ (gɪθɪŋ, gidiŋ, giθiŋ, gɪθɪn, gidin, giθin) kold (gold, gol, golt, kol, kolt)/
9	They broke all the eggs.	/ðɛɪ (dɛɪ) brok (bro, brog) al ðə (də) ɛgz (ɛgs)/
10	The car is going fast.	/ðə (də) kar (gar) ɪz (iz, ɪs, is) goʊɪŋ (goʊin) fæst (fæəst)/
11	They skated on the pond.	/ðɛɪ (dɛɪ) skɛɪdɪd (skɛɪθɪd, skɛɪdɪ, skɛɪdɪt, skɛɪdid, skɛɪdit, skɛɪdi) an ðə (də) pand (pan, pant)/
12	The oven is hot.	/ðɛ (də) əvən (əbən) ɪz (iz, ɪs, is) hat (ha)/
13	Some people are coming.	/səm (sə) pipəl ar kəmɪŋ (kəmɪn, kəmiŋ, kəmin)/
14	They met some new friends.	/ðɛɪ (dɛɪ) mɛt (mɛ) səm (sə) nu frɪndz (frɪnθz, frinθz, frɪnθs, frindz, frɪnds)/
15	They're staying for supper.	/ðɛr (dɛr) stɛɪŋ (əstɛɪŋ, əstɛɪn, stɛɪn) for səpər/
16	The football game is over.	/ðə (də) fətbal gɛɪm (gɛɪ) ɪz (iz, ɪs, is) ovɛr (obɛr)/
17	He wore his yellow shirt.	/hi wor (huor) hɪz (hiz, hɪs, his, huiz, huɪs, huis) jɛlo (dzɛlo) ʃɛrt (tʃɛrt, ʃɛr, tʃɛr)/
18	The boy slipped on the stairs.	/ðə (də) boi slɪpt (slip, əslɪpt, əslip) on ðə (də) stɛrz (əstɛrz, əstɛrs, stɛrs)/
19	The mother held her baby.	/ðə (də) məðɛr (məvɛr, mədɛr, məθɛr) hɛld (hɛl, hɛlt) hɛr bɛɪbi/
20	The apple pie was hot.	/ðə (də) æpəl paɪ wəz (wəs) hat (ha)/

Source: Reprinted with permission from Woods, A. G., Peña, E. D., & Martin, F. N. (2004). Exploring possible sociocultural bias on the SCAN-C. *American Journal of Audiology, 13,* 173–184.

Following are some commonly used spoken language assessment strategies that can also be applied to hearing assessments (Douglas, 2011a; Shi, 2013, 2014; Shi & Sanchez, 2010):

- Most people who are bilingual or multilingual will use both (all) of their languages on a regular basis; therefore, it increases face validity when administering hearing assessments in both languages spoken by the client, or in the language in which the client has the strongest proficiency.
- Keep in mind that you cannot surmise bilingual language performance from performance in only one language (Shi, 2013; Shi & Sanchez, 2010).
- The language variables most important for determining speech perception of bilinguals are: (a) phonetic differences between first and second languages; (b) a person's history with language use and proficiency; and (c) age of language acquisition.
  - Phonetic differences between languages (between Spanish and English), could cause the client to make errors in speech perception that are unrelated to audiological abilities. For example, there may be /b-v/ and /s-z/ confusions (Shi, 2014, p. 248).
  - The history of use and proficiency of a second language can affect how well the listener recognizes speech in Spanish or English.
  - The age of acquisition is a strong predictor of assessment performance (Shi, 2014). Research has found that those who developed more than one language at the same time performed better on speech recognition tasks than those who developed two languages sequentially (Shi & Shanchez, 2010; von Hapsburg, Champlin, & Shetty; 2004; von Hapsburg & Peña, 2002; Weiss & Dempsey, 2008). Simultaneous

bilingualism or dual language learning occurs when a child is exposed to and learns two languages from birth, usually before the age of 3 years (Paradis, Genesee, & Crago, 2011). Sequential bilingualism or second language learning occurs when a child learns a language other than his or her first language after 3 years of age (Paradis et al., 2011).

The language profile of a Spanish–English bilingual person is made up of language status, history, stability, competency, and use (von Hapsburg & Peña, 2002). Questions relating to these five areas are as follows (Shi, 2014, p. 247):

- Language status
  - Are you bilingual?
  - Are you native to both languages?
- Language history
  - When did you acquire each language?
  - How did you learn each language?
  - Did you receive formal education in each language?
- Language stability
  - Did you use both languages growing up?
  - Have you moved away from one language due to life events such as immigration or marriage?
- Language competency
  - Can you listen, speak, read, and write in both languages?
  - Are you equally skilled in both languages or dominant in one of them?
- Language use
  - Are you currently using both languages in everyday life?
  - Do you use one language only at work due to job requirements and the other only at home due to family needs?

A listener's ability to recognize words and process auditory information can be influenced by dialect (Shi, 2014); therefore, audiologists should expect that there will be dialectical variations on speech audiometric assessments. Let's use Spanish as an example. There are a large variety of dialects of Spanish —Mexican Spanish is different from Puerto Rican Spanish, and both are different from the Spanish spoken in Spain and Central America. Variations between languages can affect word recognition and auditory processing even if the listener is proficient in Spanish (Shi, 2014; Shi & Canizales, 2013). Shi (2014) provides a list of audiometric materials in Spanish that currently exist. That list is provided in Table 6–5. Just as we need to understand how to best provide hearing assessments, it is important to understand how to teach children with hearing impairments to listen and speak when their home language is not English (Douglas, 2011b).

Studies have shown that children with cochlear implants (CIs) are capable of being bilingual if they have adequate speech perception and access to home or school environments where oral language is the only mode of communication (Douglas, 2011b, p. 21). Research has shown that for children with hearing impairments from bilingual homes, exposure to two languages did not interrupt the acquisition of English (Douglas, 2011b; Thomas, El-Kashlan, & Zwolan, 2008; Waltzman, Robbins, Green, & Cohen, 2003). Children with CIs benefit from more than one linguistic environment—the home environment where they are communicating in their first language, and the school environment where they will typically be immersed in English (Kohnert & Derr, 2004).

The language of intervention should be "in the client's first language or in two languages" depending on whether the child is a dual language learner or a second language learner (Douglas, 2011b, p. 22). Families will make this determination based on when (and whether) they want their child with a hearing loss to be able to communicate in one or two languages. Since newborn hearing screening exists,[4] audiologists can work with families to support the development of their child with a hearing loss to become a dual language learner (acquiring two languages at the same time) (Douglas, 2011b). This decision is based on the "child's dominant language, family language use, and the child's language environments" (Douglas, 2011b, p. 23). Intervention should be provided in the child's dominant language, which allows knowledge from the child's first language to be transferred to the child's second language (Kohnert & Derr, 2004). It is also important to be cognizant of the language use in the family in order to ensure that the child with a hearing loss can communicate with his or her family members. Parents will be able to "provide rich linguistic experiences" for their child, which is necessary to build a "strong language foundation" (Douglas, 2011b, p. 24; Kohnert & Derr, 2004). The language environments to which the child with a hearing loss is exposed should be used to determine what the child needs to learn in order to participate in various contexts of his or her life, such as at home, school, and/or church (Kohnert & Derr, 2004).

CHAPTER SUMMARY

The goal of Chapter 6 was to provide information on the relationship between culture and hearing, such as variations in sign language use across cultural and racial groups. Hearing loss is one of the most prevalent communication disorders in the world, being caused by congenital diseases and preventable causes.

---

[4]Universal newborn hearing screening is mandated in some states.

TABLE 6–5. Spanish Audiometric Materials That Have Been Developed for Clinical Use

Test	Study	Target	Noise
Child speech reception			
Spanish Spondee Threshold (SST) test	Martin & Hart (1978); Schneider (1992)[a]	Bisyllabic words with pictures	
Adult speech reception			
Spanish speech reception threshold test	Spitzer (1980)[b]	Bisyllabic words	
Spanish matrix sentence test	Hochmuth et al. (2012)	Five-word sentences with a fixed syntactic structure (name + verb + numeral + object + adjective)	Speech-spectrum noise
Child word recognition			
Children's Spanish word discrimination test	Comstock & Martin (1984)	Bisyllabic words with pictures	
Pediatric Spanish–English speech perception task	Calandruccio, Gomez, Buss, & Leibold (2014)	Bisyllabic words with pictures shared by corresponding English words; specifically developed for bilingual children	Two-talker babble and speech-spectrum noise
Adult word recognition			
Spanish nonsense syllable test	Ferrer (1960)	Nonsense monosyllables (detailed characteristics not available)	
Berruecos & Rodriguez words	Berger (1977); Berruecos & Rodriguez (1967)	Bisyllabic words	
Spanish Multiple Choice Rhyme Test (SMRT)	Tosi (1969); Cooper & Langley[c] (1978)	Words (detailed characteristics not available), presented in an auditory or audiovisual mode	
Boston College Auditory test	Zubick et al. (1983)	Bisyllabic words	
Auditec word recognition test	Shi & Canizales (2013)[d]; Weisleder & Hodgson (1989)	Bisyllabic words	

continues

TABLE 6–5. *continued*

Test	Study	Target	Noise
Spanish Picture-Identification Task	McCullough & Wilson (2001); McCullough, Wilson, Birck, & Anderson (1994)[e]	Bisyllabic words with pictures, presented in an open- and closed-set format	
Comm Tech test	Roeser (1996)	Monosyllabic words	
Sentence recognition			
Spanish Synthetic Sentence Identification (SSI) test	Benitez & Speaks (1968); Lopez et al. (1997)	Nonsense sentences with minimum semantic and syntactic cues	Single-talker passage presented ipsilaterally or contralaterally to the target
Spanish Hearing in Noise Test (HINT)	Huarte (2008); Soli et al. (2002)[f]	Sentences with limited contextual cues	Speech-spectrum noise
Spanish Speech Perception in Noise (SPIN) test	Cervera & González-Alvarez (2010)	Sentences with rich vs. minimal contextual cues, generating two scores	12-talker babble
Auditory processing			
Spanish Staggered Spondaic Word (SSW) test	Ramos, Windham, & Katz (1992); Soto & Windham (1992)[g]	Spondee words presented dichotically in an overlapping manner	
Spanish adult auditory processing battery	Fuente & McPherson (2006)[h]	Monosyllabic words for the speech-in-noise, binaural fusion, and filtered speech subtests; digits for the dichotic digits subtest	White noise for the speech-in-noise subtest

Note. Tests without a formal name are referred to using the term in the published study.

[a]Schneider (1992) applied the test to children speaking the Castilian, Caribbean, and Mexican dialects. [b]Spitzer's material (1980) was also normed for children. [c]Cooper and Langley (1978) applied the test in both audio and audiovisual modes. [d]Shi and Canizales (2013) applied the test to adults speaking the Caribbean and South American Highland dialects. [e]In their response to a letter to the editor that discussed the selection of some of the test words, the authors pointed out that the test was designed for evaluating adults more than children. [f]Huarte (2008) is a Castilian Spanish version of the HINT; Soli et al. (2002) is an American Spanish version. [g]This test has been incorporated into the Spanish adult auditory processing battery by Fuente and McPherson (2006). Fuente and McPherson (2006) referenced the manual of the test released by the manufacturer (Soto & Windham, 1992). [h]This test also includes nonspeech subtests such as pitch pattern sequence, duration pattern sequence, masking level difference, and random gap detection.

Source: Reprinted with permission from Shi, L. F. (2014). Speech Audiometry and Spanish-English bilinguals: Challenges in clinical practices. *American Journal of Audiology, 23*, 243–259.

This chapter underscored the importance of audiologists being proactive in gaining knowledge about assessment and intervention with individuals from cultural and linguistic backgrounds different than their own. Some literature shows the differences in hearing loss, as well as hearing aid use and hearing health outcomes, among African Americans, Latin@s/Hispanics, and Caucasians in the United States. Several models were presented that could be used for providing culturally responsive hearing services. Several factors can affect the help-seeking behavior of those with hearing impairments, including cultural beliefs about hearing loss, stigma about hearing loss, and health literacy. It is important for SLPs and audiologists to be knowledgeable about the beliefs and stigmas held by cultural groups in order to provide culturally responsive services.

EXTENDED LEARNING

The following activities will facilitate your continued learning about hearing and culture.

1. Review the American Academy of Audiology (AAA) and the ASHA code of ethics, and identify issues that may affect your work with people from culturally and linguistically diverse backgrounds.[5]
2. Develop a hearing assessment and intervention plan for Fatimatou, the young child who was the subject of the case presented at the beginning of this chapter. Include in the plan what assessment tools you would use and why. Also include which language intervention would be offered and why.

FURTHER READING

Calandruccio, L., & Smiljanić, R. (2012). New sentence recognition materials developed using a basic non-native English lexicon. *Journal of Speech, Language, and Hearing Research, 55,* 1342–1355.

Lin, F. R., Maas, P., Chien, W., Carey, J. P., Ferrucci, L., & Thorpe, R. (2012). Association of skin color, race/ethnicity and hearing loss among adults in the USA. *Journal of Association for Research in Otolaryngology, 13*(1), 109–117.

Lucas, C., Bayley, R., McCaskill, C., & Hill, J. (2015). The intersection of African American English and Black American Sign Language. *International Journal of Bilingualism, 19*(2), 156–168.

Shi, L. F., & Canizales, L. A. (2013). Dialectal effects on a clinical Spanish word recognition test. *American Journal of Audiology, 21,* 74–83.

REFERENCES

Agrawal, Y., Platz, E. A., & Niparko, J. (2009). Risk factors for hearing loss in U.S. Adults: Data from the national health and nutrition examination survey 1999–2002. *Otology and Neurotology, 30,* 139–145.

American Speech-Language-Hearing Association (ASHA). (2017a). *Adult aural/audiologic rehabilitation.* Retrieved from http://www.asha.org/public/hearing/Adult-Aural-Rehabilitation/

American Speech-Language-Hearing Association (ASHA). (2017b). *Child aural/audiologic rehabilitation.* Retrieved from http://www.asha.org/public/hearing/treatment/child_aur_rehab.htm

American Speech-Language-Hearing Association (ASHA). (2017c). *Conductive hearing loss.* Retrieved from http://www.asha.org/public/hearing/Conductive-Hearing-Loss/

American Speech-Language-Hearing Association (ASHA). (2017d). *Demographic profile of ASHA*

---

[5]The idea for this activity came from Lubinski, R., & Hudson, M. W. (2012). *Professional issues in speech-language pathology and audiology* (4th ed.). Clifton Park, NY: Delmar.

members providing bilingual services. Retrieved from http://www.asha.org/uploadedFiles/Demo graphic-Profile-Bilingual-Spanish-Service-Members.pdf

American Speech-Language-Hearing Association (ASHA). (2017e). *Hearing loss—Beyond early childhood.* ASHA Practice Portal. Retrieved from http://www.asha.org/Practice-Portal/Clinical-Topics/Hearing-Loss/

American Speech-Language-Hearing Association (ASHA). (2017f). *Mixed hearing loss.* Retrieved from http://www.asha.org/public/hearing/Mixed-Hearing-Loss/

American Speech-Language-Hearing Association (ASHA). (2017g). *Sensorineural hearing loss.* Retrieved from http://www.asha.org/public/hearing/Sensorineural-Hearing-Loss/

Auinger, P., Lanphear, B. P., Kalkwarf, H. J., & Mansour, M. E. (2003). Trends in otitis media among children in the United States. *Pediatrics, 112*(3), 514–520.

Bainbridge, K. E., & Ramachandran, V. (2014). Hearing aid use among older U.S. adults: The National Health and Nutrition Examination Survey, 2005–2006 and 2009–1010. *Ear and Hearing, 35,* 289–294.

Benitez, L., & Speaks, C. (1968). A test of speech intelligibility in the Spanish language. *International Journal of Audiology, 7,* 16–22.

Berger, K. W. (1977). *Speech audiometry materials.* Kent, OH: Herald.

Berruecos, P. T., & Rodriguez, J. L. (1967). Determination of the phonetic percent in the Spanish language spoken in Mexico City, and formation of P. B. lists of trochaic words. *International Journal of Audiology, 6,* 211–216.

Borrell-Carrió, F., Suchman, A. L., & Epstein, R. M. (2004). The biopsychosocial model 25 years later: Principles, practice, and scientific inquiry. *Annals of Family Medicine, 2*(6), 576–582.

British Deaf Association. (2017). *What is Deaf culture?* Retrieved from https://www.bda.org.uk/what-is-deaf-culture

Calandruccio, L., Gomez, B., Buss, E., & Leibold, L. J. (2014). Developmental and preliminary evaluation of a pediatric Spanish-English speech perception task. *American Journal of Audiology, 23,* 158–172.

Centers for Disease Control and Prevention (CDC). (2016a). *Cytomegalovirus (CMV) and congenital CMV infection.* Retrieved from https://www.cdc.gov/cmv/overview.html

Centers for Disease Control and Prevention (CDC). (2016b). *What is health literacy.* Retrieved from https://www.cdc.gov/healthliteracy/learn/index.html

Centers for Medicare and Medicaid (2016). *Medicare benefit policy manual, Chapter 15: Medicare coverage of audiologic diagnostic testing.* Retrieved from https://www.cms.gov/Regulations-and-Guidance/Guidance/Manuals/downloads/bp102c15.pdf

Cervera, T., & González-Alvarez, J. (2010). Lists of Spanish sentences with equivalent predictability, phonetic content, length, and frequency of the last word. *Perceptual and Motor Skills, 111,* 517–529.

Champion, V. L., & Skinner, C. S. (2006). The health belief model. In K. Glanz, B. K. Rimer, & K. Viswanath (Eds.), *Health behavior and health education: Theory, research and practice.* 4th ed. (pp. 45–65). San Francisco, CA: Jossey-Bass.

Comstock, C. L., & Martin, F. N. (1984). A children's Spanish word discrimination test for non-Spanish-speaking audiologists. *Ear and Hearing, 5,* 166–170.

Cooper, J. C., & Langley, L. R. (1978). Multiple choice speech discrimination tests for both diagnostic and rehabilitative evaluation: English and Spanish. *Journal of the Academy of Rehabilitative Audiology, 11,* 132–141.

Cruickshanks, K. J., Dhar, S., Dinces, E., Fifer, R. C., Gonzalez, F., Heiss, G., . . . Tweed, T. S. (2015). Hearing impairment prevalence and associated risk factors in the Hispanic community health study/study of Latinos. *JAMA Otolaryngology–Head and Neck Surgery, 14*(7), 641–648.

Diala, C. C., Mutaner, C., Walrath, C., Nickerson, K., LaVeist, T., & Leaf, P. (2001). Racial/ethnic differences in attitudes toward seeking professional mental health services. *American Journal of Public Health, 91,* 805–807.

Dollard, S. C., Staras, S. A. S., Amin, M. M., Schmid, D. S., & Cannon, M. (2011). National prevalence estimates for cytomegalovirus IgM and IgG avidity and association between high IgM antibody titer and low IgG avidity. *Clinical and Vaccine Immunology, 18*(11), 1895–1899.

Douglas, M. (2011a). Spoken language assessment considerations for children with hearing impairment when the home language is not English. *SIG 9 Perspectives on Hearing and Hearing Disorders in Childhood, 21*, 4–19.

Douglas, M. (2011b). Teaching children with hearing impairment to listen and speak when the home language is not English. *SIG 9 Perspectives on Hearing and Hearing Disorders in Childhood, 21*, 20–30.

Duncan, J., Rhoades, E. A., & Fitzpatrick, E. M. (2014). *Auditory [re]habilitation for adolescents with hearing loss: Theory and practice.* Oxford, UK: Oxford University Press.

Engel, G. L. (1980). Clinical application of the biopsychosocial model. *American Journal of Psychiatry, 137*, 535–544.

Fernandes, J. K., & Myers, S. S. (2010). Inclusive deaf studies: Barriers and pathways. *Journal of Deaf Studies and Deaf Education, 15*, 17–29.

Ferrer, O. (1960). Speech audiometry: A discrimination test for Spanish language. *Laryngoscope, 70*, 1541–1551.

Fuente, A., & McPherson, B. (2006). Auditory processing tests for Spanish-speaking adults: An initial study. *International Journal of Audiology, 45*, 645–659.

Givens, J. L., Katz, I. R., Bellamy, S., & Holmes, W. C. (2007). Stigma and the acceptability of depression treatments among African Americans and Whites. *Journal of General Internal Medicine, 22*, 1292–1297.

Glanz, K., Rimer, B. K., & Lewis, F. M. (2002). *Health behavior and health education: Theory, research, and practice* (3rd ed.). San Francisco, CA: Jossey-Bass.

Goffman, E. (1963). *Stigma: Notes on the management of spoiled identity.* New York, NY: Simon & Schuster.

Goldstein, B., & Iglesias, A. (2001). The effect of dialect on phonological analysis: Evidence from Spanish-speaking children. *American Journal of Speech-Language Pathology, 10*, 394–406.

Green, L. J. (2002). *African American English: A linguistic introduction.* Cambridge, UK: Cambridge University Press.

Hardie, N. A., Kyanko, K., Busch, S., Losasso, A. T., & Levin, R. A. (2011). Health literacy and health care spending and utilization in a consumer-driven health plan. *Journal of Health Communication, 16*(Suppl. 3), 308–321.

Harris, J. L., Fleming, V. B., & Harris, C. L. (2012). A focus on health beliefs: What culturally competent clinicians need to know. *SIG 14 Perspectives on Communication Disorders and Sciences in Culturally and Linguistically Diverse (CLD) Populations, 19*, 40–48.

Hasseikus, A., & Moxley, A. (2009). Health literacy at the intersection of cultures. *ASHA Leader, 14*, 30–31.

Helzner, E. P., Cauley, J. A., Pratt, S. R., Wisniewski, S. R., Zmuda, J. M., Talbott, E. O., . . . Newman, A. B. (2005). Race and sex differences in age-related hearing loss: The health, aging and body composition study. *Journal of American Geriatric Society, 53*(12), 2119–2127.

Hochmuth, S., Brand, T., Zokoll, M. A., Castro, F. Z., Wardenga, N., & Kollmeier, B. (2012). A Spanish matrix sentence test for assessing speech reception threshold in noise. *International Journal of Audiology, 51*, 536–544.

Holcomb, T. K. (2013). *Introduction to American Deaf culture.* Oxford, UK: Oxford University Press.

Howarth, C. (2001). Towards a social psychology of community: A social representations perspective. *Journal for the Theory of Social Behaviour, 31*(2), 223–238.

Howe, T. (2008). The ICF contextual factors related to speech-language pathology. *International Journal of Speech-Language Pathology, 10*(1–2), 27–37.

Huarte, A. (2008). The Castilian Spanish Hearing in Noise Test. *International Journal of Audiology, 47*, 369–370.

Hult, F. M., & Compton, S. E. (2012). Deaf education policy as language policy: A comparative analysis of Sweden and the United States. *Sign Language Studies, 12*(4), 602–620.

Keith, R. W. (2000). *SCAN-C: A Test for Auditory Processing Disorders in Children-Revised.* San Antonio, TX: Psychological Cooperation.

Kleinman, A. (1978). Culture, illness and care: Clinical lessons from anthropologic and cross-cultural research. *Annals of Internal Medicine, 88*(2), 251–258.

Kleinman, A., & Benson, P. (2006). Anthropology in the clinic: The problem with cultural competence and how to fix it. *PLOS Medicine, 3*(10), e294.

Kleinman, A., Eisenberg, L., & Good, B. (2006). Culture, illness, and care: Clinical lessons from anthropologic and cross-cultural research. *Journal of Lifelong Learning in Psychiatry, IV*(1), 140–149.

Knoors, H., & Marschark, M. (2014). *Teaching Deaf learners: Psychological and developmental foundations.* Oxford, UK: Oxford University Press.

Knudsen, L. V., Oberg, M., Nielsen, C., Naylor, G., & Kramer S. E. (2010). Factors influencing help seeking, hearing aid uptake, hearing aid use and satisfactions with hearing aids: A literature review. *Trends in Amplification, 14*(3), 127–154.

Kohnert, K., & Derr, A. (2004). Language intervention with bilingual children. In B. Goldstein (Ed.), *Bilingual language development and disorders in Spanish-English speakers* (pp. 311–338). Baltimore, MD: Paul H. Brookes.

Lamble, L. (2016, April 21). "It's a disaster": Children bear brunt of southern Africa's devastating drought. *The Guardian.* Retrieved from https://www.theguardian.com/global-development/2016/apr/21/drought-southern-africa-heavy-toll-students-fainting-malawi-zimbabwe

LaVigne, M., & Vernon, M. (2003). An interpreter isn't enough: Deafness, language and due process. *Wisconsin Law Review, 5,* 844–936.

Lee, D. J., Carlson, D. L., Lee, H. M., Ray, L. A., & Markides, K. S. (1991). Hearing loss and hearing aid use in Hispanic adults: Results from the Hispanic health and nutrition examination survey. *American Journal of Public Health, 81*(1), 1471–1474.

Lin, F. R., Thorpe, R., Gordon-Salant, S., & Ferrucci, L. (2011). Hearing loss prevalence and risk factors in adults in the United States. *Journal of Gerontology: Series A–Biological Sciences, 66A*(5), 582–590.

Lin, F. R., Yaffe, K., Xia, J., Qian-Li, X., Harris, T., Purchase-Helzner, E., . . . Simonsick, E. M.; for the Health ABC Study Group. (2013). Hearing loss and cognitive decline in older adults. *JAMA Internal Medicine, 173*(4), 293–299.

Lonka, E., Hasan, M., & Komulainen, E. (2011). Spoken language skills and educational placement in Finnish children with cochlear implants. *Folia Phoniatrica et Logopaedica, 63,* 296–304.

Lopez, S. M., Martin, F. N., & Thibodeau, L. M. (1997). Performance of monolingual and bilingual speakers of English and Spanish on the Synthetic Sentence Identification test. *American Journal of Audiology, 6,* 33–38.

Lubinski, R., & Hudson, M. W. (2012). *Professional issues in speech-language pathology and audiology* (4th ed.). Clifton Park, NY: Delmar.

Lucas, C., Bayley, R., McCaskill, C., & Hill, J. (2015). The intersection of African American English and Black American Sign Language. *International Journal of Bilingualism, 19*(2), 156–168.

Manchaiah, V., Danermark, B., Ahmadi, T., Tome, D., Zhao, F., Li, Q., . . . Germundsson, P. (2015). Social representation of "hearing loss": Cross-cultural exploratory study in India, Iran, Portugal, and the UK. *Clinical Interventions in Aging, 10,* 1857–1872.

Martin, F. N., & Hart, D. B. (1978). Measurement of speech thresholds of Spanish-speaking children by non-Spanish-speaking audiologists. *Journal of Speech and Hearing Disorders, 43,* 255–261.

McCullough, J. A., & Wilson, R. H. (2001). Performance on a Spanish picture-identification task using a multimedia format. *Journal of American Academy of Audiology, 12,* 254–260.

McCullough, J. A., Wilson, R. H., Birck, J. D., & Anderson, L. G. (1994). A multimedia approach for estimating speech recognition of multilingual clients. *American Journal of Audiology, 3,* 19–22.

McPherson, B., & Swart, S. M. (1997). Childhood hearing loss in sub-Saharan Africa: A review and recommendations. *International Journal of Pediatric Otorhinolaryngology, 40,* 1–18.

Mick, P., Kawachi, I., & Lin, F. R. (2014). The association between hearing loss and social isolation in older adults. *Otolaryngology–Head and Neck Surgery, 150*(3), 378–384.

Miller, K. R., & Vernon, M. (2001). Linguistic diversity in Deaf defendants and due process rights. *Journal of Deaf Studies and Deaf Education, 6*(3), 226–234.

Mocarski, E. S., Shenk, T., & Pass, R. F. (2007). Cytomegaloviruses. In D. M. Knipe & P. M. Howley (Eds.), *Fields virology* (Vol. 2, 5th ed., pp. 2701–2772). Philadelphia, PA: Lippincott, Williams and Wilkins.

Moscovici, S. (1963). Attitudes and opinions. *Annual Review of Psychology, 14,* 231–260.

Mwaanza, N., Chilukutu, L., Tembo, J., Kabwe, M., Musonda, K., Kapasa, M., . . . Bates, M. (2014). High rates of congenital cytomegalovirus infection linked with maternal HIV infection among neonatal admissions at a large referral center in sub-Saharan Africa. *Clinical Infection Diseases, 58*, 728–735.

Nash, S. D., Cruickshanks, K. J., Huang, G. H., Klein, R., Nieto, F. J., & Tweed, T. S. (2013). Unmet hearing care needs: The Beaver Dam offspring study. *American Journal of Public Health, 103*, 1134–1139.

National Institute on Deafness and Other Communication Disorders (NIDCD). (2016a). *Quick statistics about hearing.* Retrieved from https://www.nidcd.nih.gov/health/statistics/quick-statistics-hearing

National Institute on Deafness and Other Communication Disorders (NIDCD). (2016b, December 15). *Quick statistics about hearing.* Retrieved from https://www.nidcd.nih.gov/health/statistics/quick-statistics-hearing

Nicholson, N., Martin, P. F., & Munoz, K. (2015). *SIG 9 Perspectives of Hearing and Hearing Disorders in Childhood, 25*, 70–82

Nieman, C. L., Marrone, N., Szanton, S. L., Thorpe, R. J., & Lin, F. R. (2016). Racial/ethnic and socioeconomic disparities in hearing health care among older Americans. *Journal of Aging Health, 28*(1), 68–94.

Paradis, J., Genesee, F., & Crago, M. B. (2011). *Dual language development and disorders: A handbook on bilingualism and second language learning* (2nd ed.). Baltimore, MD: Paul H. Brookes.

Peat, J., Barton, B., & Elliott, E. (2008). *Statistics workbook for evidence-based health care.* Hoboken, NJ: John Wiley & Sons, Ltd.

Pray, J. L., & Jordan, I. K. (2010). The deaf community and culture at a crossroads: Issues and challenges. *Journal of Social Work in Disability and Rehabilitation, 9*(2–3), 168–193.

Ramkissoon, I., Proctor, A., Lansing, C. R., & Bilger, R. C. (2002). Digit speech recognition thresholds (SRT) for non-native speakers of English. *American Journal of Audiology, 11*, 23–28.

Ramos, H. S., Windham, R. A., & Katz, J. (1992). Introducing a Spanish-language version of the Staggered Spondaic Word test. *Hearing Journal, 45*(9), 39–43.

Rhoades, E. A., Perusse, M., Douglas, W. M., & Zarate, C. M. (2008). Auditory based bilingual children in North America: Differences and choices. *Volta Voices, September/October, 15*(5), 20–22.

Rhoades, E. A., Price, F., & Perigoe, C. B. (2004). The changing American family and ethnically diverse children with hearing loss and multiple needs. *The Volta Review, 104*(4), 285–305.

Roeser, R. J. (1996). Audiological procedures/materials. In R. J. Roeser (Ed.), *Audiology desk reference: A guide to the practice of audiology* (pp. 161–256). New York: Thieme.

Salas-Provance, M. B., Good Erickson, J., & Reed, J. (2002). Disabilities as viewed by four generations of one Hispanic family. *American Journal of Speech-Language Pathology, 11*, 151–162.

Schneider, B. S. (1992). Effect of dialect on the determination of speech-reception thresholds in Spanish-speaking children. *Language, Speech, and Hearing Services in Schools, 23*, 159–162.

Shi, L. F. (2013). How "proficient" is proficient? Comparison of English and relative proficiency rating as a predictor of bilingual listeners' word recognition. *American Journal of Audiology, 21*, 40–52.

Shi, L. F. (2014). Speech audiometry and Spanish-English bilinguals: Challenges in clinical practices. *American Journal of Audiology, 23*, 243–259.

Shi, L. F., & Canizales, L. A. (2013). Dialectal effects on a clinical Spanish word recognition test. *American Journal of Audiology, 21*, 74–83.

Shi, L. F., & Sanchez, D. (2010). Spanish/English bilingual listeners on clinical word recognition tests: What to expect and how to predict. *Journal of Speech, Language, and Hearing Research, 53*, 1096–1110.

Shrestha, L. B., & Heisler, E. J. (2011). *The changing demographic profile of the United States.* Washington, DC: Congressional Research Service.

Soli, S. D., Vermiglio, A., Wen, K., & Filesari, C. A. (2002). Development of the Hearing In Noise Test (HINT) in Spanish. *Journal of the Acoustical Society of America, 112*, 2384.

Soman, U. G., Kan, D., & Tharpe, A. M. (2012). Rehabilitation and educational considerations for children with cochlear implants. *Otolaryngologic Clinics of North America, 45*, 141–153.

Soto, H., & Windham, R. A. (1992). *El test SSW. Manual de la versión en español* [The SSW test: Manual for the Spanish version.]. St. Louis, MO: Auditec.

Spitzer, J. B. (1980). The development of a picture speech reception threshold test in Spanish for use with urban U.S. residents of Hispanic background. *Journal of Communication Disorders, 13,* 147–151.

Stevens, G., Flaxman, S., Brunskill, E., Mascarenhas, M., Mathers, C. D., & Finucane, M. (2011). Global and regional hearing impairment prevalence: An analysis of 42 studies in 29 countries. *European Journal of Public Health, 23*(1), 146–152.

Tabak, J. (2006). *Significant gestures: A history of American Sign Language.* Westport, CT: Praeger.

Thomas, E., El-Kashlan, H., & Zwolan, T. A, (2008). Children with cochlear implants who live in monolingual and bilingual homes. *Otology and Neurotology, 29,* 230–234.

Tosi, O. E. (1969). Estudio experimental sobre la inteligibilidad de un test de multiple eleccion en idioma español [An experimental study on the intelligibility of a multiple choice test in the Spanish language.]. *Fonoaudiología, 15,* 28–35.

Trefil, J., & Hazen, R. M. (2004*). Physics matters: An introduction to conceptual.* Hoboken, NJ: John Wiley & Sons.

U.S. Department of Health and Human Services, Office of Disease Prevention and Health Promotion. (2010). *National Action Plan to improve health literacy.* Washington, DC: U.S. Government Printing Office.

von Hapsburg, D., Champlin, C. A., & Shetty, S. R. (2004). Reception thresholds for sentences in bilingual (Spanish/English) and monolingual (English) listeners. *Journal of the American Academy of Audiology, 15,* 88–98.

von Hapsburg, D., & Peña, E. D. (2002). Understanding bilingualism and its impact on speech audiometry. *Journal of Speech, Language, and Hearing Research, 45,* 202–213.

Wagner, W., Duveen, G., Farr, R., Jovchelovitch, S., Lorenzi-Cioldi, F., Markova, I., & Rose, D. (1999). Theory and method of social representations. *Asian Journal of Social Psychology, 2,* 95–125.

Wallhagen, M. I. (2010). The stigma of hearing loss. *The Gerontologist, 50,* 66–75.

Waltzman, S. B., Robbinsm, A. M., Green, J., & Cohen, N. (2003). Second oral language capabilities in children with CI's. *Otology and Neurotology, 24*(5), 757–763.

Weisleder, P., & Hodgson, W. R. (1989). Evaluation of four Spanish word-recognition-ability lists. *Ear and Hearing, 10,* 388–392.

Weiss, D., & Dempsey, J. J. (2008). Performance of bilingual speakers on the English and Spanish versions of the Hearing in Noise Test (HINT). *Journal of the American Academy of Audiology, 19,* 5–17.

Wolf, M. S., Gazmararian, J. A., & Baker, D. W. (2005). Health literacy and functional health status among older adults. *Archives of Internal Medicine, 165,* 1946–1952.

Woll, B., & Ladd, P. (2011). Deaf communities. In M. Marschark & P. E. Spencer (Eds.), *The Oxford handbook of deaf studies, language and education* (Vol. 1, 2nd ed., pp. 159–172). Oxford, UK: Oxford University Press.

Woods, A. G., Peña, E. D., & Martin, F. N. (2004). Exploring possible sociocultural bias on the SCAN-C. *American Journal of Audiology, 13,* 173–184.

World Health Organization (WHO). (2001). *International classification of functioning, disability and health (ICF).* Geneva, Switzerland: Author.

World Health Organization and World Bank. (2011). *World report on disabilities.* Malta: Author.

World Health Organization (WHO). (2012). *WHO global estimates on prevalence of hearing loss.* Retrieved from http://www.who.int/pbd/deafness/WHO_GE_HL.pdf?ua=1

World Health Organization (WHO). (2017). *Deafness and hearing loss.* Retrieved from http://www.who.int/mediacentre/factsheets/fs300/en/

Zubick, H. H., Irizarry, L. M., Rosen, L., Feudo, P., Jr., Kelly, J. H., & Strome, M. (1983). Development of speech-audiometric materials for native Spanish-speaking adults. *Audiology, 22,* 88–102.

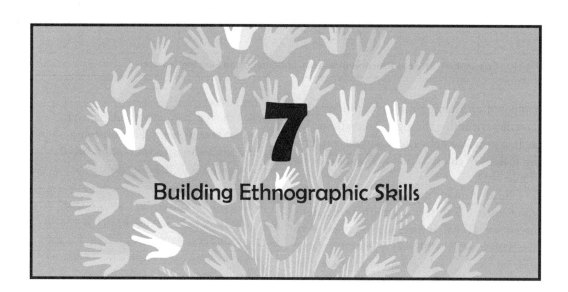

7

Building Ethnographic Skills

Ethnographic skills are used widely in the field of anthropology (Neuman, 2003) but can also be appropriate for other disciplines. In speech, language, and hearing sciences, for example, a method called *ethnographic interviewing*, a highly valued interviewing technique, is used widely to learn how the client and his or her family members conceptualize and understand their communication needs, strengths, and challenges (Westby, Burda, & Mehta, 2003). The goal of Chapter 7, Building Ethnographic Skills, is to provide guidance in developing ethnography skills, which are important for understanding how others make meaning of their circumstances, diverse cultural practices, and the beliefs, values, and assumptions that support those practices.

LEARNING OBJECTIVES

After reading, discussing and processing the information presented in this chapter, you will be able to demonstrate the following knowledge, skills, and attitudes:

1. Knowledge
   a. Define ethnography

   b. List the assumptions associated with the theory of ethnography
   c. Identify and define ethnographic methods associated with data collection, review, and analysis
2. Skills
   a. Conduct ethnographic interviews
   b. Engage in analysis of cultural artifacts
   c. Conduct document review and analysis
3. Attitudes
   a. Demonstrate comprehension of the value of ethnographic interviews, and the analysis of cultural artifacts and documents in weekly journals
   b. Demonstrate willingness to approach information gathering from a posture of collaboration and learning

KEY CONCEPTS

To build ethnographic skills it is important to understand concepts associated with these skills. Concepts introduced in this chapter are those that provide a basic foundational knowledge of ethnography, and its corresponding methods composed of listening through ethnographic interviews; learning through observations (including participant observations); and conducting analyses of cultural artifacts and documents (Table 7–1).

Read through the following case about Ms. Cadence Ramsey. A health professions interviewer (I) will initiate the interview with Ms. Ramsey (CR) with one type of *descriptive question* used in ethnographic interviewing called an *experience question*, which focuses on the interviewee's experience or experiences with a certain issue or event (Spradley, 1979). When reading the following case, make a note of the comments that the interviewee makes identifying topics that she determines to be most important to her. These are important points and/or statements (*markers*) and are often repeated or stand out in the interviewee's responses to questions.[1]

Box 7–1
Case: Cadence Ramsey

Cadence is being interviewed by a medical professional about the head-

---

TABLE 7–1. Key Concepts

Cultural artifacts	Thin description
Document analysis	Participant observations
Ethnography	
Descriptive questions	Markers
Beliefs	Structural questions
Norms	Values
Thick description	Social practices

aches she has been experiencing over the past several years. The following transcript picks up about one-third of the way through the interview:

I: I understand, Ms. Ramsey, that you have been having headaches for a number of years now. Please tell me more about your experiences with headaches.

CR: Well, they actually started when I was 7 years old. At least that is what I remember. They could have been occurring before then, but 7 years of age was the time that I am conscious of having headaches. I remember going to the doctor with my mother and the doctor told my mother that I needed to relax more—to not be so stressed. That would turn out to be the comment that I would hear at every doctor's visit that I went to from the time I was 7 until I was 52. "Relax Cadence." "Stop putting so much pressure on yourself Cadence." "Calm down Cadence." "You need to find more ways to relax, Cadence." That was the mantra I heard all of my life—just relax. That's a long time to suffer from what I now know are migraines without any relief. The headaches would be so intense I would vomit—that's the level of pain I was in and without any relief. When I was in college, the medicine that the health center gave me was so powerful, I would zone out and lose several days; I'd take the medicine and then wake up a couple of days

---

[1] On the PluralPlus companion website there are extension activities where the students will be given a case specific to speech-language pathology (SLP) and audiology to complete in class, and then an outside assignment to complete regarding this topic of ethnographic interviewing.

later. I had some relief but it was costing me in other ways. You can't be successful in college and miss several days because of sleeping off a bad headache. I must have awakened to go to the bathroom, but the point is that I didn't remember anything other than sleeping. So I was not able to use that medicine for very long. I became very good at just working through the pain—no matter how bad or intense, I'd do what I needed to do—particularly since I believed I had the bad headaches because I "wouldn't just relax," as I was told constantly. My shortest headache was 7 days long, and my longest was 27 days. So when I was 52 years old I finally found a specialty clinic in my area—well it's a 2-hour drive from where I live. I went there—to this specialty clinic —and was officially diagnosed with migraines. I had to take a class about why people get migraines, what causes them, and what are the triggers for a migraine. I was in tears after the class because I finally realized after 45 years of pain, that "just relaxing" as I was always told, is not the solution to migraines.

Activity 7–1

In Table 7–2, list some of the markers that you identified in Cadence Ramsey's response to the experience question that was asked of her.

ETHNOGRAPHY

Ethnography is a qualitative method of social research used to study and learn about social life from the people who are living that life (Fetterman, 2010). It falls within the interpretivist tradition of how things work in the world, and why they work in a particular way. As presented in Chapter 3, proponents of interpretivist explanations focus on identifying the underlying meaning of such things as a behavior, a statement, a way of life, an event, or a point of view (Neuman, 2003; Spradley, 1979). Ethnography has been called a field research method and is used to examine social settings, cultural groups, and daily social life in response to questions such as, "How does person X see the world?" "What is person Y's world view?" or "Why does group A do x, y, and z?"

The practice that characterizes ethnography is known as a *thick description* (Geertz, 1973, p. 6), a concept borrowed from Ryle

TABLE 7–2. Markers

1.
2.
3.
4.
5.

(cited in Geertz, 1973), which is a very detailed and specific description of something. Specifically, a thick description is the detailed, contextualized account of an event, perception, or point of view that also includes an interpretation of it, allowing the description to gain meaning (Hengst, Devanga, & Mosier, 2015). *Thin descriptions* include isolated, decontextualized characterizations (Hengst et al., 2015). Consider the contrasting descriptions of the same event in Table 7–3. You will see that the thick description in Table 7–3 more closely resembles the reality of daily life (Hengst et al., 2015).

Ethnographic Methods

Some of the methods associated with ethnography are the ethnographic interview, participant observation, and artifact and document analyses. These methods are discussed next.

The Ethnographic Interview

The ethnographic interview is an invaluable tool for learning from the perspectives of others. An ethnographic interview is a collaborative endeavor between the interviewer and the interviewee. It is a method that can be used to facilitate the acquisition of information in a culturally responsive manner. Inherent in this process is the ability to value, respect, and learn from persons who may have practices and beliefs different from your own. It is important to note that this method of gathering information is not only useful with those who are from cultural, linguistic, or ethnic backgrounds different than your own, it can be used with anyone, especially if we keep in mind that any interaction has the potential to be an intercultural one.[2] Social life of any human being is composed of beliefs, values, norms (*culture*), and social practices (which are driven by culture). When engaged in an

TABLE 7–3. Examples of Thin and Thick Descriptions

Thin Description	Thick Description
During free choice time, Child A took Child B's truck without asking, and then started playing with it.	During free choice time, Child A typically chooses to play with the red truck. During this particular morning, however, Child B obtained the truck from the toy box before Child A was able to get it. Child A began to play with the blocks when he heard a great deal of noise. He directed his eyes toward the noise and Child B, who at the time was handling the red truck. Child B threw the truck, retrieved it, banged the truck against the wall, and then dropped it in the toy bin before picking up the truck again and banging it against the tile floor. Child A, having witnessed the recurring treatment of the truck, went up to Child B and forcefully took the red truck without saying a word, as if to rescue the red truck from the bad treatment being imposed on it from Child B.

---

[2]At an ASHA conference in the 1980s, Dr. Orlando L. Taylor, one of the leaders in the field of communication sciences and disorders and one of the founders of the National Black Association of Speech Language and Hearing, stated that every clinical interaction has the potential to be a cross-cultural interaction.

ethnographic interview, you want to remember that you are trying to learn about the interviewee's beliefs, values, norms, and social practices, and/or the interviewees' concerns about language, speech, or hearing.

A traditional interview is usually conducted when the interviewer has a list of questions he or she wants to ask the interviewee. The underlying assumption of this traditional interview process is that the interviewer knows what questions are important to ask, and that the interviewee responds to them (Westby et al., 2003). I have, unfortunately, heard clinicians often say that the client "was not giving me the answers I wanted." In a traditional interview, the interviewee may indeed be hoping to acquire specific types of responses to particular questions. Thus, the interviewer receives the type of information the *interviewer* wants to obtain, potentially limiting important information from the interviewee. If we use the case of Ms. Ramsey as an example, some of the traditionally organized interview questions may have been questions such as, "At what age did your headaches begin?" "How many hours do they typically last?" or "When experiencing a migraine, do you get pain behind your eyes?" If a traditionally organized interview was used with Ms. Ramsey, it is likely that we would not have known about the rich and deep contexts in which she experienced and lived with migraines. An underlying assumption of an ethnographic interview is that the *interviewee knows* what is important to tell about his or her own experiences, or perspectives. It is the responsibility of the interviewer to create the conditions that will elicit information from the interviewee that the interviewee believes is important to share. Westby et al. (2003) call this process, "Asking the right questions in the right ways" (p. 1).

There are two basic types of questions to ask during an ethnographic interview: descriptive questions and structural questions. Descriptive questions are asked in a way

that encourages the interviewee to talk about broad experiences, perceptions, and relationships with others in their environment. These questions are used in the first phase of the ethnographic interview; the goal is to learn about the interviewee's broad experiences. There are several types of descriptive questions listed in Table 7–4. Spradley (1979) advised that ethnographic interviews begin with descriptive questions, such as a grand tour question. The interviewer then needs to engage active listening skills to identify the markers that are expressed in the response of the interviewee. Returning to the example of Ms. Ramsey, one marker that stands out is her repeated use of "relax."

Generally, to conduct an ethnographic interview one would do the following:

1. **Provide an ethnographic explanation** (Spradley, 1979; Westby et al., 2003). An ethnographic explanation informs the interviewee of the purpose of the interview, how the interview will be structured, and the reasons that the interviewer is asking the types of questions being asked. An ethnographic interview has a specific purpose (Neuman, 2003; Spradley, 1979), which is to "understand the lived experience" of the interviewee "by asking about and closely listening to the beliefs, values, material conditions, and structural forces that underwrite socially patterned behaviors" (Hockey & Forsey, 2012, p. 83). An ethnographic explanation may sound something like, "Thank you for agreeing to talk with me today. I am interested in learning more about your headaches, what causes them, how they are treated and how you responded to having them. This information will help me learn how we can work together to solve the issue of your headaches. I'd like to tape this conversation or write

TABLE 7–4. Definitions and Examples of Descriptive Questions for an Ethnographic Interview

Question Type	Example
Grand tour questions focus on broad experiences and perceptions and elicit detailed descriptions of events or issues.	"Tell me about growing up in Senegal."
Mini-tour questions focus on a more confined or specific experience, perception, event, or issue. One way to think of a mini-tour question is as a subset of a grand tour question.	"Tell me about attending school in Senegal."
Example questions ask the interviewee to provide an example of an experience, event, perspective, or issue.	"Give me an example of what you told the doctors to help them understand the severity of your headaches."
Experience questions ask the interviewee to share their experience with a particular event or issue.	"Tell me about your experience with Imitrex*."
Native language questions are used to make meaning of the way the interviewee is using a particular concept or statement.	"What does 'relaxing' look like?" "What do you do when you 'zone out'?"

Note. *Imitrex is a brand of sumatriptan used to treat migraines and cluster headaches.
Source: Based on Spradley (1979) and Westby et al. (2003).

a few notes as we talk. Is that ok? Feel free to take your own notes, too. As we are talking today, I will be inviting you to share information with me about your headaches. Just answer with as much detail as you would like . . . I am interested in *learning* about headaches from you. We'll talk about 30 minutes and then I'll check in with you to see if you want to continue or stop. Is this plan ok?"

2. **Initiate the interview with a grand tour question.** Remember that a grand tour question asks about broad experiences, events, and/or perceptions. Such a grand tour question could be, "Tell me what a typical headache is like for you."

3. **Ask follow-up questions based on markers presented in the interviewee's response to the questions.** The follow-up questions compose what we can call the second phase of the ethnographic interview. These follow-up questions should be formulated as other types of descriptive questions (mini-tour, example, experience, and native language questions). A mini-tour question that might be asked following the grand tour question mentioned in number 2 could be, "Tell me more about the headaches you have in the evenings."

4. **Ask structural questions, which comprise the third phase of the interview.** Structural questions allow the interviewer to delve deeper into a topic originally raised by the descriptive questions. These questions are more explicit

or direct and focus on the interviewee's motives and thinking (Spradley, 1979; Svasek & Domecka, 2012; Westby, 2003). Examples of these more specific structural questions are presented in Table 7–5.

Westby et al. (2003, pp. 6–7) provide some important "question-asking" practices to remember when engaged in ethnographic interviewing. These important practices to remember are listed below:

1. **Ask for behavior instead of meaning.** Asking for behavior may result in a more meaningful response. For example, asking, "What do you mean you are getting forgetful?" may result in a response such as, "I just don't remember things like I used to." But, asking,

TABLE 7–5. Structural Questions

Structural Question	Example
Inclusion questions encourage the interviewee to describe *types* of events, experiences, or information.	What kind of information have you been told about migraines?
Spatial questions are about the locations of events or experiences.	Tell me where in your head you experience a migraine.
Cause-and-effect questions prompt discussions about causes of things and their relative consequences.	What are the causes of your migraines?
Rationale questions encourage the interviewee to give a reason for some behavior or perspective.	Tell me about the reasons you take Imitrex instead of Midrin.*
Location questions ask about the place that something occurred.	Tell me about the places you go in order to reduce the intensity of your migraines.
Function questions ask about the purpose of certain actions.	You mentioned that you use "soft lighting." What role does soft lighting play in your daily life?
Means–end questions prompt the interviewee to describe a particular way he or she does something in order to get some sort of outcome.	Tell me what types of things you do to prevent migraines.
Sequence questions ask the interviewee to give a step-by-step description of some event.	Tell me about the stages of a migraine.
Attribution questions request characteristics of an event, perspective, or behavior.	List the characteristics of a migraine attack.

Note. *Midrin is a combination of the drugs acetaminophen, dichloralphenazone, and isometheptene, and it is used to treat migraines.

Source: Based on Westby et al. (2003).

"Tell me what you do when you forget things" may elicit information about what she forgets, when she forgets, and the type of information that is forgotten (Westby et al., 2003, p. 6).

2. **Use open-ended questions rather than dichotomous questions.** Dichotomous questions can elicit a yes/no response rather than a more detailed response (Westby et al., 2003, p. 6). For example, asking, "Do your migraines prevent you from working?" may elicit a simple *yes* or *no* response. Saying, "Tell me about the ways that migraines affect your life," may yield a more descriptive response.

3. **Restate what the client says by repeating the client's exact words; do not paraphrase or interpret** (Westby et al., 2003, p. 6). Using the interviewee's own words demonstrates that the interviewer is actively listening, and it prevents the interviewer from interpreting what the interviewee says through the interviewer's own cultural lens. For example, if the interviewee says, "The doctors blamed me for my migraines." You may want to respond with, "That experience must have been difficult for you." It is likely the interviewee would respond with, "Well . . . I guess so." You would, however, be imposing your own interpretations and lived experiences onto the interviewee. Rather, if you respond by mirroring what the interviewee said, "The doctors blamed you for your migraines," the interviewee may expand on that thought with something like, "They probably didn't mean to, and I am sure they were not acting with malice, but the effect of spending most of my life thinking that

I somehow had more control over my migraines than I did, really affected my mind and outlook on life."

4. **Summarize the [*interviewee's*] statements and give him or her the opportunity to correct you if you have misunderstood something he or she has said** (Westby et al., 2003, p. 6). Summarizing the interviewee's statements periodically can be used to facilitate a change in the topic. For example, this summarization might look like this, as reported in Westby et al. (2003): "Before we talk about your work as a storyteller, I want to make certain I understand what you've told me about feeling overtaxed. You mentioned that you were overtaxed because *the migraines*[3] make you feel weak, you must make certain your mother is being cared for, and because of your husband's illness, he isn't able to help you like he used to" (p. 6).

5. **Avoid multiple questions** (Westby et al., 2003, p. 7). Asking multiple questions at once makes it difficult for the interviewee to focus on a response. It is likely that if asked multiple questions at once, the interviewee will only respond to the last question that was asked. Questions such as this should be avoided, "Ms. Ramsey, what do you do to minimize the number of times you get a migraine in a month? What do you do once you get a migraine? And, please give me some examples of the ways your family members respond to you when you have a migraine." It is likely that the interviewee would respond only to the last question asked.

6. **Avoid leading questions that tend to orient the interviewee to respond**

---

[3] The italicized phrase was added by the authors.

in a particular way (Westby et al., 2003, p. 7). A leading question is one such as, "What do you dislike about the doctors?" Asking this question suggests that there is something to dislike. A more neutral question would be something like, "Tell me about your experiences with doctors."

7. **Avoid using *why* questions because such questions tend to sound judgmental and assume that the person knows why** (Westby et al., 2003, p. 7). Rather than asking why questions, a rationale structural question would be better. A why question might be, "Why don't you still go to medical doctors?" Whereas a rationale structural question could be, "Tell me your reasons for no longer going to medical doctors."

In addition to conducting an ethnographic interview, you might also benefit from observations. The discussion of observations below is focused on participant observations.

Learning Through Observations

Another field research method that is useful for learning about the lived experiences of others is the tool of observations. There are different types of observations. One is the observation of a natural environment where the examiner does not make any changes and does not attempt to interact with the people in the environment where the observation is taking place. This naturalistic observation can be designed in a way such that a certain set of *a priori* behaviors are identified and then imposed on the context. This type of *a priori* observation is considered an etic observation—where observations from outside of a cultural context are imposed onto the cultural context. For example, several diagnostic checklists (Pragmatic Protocol [Prutting &

Kirchner, 1987]; Social Interactive Coding System [Rice, Sell, & Hadley, 1990]) require the observer to first review the observation form, and then note whether the child being observed engaged in the behavior listed on the observation form. Participant observation, on the other hand, is not the same as an etic observation in natural contexts, but is an emic approach. An emic approach "is an 'inside-out' approach" (DeJarnette, Rivers, & Hyter, 2015, p. 67), which is an examination of behavior (events, ideas, etc.) from the perspective of those who are engaged in that behavior. It is an *intra*cultural (within culture) perspective rather than an *inter*cultural (between culture) one. A speech-language pathologist (SLP) may want to use participant observation (which speech acts *emerge* from a child's [or adolescent's or adult's] interactions with others).

Participant observation is a systematic "form of engagement" (Gunn & Logstrup, 2014, p. 431) that occurs when the examiner or observer is involved with the groups being observed, and in the ongoing actions or events that are being observed (Dewalt & Dewalt, 2011). This type of observation results in qualitative and descriptive data and comes out of the field of anthropology (Dahlke, Hall, & Phinney, 2015; Polit & Beck, 2010). In Participant Observation, the researcher/examiner is the instrument in the research and must focus on the context in which the events are taking place, the activities of the people involved in the events, and how those involved in the events communicate, for example. Participant observations can serve to confirm information provided in interviews, just like interviews can confirm or clarify events and behaviors that have been observed. To be a successful participant observer, one must acquire skills, such as knowledge of the language in which the observations take place, being able to attend to the commonplace activities that occur in everyday life, being able to remember what happens (facilitated by writing field notes), as well as maintaining a posture of humility and the ability to keep one's own assumptions and interpretations in check (Bernard, 1988).

There are several frameworks discussed in the literature that focus on what to observe when engaged in a participant observation endeavor; however, we focus on only three such frameworks in this chapter. One framework, the KEEPRAH Holistic Model, was introduced to us by a doctoral student whose teaching practicum was supervised by Dr. Hyter in 2012. This framework was used by the U.S. Peace Corps (1985). The original framework, as outlined by the Peace Corps, was composed of some of the following categories, which have been redefined based on the conceptual framework used in this book:

- **K**inship—Relationships among members of the group being observed
- **E**conomics—Production and distribution of goods, services, and resources
- **E**ducation—Knowledge, skills, values of the group
- **P**olitics—Exercise of power from above and below; instruments of coercion and consensus
- **R**eligion—Belief systems
- **A**ssociation—Groupings within the cultural group (committees or clubs)
- **H**ealth—Wellness/illness models and practices

Hyter (2013) added three other categories to this framework:

- **L**eisure—Unscheduled time
- **T**ransportation—Movement from one location to another
- **C**ommunication systems—Ways to transmit and/or share information

We are calling this adapted framework the KEEPRAH+LTC framework (Hyter, 2013). Things to think about during engaged observations while using this model are provided in Table 7–6. An exercise that will facilitate your learning on how to engage in an observation using the KEEPRAH+LTC framework is explained on the PluralPlus companion website.

Another framework, also promoted by the Peace Corps, is one that focuses on local knowledge—that is, knowledge held by people who are part of a group or that has been developed or is developing within a group of people (Peace Corps, 2002, pp. 7–9). Types of knowledge that already exist in communities and among groups of people are provided in Table 7–7.

The third framework that we discuss is SPEAKING, which was developed by Dell Hymes (1972) and simplified by Daas and McBride (2014). This framework primarily focuses on language and the structure of communication interactions, but can be used in a variety of contexts. The SPEAKING framework includes the following categories:

- **S**etting and scene—The setting is the time and place in which the communicative interaction takes place. The scene refers to the "cultural definition" or local perspective about the context in which the communicative interaction takes place (Hymes, 1973, p. 60).
- **P**articipation and purposes—Descriptions of those who are participating in the communicative interaction, including as much detail as possible, such as gender, who was talking to whom, and clothing (Daas & McBride, 2014, p. 15).
- **E**nds—This refers to the inferred goals of the interlocutors, such as "why the participants in the setting" are "acting a particular way" (Daas & McBride, 2014, p. 15; Hymes, 1973).

TABLE 7–6. KEEPRAH+LTC Observational Categories

Observational Categories	Think About
KINSHIP *Relationships among group members*	Who makes the decisions? What is the role of adults, children, and the elderly? What are the responsibilities of the group members? What types of interactions occur between members of the group? What are some of the values in which the group members are socialized? What assumptions might scaffold kinship relations?
ECONOMICS *Production and distribution of goods, services, and resources*	What goods and services are produced and distributed? What assumptions might scaffold the production, management, distribution, and use of goods and services? How are goods and services produced and distributed? (what process using which mechanism) What is the level of availability of goods and services in the group? What is the role of land? How is land obtained? Who has access and who uses land? What institutions exist? What are their functions? Who has access to these institutions?
EDUCATION *Knowledge, skills, values of the group*	What is taught—content? What processes are used in education? What assumptions might scaffold the educational processes and content? What are the teaching methods? Who benefits from the teaching methods and content? Who has responsibility for teaching? What is the role or goals of education? Who has access to education? In which languages is education occurring? Who uses which languages? What role does literacy play in the group/society/family/culture?
POLITICS *Exercise of power from above and below* *Instruments of coercion and consensus*	How is power distributed? What assumptions might scaffold this distribution process? Who has power? What are the decision-making processes? Who participates? How are they organized? Who benefits from decision-making processes and outcomes? Who participates in the carrying out or execution of decisions?
RELIGION *Belief systems*	What are the belief-based practices? What assumptions might scaffold these beliefs? What role does religion play in daily life?
ASSOCIATIONS *Grouping within the cultural group (e.g., clubs)*	What groups exist in the society/community/culture? How did these groups form? Why did they form? What is the relationship between/among groups? Who benefits from intergroup associations? What role do these groups play in the larger society/community/culture?
HEALTH *Wellness/illness models*	What diseases exist? Why do they exist? What are health practices? What is considered health? Who benefits from health practices? Who has access to health practices? Who administers health care? How is food developed and distributed? Who has access to food? What assumptions undergird health and food practices?

continues

155

TABLE 7–6. *continued*

Observational Categories	Think About
LEISURE *Unscheduled time*	What leisure activities occur? Who participates in leisure activities? Who benefits from these activities? What assumptions undergird the leisure activities?
TRANSPORTATION *Movement from one location to another*	What are the means of transportation? Who benefits from transportation? Who does the transporting? Who gets transported? What are the underlying assumptions about the relevance/importance/use of transportation? What role does transportation play?
COMMUNICATION SYSTEMS *Information transmission and sharing*	How is communication conveyed? What is communicated? What languages are used? Who can communicate on a wide scale? Who benefits from what is communicated and the communication process?

Source: Based on Peace Corps (1985).

TABLE 7–7. Types of Local Knowledge in Communities

Observational Categories	Think About
Information	How to live life in the group/community
Practices and technologies	Healing practices, how to grow food
Beliefs	Life, death, health, and illness
Tools	Instruments used to make items (e.g., cookware, plow)
Materials	Elements from which items (e.g., supplies, housing) are made
Experimentation	Testing/trying out new processes
Biological resources	Local animals, land, and crops
Human resources	Specialized skills held by members of the group or community
Education	Teaching and learning practices
Communication	Exchange of information

Source: Based on Peace Corps (2002, pp. 7–9).

- Act sequence—The content and form of a message is the focus here; in other words, note not only what is said but how it is stated. Hymes (1973) states that "*how* something is said, is part of *what* is said" (p. 59).
- Key—The manner in which a communicative interaction occurs—whether something is said jokingly or seriously, formally or informally (Daas & McBride, 2014; Hymes, 1973).
- Instrumentalities—These are language variations or dialects, mutual intelligibility, and registers used to communicate (Hymes, 1973, p. 63)
- Norms of interaction and interpretation—These are the perceived rules of the interaction (Hymes, 1973; Daas & McBride, 2014, p. 15).
- Genres—Categories of discourse such as a poem, riddle, prayer, etc. (Hymes, 1973, p. 65).

Classroom activities that can be used to facilitate and enhance participant observation skills are available on the PluralPlus companion website. An observation form is provided in Appendix 7–1. The third ethnographic method discussed in this chapter is the analysis of cultural objects.

Analyzing Cultural Artifacts

Artifacts refer to objects used within the context of a given culture (Hoskins, 1998). Analyzing cultural artifacts facilitates learning about the history of the cultural group that made or uses the object. They are also examples of the ways groups of people who share cultural values, beliefs, and assumptions think (Sheumaker, & Vajda, 2008). These objects can have a variety of uses and meanings among groups that use them. It is

difficult to learn about the life, beliefs, and values of groups of people (or even one person), without also understanding the objects that make that group's or person's life meaningful (Hoskins, 1998). Let's consider an example of an artifact created and used in the United States—the typewriter. There may be people who are living now, who have never used (or perhaps have never even seen) a typewriter. Computers, smartphones, and iPads now are used by many people in the United States and in other countries, although the typewriter may still be useful in some industries.

The typewriter demonstrates the change in employment history in the United States. At the time that the typewriter was created, it was considered a technological innovation. It was also produced at the time when women in the United States were beginning to work outside of the home—in this way it had an impact on how work was organized. Although the idea of a typewriter emerged in 1714 (Allan, 2015; Polt, 2015), the typewriter as we know it was developed in the latter part of the 19th century (1874) (Allan, 2015; Polt, 2015). In much of the early 19th century, work was primarily composed of physical laborers. When there were office workers, persons working with their heads rather than their hands, those workers were primarily men (Sheumaker & Wajda, 2008). By the 1880s, however, business colleges were emerging and women were enrolling in those colleges. When these women graduated from the business colleges there was a demand for work, which resulted in men being promoted to managers and women being hired to type and serve as "secretaries, receptionists, accounting clerks, and book keepers" (Sheumaker & Wajda, 2008, p. 331).

Let's consider another object, found in West Africa—a piece of cloth called bazin, which is depicted in Figure 7–1.

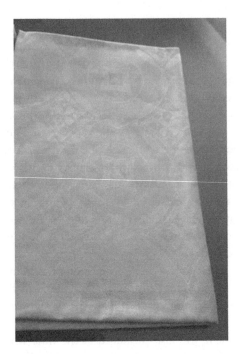

FIGURE 7–1. Bazin fabric from Mali. Fabric courtesy of W. F. Santiago-Valles, photo by Yvette D. Hyter.

This cloth tells a story of globalization, which, for our purposes here, is defined as the interdependence among nation-states (Santiago-Valles, 2016, personal communication; Steger, 2010). Bazin is a fabric made of heavy cotton, silk, or wool that has a distinctive sheen. In some parts of Europe this material is called "damask," and in French it is referred to as "brocade." This material is sold in countries such as Mali, Niger, Senegal, and Morocco, and it competes with the rich embroidered cloth for which Nigeria is famous. Bazin tells the story of globalization on at least four levels.[4]

On one level, cotton fabric is imported into African countries from Germany, Holland, Austria, and China. One of the consequences of globalization includes the conditions imposed on nation-states, particularly those in the global south.[5] One condition imposed by the International Monetary Fund and the World Bank was that countries needed to privatize government-owned institutions, engage in trade and financial liberalization, and deregulate their economy (Akindele, Gidado, & Olaopo, 2002; Kentikelenis, Stubbs, & King, 2016). One such requirement was to reduce tariff walls (Akindele et al., 2002), making imports plentiful and cheap in such countries as Senegal, for example, and lucrative for the importing country. Another example of the connection between globalization and bazin, is that the dyeing of the cloth is done primarily by women who work in collectives; however, the chemicals used in the dye (sulfur) often create illnesses in the women.[6] Dangerous chemicals are more easily imported into countries in the Global South due to the requirement to reduce environmental protections—another condition imposed by lending agencies (Akindele et al., 2002). The countries in the Global South often do not have resources for safe disposal of the leftover water from dyeing the cloth, which ends up in women's bodies, and in water sources (Larsson, 2009). A third level of this relationship between bazin and globalization is the trans-

---

[4]The discussion about examining the effects of globalization by understanding the history of bazin was told to Dr. Hyter by W. F. Santiago-Valles, emeritus professor with doctorates in cultural communication and political economy, and has studied the causes and consequences of globalization for over 40 years.

[5]The Global South refers more to the income of countries than to the location. Global South and majority world countries (where most of the people in the world live) refer to countries with low incomes such as those in sub-Saharan Africa. On the other hand, the Global North or minority world countries (where the least number of the people in the world live), refer to high-income countries of the world such as the United States, Europe, Australia, Israel, parts of China, and New Zealand.

[6]The most famous neighborhood in Mali for production of bazin is Badalodougou West.

national networks that are created among the cotton importers, sellers of the dye, the fabric dyers, tailors who transform the fabric into clothing, the nongovernmental organizations (NGOs) that provide microloans to those selling the fabric, bankers, local consumers who buy and wear the fabric, and the tourists who purchase the fabric for personal use. Bazin in Senegal, for example, is largely worn on Fridays to go to the Mosque or on Sundays for weddings. The final connection between bazin and globalization is that due to the level of impoverishment and number of wars on the African continent, some Malians and persons from Senegal, for example, have immigrated to Europe and North America. As a result, there are boutiques in the United States where bazin is readily available, such as in Harlem on 116th street in a neighborhood called "Little Senegal."

We can begin to understand the role of artifacts by asking questions about them during an ethnographic interview. Artifacts can be used to communicate ideas, convey emotions, symbolize values and beliefs, and enter into a deeper conversation.

There are different models that are used to understand cultural artifacts. Pearce (1993) suggests that there are common properties, and all artifacts can be classified based on these properties (history, material, construction, design, and function). Also, she asserts that all artifacts can be used for four basic activities —identification (authentication of an object), evaluation (comparison of the object with other similar objects), cultural analysis (analyzes the relationship between the object and the culture in which it is used), and interpretation (meaning and significance of the object in its cultural context) (Cauvin, 2016, p. 40).

Prown (1982) states that there are three general principles for understanding the role of artifacts in culture: descriptions, deductions, and speculations. Descriptions of artifacts require the analyzer to examine the artifacts with the awareness that they have different properties and can be used for different purposes. Specifically, each artifact has a history, is made of certain material, has been constructed in a particular manner, has a certain design, and has a specific function. Deductions are made about what the object is and how it is used. This stage of artifact analysis focuses on the relationship between the object and the analyzer in that the analyzer deduces the purpose of the artifact (p. 8). Speculations result from imagining the purpose and utility of the object, and its role in culture. An artifact analysis form is located in Appendix 7–2.

In partnership with the analysis of cultural artifacts, one can also learn a great deal by analyzing key words, as the relationship between a culture and the words used in the cultural group's language is extremely close (Wierzbicka, 1997). When Dr. Hyter's mother-in-law, a Puerto Rican woman whose first language was Spanish, was alive, she used to say that the plants were "*sleeping*" during the winter. Dr. Hyter never once thought about plants sleeping. Until she heard her mother-in-law say that particular phrase, Dr. Hyter could only think of plants as *dying* during the winter. Let's examine another example of the importance of key words from Senegal. There is a concept in Wolof, the lingua franca in Senegal, called *Mbokk*. This word means "family," but it is more than a biological family. It is a group of people who struggle together, who support each other, who walk through life together. This conceptualization of family is evident in the way many living in Senegal refer to people with whom they are connected as mother, father, brother, or sister. In many parts of the United States, a significant word is "independence," which is a word that undergirds the cultural perspective that people strive to be "self-sufficient" or to make their way through life *individually*, and that a valid goal of young people is to live alone and separate from other members of their families.

What is important to keep in mind about artifact and key word analyses is that these are processes for understanding others better, and can be completed in concert with other processes, such as the ethnographic interviewing and participant observations (Bowen, 2009). The final ethnographic method discussed in this chapter is the analysis of documents.

Analyzing Documents

Document analysis is systematic and can be focused on printed documents as well as electronic ones, and the analysis can target the text and/or pictures (Bowen, 2009). To engage in document analysis, one needs to find, select, evaluate, and synthesize data within the documents (Bowen, 2009). The type of data that one extracts from documents usually includes quotes, pictures, ideas, or paragraphs that are organized into categories or themes (Labuschagne, 2003; Rasmussen, Muir-Cochrane, & Henderson, 2012). Some of the qualitative research techniques that can be used to analyze documents include, but are not limited to, thematic/content analyses, comparing themes across documents, key word analysis, and number of words and number of different words (Leech & Onwuegbuzie, 2008). For our purposes in this chapter, we focus on content analysis and thematic analyses—processes that are typically used in a range of disciplines including education, journalism, political science, psychology, sociology, and speech-language pathology.

Content analysis "systematically describes, categorizes and/or makes inferences about" any form of text, widely defined as anything that is written, presented in pictures or spoken (Croucher & Cronn-Mills, 2015, p. 206; Neuman, 2006). The first step of content analysis is to determine what question you will be asking of the data, such as, "What are the underlying assumptions inherent in the Individuals with Disabilities Education Improvement Act (IDEA, 2004)?" or "What dispositions do people with migraines exhibit?"

Second, determine if the analysis will be deductive (or etic)—imposed onto the data from the outside—or inductive (emic)—emerging from inside the data (DeJarnette et al., 2015; Neuman, 2003). The focus of the questions above suggests using an emic rather than an etic analysis.

The third step is to determine which document will be examined. For our purposes here, we use the transcript from Ms. Ramsey's interview, presented earlier in this chapter. The fourth step is to determine what will be the unit of analysis or the scope of the data being analyzed. Another way to think of unit of analysis is the smallest meaningful unit of content that will be coded—such as individual words, a theme, entire passages, or pictures. In other words, determine the specific component or components being analyzed. Let's focus on determining themes that emerge from Mrs. Ramsey's interview. Table 7–8 illustrates how we coded and then identified categories and themes for some parts of Ms. Ramsey's interview text.

a. We begin by simply reading through Ms. Ramsey's interview text (Guest, McQueen, & Namey, 2012; Neuman, 2006). This first reading is called a first pass.

b. Then, write down codes while the text is read. Codes are labels or names that are given to the statements (timeline, memories). A code should have a name, be defined so that it can be identified in the text, and have an example (Guest, McQueen, & Namey, 2012). An example of the code definitions is provided in Table 7–9. Although the codes in Table 7–8 are presented in table form, we suggest handwriting the codes that emerge from the text while reading through it. Codes could also be color coded; that is, each code could be highlighted with a different color marker.

TABLE 7–8. Coding, Categorizing Data, and Identifying Overall Themes That Emerge From the Data

Excerpt From Ms. Ramsey's Interview Text	Emic or Emergent Code	Category	Theme
That's a long time to suffer from what I now know are migraines without any relief	*No relief*	Effects of migraine	*Negative impact on daily life*
. . . the medicine that the health center gave me was so powerful, I would zone out and lose several days	*Loss of time*		
I became very good at just working through the pain—no matter how bad or intense, I'd do what I needed to do	*Working through pain*	Doing what is necessary	*Perseverance*
. . . a specialty clinic in my area . . . it's a 2-hour driving distance from where I live	*Traveling to clinic*		

TABLE 7–9. Ms. Ramsey's Statements With Thematic Codes

Example Statements From Ms. Ramsey's Interview	Thematic Code Name	Definition	Ways to Identify	What It Is Not
. . . they actually started when I was 7 years old.	Timeline	When some event occurred	Includes a reference to age range or years that some event occurred	Does not refer to the respondent's report of his or her age

c. After writing down the codes, put all of the same codes into one page, and then review the text again to see if the codes could be organized into a more cohesive category.

d. Then, in a final review, determine if the categories are part of a higher-level theme that seems to characterize the text.

If we interviewed several people with a history of migraines, we would follow the same procedure with each text. Once we have the texts coded, we might discover that the codes could be part of a larger category. Imag-ine that several interviewees said the following statements:

- Interviewee 1: "I became very good at just working through the pain—no matter how bad or intense, I'd do what I needed to do." [*Working through the pain*]
- Interviewee 2: "I had to push through it . . . I just had to keep moving." [*pushing through*]
- Interviewee 3: "Sometimes the pain was so severe, I thought I was going to faint, but I couldn't cancel my classes. I never miss a day of class." [*cannot miss a day*]

All of these codes could be collapsed into one category called, "*doing what is necessary*," that has the overarching theme of "*perseverance*."

CHAPTER SUMMARY

The goal of Chapter 7 was to provide information about ethnographic processes and to help you develop ethnographic skills. In this chapter, we highlighted the value of using ethnographic interviewing to be able to learn from the clients about their concerns from their own cultural and/or familial perspective. Thin and thick descriptions were differentiated, and these descriptions serve to contextualize the behaviors or skills that we will be concerned about when working with individuals who have disabilities and their family members. You learned about the differences between traditional and ethnographic interviews, how to formulate ethnographic questions, and how to implement an ethnographic interview. Participant observation and artifact analysis were also addressed. SLPs and audiologists have ample opportunities to learn more about the people we serve by using observation and artifact analysis skills. Participant observation, artifact analysis as well as understanding key words within cultural groups, and the analyses of documents are additional ways to understand the cultural worldview of those being served by SLPs and audiologists.

EXTENDED LEARNING

Below are some activities that are designed to help you continue to learn about the topics discussed in this chapter, and to apply some of them in realistic contexts.

1. Form groups of three. One person will be the interviewer, one will be the interviewee, and another will be the interviewer's helper in identifying and formulating ethnographic questions to ask the interviewee.
   a. The interviewer is a preschool classroom teacher who works at Morning Glory Preschool in a small rural Midwestern town. As an interviewer, utilize ethnographic questions to find out more about Michael, his strengths, his challenges, and his mother's concerns and hopes for him.
   b. The interviewee is a parent of a preschooler who is looking for a preschool experience for her child, Michael. Michael has cried for up to 2 hours in previous preschools. If he is not crying, teachers have reported that he pulls toys from the shelves and steps on them. He has been expelled from several preschools due to his "unmanageable behavior." Michael's mother is concerned that Morning Glory is Michael's last option for early education. As the interviewee, build on Michael's case, filling in plausible information from the perspective of the mother during the interview.

2. Next, formulate ethnographic follow-up questions that will help you understand the points that Ms. Ramsey was making in her responses at the beginning of the chapter. Work with two other classmates. Have one classmate take on the role of Ms. Ramsey and respond to questions in a plausible manner considering Ms. Ramsey's background and experiences. The other classmate can serve as a support to you (interviewer) in developing and formulating ethnographic questions.

FURTHER READING

Consider reading these additional works regarding ethnographic skills.

Bowen, G. A. (2009). Document analysis as a qualitative research method. *Qualitative Research Journal, 9*(2), 27–40.

Hsieh, H-F., & Shannon, S. E. (2005). Three approaches to qualitative content analysis. *Qualitative Health Research, 15*(9), 1277–1288.

Spradley, J. P. (1979). *The ethnographic interview.* Belmont, CA: Wadsworth.

Westby, C. E., Burda, A., & Mehta, Z. (2003). Asking the right questions in the right ways: Strategies for ethnographic interviewing. *ASHA Leader, 8*, 4–17.

REFERENCES

Akindele, S. T., Gidado, T. O., & Olaopo, O. R. (2002). Globalisation: Its implications and consequences for Africa. *Journal of Social Sciences, 5*(4), 221–230.

Allan, T. (2015). *Typewriter: The history, the machines, the writers.* New York, NY: Shelter Harbor Press.

Bernard, R. (1988). *Research methods in cultural anthropology.* Newbury Park, CA: Sage Publications.

Bowen, G. A. (2009). Document analysis as a qualitative research method. *Qualitative Research Journal, 9*(2), 27–40.

Cauvin, T. (2016). *Public history: A textbook of practice.* New York, NY: Routledge.

Croucher, S. M., & Cronn-Mills, D. (2015). *Understanding communication research methods: A theoretical and practical approach.* New York, NY: Routledge.

Daas, K. L., & McBride, M. C. (2014). Participant observation: Teaching students the benefits of using a framework. *Communication Teacher, 28*(1), 14–19.

Dahlke, S., Hall, W., & Phinney, A. (2015). Maximizing theoretical contributions of par-tic-ipant observation while managing challenges. *Qualitative Health Research, 25*(8), 1117–1122.

DeJarnette, G., Rivers, K. O., & Hyter, Y. D. (2015). Ways of examining speech acts in young African American children: Considering inside-out and outside-in approaches. *Topics in Language Disorders, 35*(1), 61–75.

Dewalt, K. M., & Dewalt, B. R. (2011). *Participant observation: A guide for fieldworkers* (2nd ed.). Plymouth, UK: AltaMira Press.

Fetterman, D. M. (2010). *Ethnography: Step by step* (3rd ed.). Los Angeles, CA: Sage.

Geertz, C. (1973). Thick description: Toward an interpretive theory of culture. In C. Geertz, *The interpretation of cultures: Selected essays* (pp. 3–30). New York, NY: Basic Books.

Guest, G., McQueen, K. M., & Namey, E. E. (2012). *Applied thematic analysis.* Los Angeles, CA: Sage.

Gunn, W., & LØgstrup, L. B. (2014). Participant observation, anthropology methodology and design, anthropology research inquiry. *Arts and Humanities in Higher Education, 13*(4), 428–442.

Hengst, J. A., Devanga, S., & Mosier, H. (2015). Thin vs. thick description: Analyzing representations of people and their life worlds in the literature of Communication Sciences and Disorders. *American Journal of Speech-Language Pathology, 24*, 838–853.

Hockey, J., & Forsey, M. (2012). Ethnography is not participant observation: Reflections on the interview as participatory qualitative research. In J. Skinner (Ed.), *The interview: An ethnographic approach* (pp. 68–87). New York, NY: BERG.

Hoskins, J. (1998). *Biographical objects: How things tell the stories of people's lives.* New York, NY: Routledge.

Hymes, D. (1972). Models of the interaction of language and social life. In J. Gumperz & D. Hymes (Eds.), *Directions in sociolinguistics: The ethnography of communication* (pp. 35–71). New York, NY: Holt, Reinhart & Winston.

Hyter, Y. D. (2013). *Hyter adaptations to the Peace Corp's KEEPRAH framework: Leisure, transportation, and communication systems* (Unpublished document). Western Michigan University, Kalamazoo, MI.

Hyter, Y. D., & Applegate, E. B. (2012). *Assessment of pragmatic language and social communication: Research version.* Unpublished document. Western Michigan University, Kalamazoo, MI.

Kentikelenis, A. E., Stubbs, T. H., & King, L. P. (2016). IMF conditionality and development policy space, 185–2014. *Review of International Economy, 23*(4), 543–582.

Labuschange, A. (2003). Qualitative research: Airy fairy or fundamental? *The Qualitative Report, 8*(1), 100–103. Retrieved from http://insuworks.nova.edu/tqr/vol8/iss1/7

Larsson, H. (2009). *Textile dying in Mali: Possibilities for small scale effluent treatment. Master's thesis in soil science.* Swedish University of Agricultural Sciences. Retrieved from http://stud.epsilon.slu.se/594/1/larsson_h_091105.pdf

Leech, N., & Onwuegbuzie, A. J. (2008). Qualitative data analysis: A compendium of techniques and a framework for selection for school psychology research and beyond. *School Psychology Quarterly, 23*(4), 587–604.

Neuman, W. L. (2003). *Social research methods: Qualitative and quantitative approaches* (5th ed.). Boston, MA: Allyn & Bacon.

Neuman, W. L. (2006). *Social research methods: Qualitative and quantitative approaches* (6th ed.). Boston, MA: Pearson/Allyn & Bacon.

Peace Corps. (1985). A training manual for combating childhood communicable diseases: Volume I. *Peace Corps Information Collection and Exchange Training Manual No. T039.* Washington, DC: Peace Corps ED288055. Retrieved from http://www.nzdl.org/gsdlmod?e=d-00000-00---off-0hdl--00-0----0-10-0---0---0direct-10---4-------0-1l--11-en-50---20-about---00-0-1-00-0-0-11-1-0utfZz-8-00-0-0-11-10-0utfZz-8-00&a=d&c=hdl&cl=CL1.17&d=HASH01100bdcb8601754fcce12d1.8.pr

Peace Corps. (1986). *The Peace Corps small enterprise development pre-service training manual.* Washington, DC: ED2880555.

Peace Corps. (2002). *Roles of the volunteer in development: Toolkits for building capacity.* Information Collection and Exchange Publication No: T0005. Washington, DC: Peace Corps. Re-trieved from http://files.peacecorps.gov/multimedia/pdf/library/T0005_rvidcomplete.pdf

Pearce, S. (1993). *Museums, objects, and collections.* Washington, DC: Smithsonian Press.

Polit, D. F., & Beck, C. T. (2010). *Essentials of nursing research: Appraising evidence for nursing practice* (7th ed.). Philadelphia, PA: Lippincott.

Polt, R. (2015). *The typewriter revolution: A typist's companion for the 21st century.* New York, NY: Countryman Press.

Prown, J. (1982). Mind and matter: An introduction to material culture theory and method. *Winterthur Portfolio, 17*(1), 1–19.

Prutting, C., & Kirchner, D. M. (1987). A clinical appraisal of the pragmatic aspects of language. *Journal of Speech and Hearing Disorders, 52,* 105–119.

Rasmussen, P., Muir-Cochran, E., & Henderson, A. (2012). Document analysis using an aggregative and iterative process. *International Journal of Evidenced-Based Healthcare, 10,* 142–145.

Rice, M. L., Sell, M. A., & Hadley, P. A. (1990). The social interactive coding system (SICS): On-line, clinically relevant descriptive tool. *Language, Speech, and Hearing Services in Schools, 21*(1), 2–14.

Sheumaker, H., & Wajda, S. T. (2008). *Material culture in America: Understanding everyday life.* Santa Barbara, CA: ABC-CLIO.

Spradley, J. P. (1979). *The ethnographic interview.* Belmont, CA: Wadsworth.

Steger, M. (2010). *Globalization: A brief insight.* New York: Sterling.

Svasek, M., & Domecka, M. (2012). The autobiographical narrative interview: A potential arena of emotional remembering, performance and reflection. In J. Skinner (Ed.), *The interview: An ethnographic approach* (pp. 106–125). New York, NY: BERG.

Westby, C. E., Burda, A., & Mehta, Z. (2003). Asking the right questions in the right ways: Strategies for ethnographic interviewing. *ASHA Leader, 8,* 4–17.

Wierzbicka, A. (1997). *Understanding cultures through their key words: English, Russian, Polish, German, and Japanese.* Oxford, UK: Oxford University Press.

Appendix 7-1
Ethnographic Participant Observation Form

Observation Context →		
Category	**Think About . . .**	**My Observations**
KINSHIP *Relationships among group members*	Who makes the decisions? What is the role of adults, children, and the elderly? What are the responsibilities of the group members? What types of interactions occur between members of the group? What are some of the values in which the group members are socialized? What assumptions might scaffold kinship relations?	
ECONOMICS *Production and distribution of goods, services, and resources*	What goods and services are produced and distributed? What assumptions might scaffold the production, management, distribution, and use of goods and services? How are goods and services produced and distributed? (what process using which mechanism) What is the level of availability of goods and services in the group? What is the role of land? How is land obtained? Who has access and who uses land? What institutions exist? What are their functions? Who has access to these institutions?	
EDUCATION *Knowledge, skills, values of the group*	What is taught—content? What processes are used in education? What assumptions might scaffold the educational processes and content? What are the teaching methods? Who benefits from the teaching methods and content? Who has responsibility for teaching? What is the role or goals of education? Who has access to education? In which languages is education occurring? Who uses which languages? What role does literacy play in the group/society/family/culture?	
POLITICS *Exercise of power from above and below* *Instruments of coercion and consensus*	How is power distributed? What assumptions might scaffold this distribution process? Who has power? What are the decision-making processes? Who participates? How are they organized? Who benefits from decision-making processes and outcomes? Who participates in the carrying out or execution of decisions?	

continues

Observation Context →		
Category	**Think About . . .**	**My Observations**
RELIGION *Belief systems*	What are the belief-based practices? What assumptions might scaffold these beliefs and practices? What role does religion play in the daily life?	
ASSOCIATIONS *Grouping within the cultural group (e.g., clubs)*	What groups exist in the group/society/community/culture? How did these groups form? Why did they form? What is the relationship between/among groups? Who benefits from intergroup associations? What role do these groups play in the larger group/society/community/culture?	
HEALTH *Wellness/illness models*	What diseases exist? Why do they exist? What are health practices? What is considered health? Who benefits from health practices? Who has access to health practices? Who administers health care? How is food developed and distributed? Who has access to food? What assumptions undergird health and food practices?	
LEISURE *Unscheduled time*	What leisure activities occur? Who participates in leisure activities? Who benefits from these activities? What assumptions undergird the leisure activities?	
TRANSPORTATION *Movement from one location to another*	What are the means of transportation? Who benefits from transportation? Who does the transporting? Who gets transported? What are the underlying assumptions about the relevance/importance/use of transportation? What role does transportation play?	
COMMUNICATION SYSTEMS	How is communication conveyed? What is communicated? What languages are used? Who can communicate on a wide scale? Who benefits from what is communicated and the communication process?	

Source: Based on Peace Corps (1986).

Appendix 7–2
Artifact Analysis Form

MATERIAL

1.	What is the artifact?	
2.	What is it made of/from?	
3.	How is it constructed?	

HISTORY

4.	Who made the artifact?	
5.	When was it made?	
6.	When was it used?	
7.	Why was it made?	
8.	Who is/was the intended user?	
9.	Where did it come from?	
10.	What is an item with which you are familiar that is similar to this artifact?	
11.	How did/does the artifact connect groups of people?	
12.	What values are reflected in this artifact?	

ENVIRONMENT

13.	What meaning does this artifact acquire in the micro context of its existence?	
14.	What meaning does this artifact acquire in the macro context of its existence?	
15.	What does this artifact tell us about those who use/made this artifact?	
16.	What does this artifact tell us about the technology of the time in which the artifact was made/used?	

continues

SIGNIFICANCE

17.	How significant is this artifact in the life of those who made/used it?	
18.	What values are reflected through this artifact?	
19.	How did the meaning of the artifact change over time?	

INTERPRETATION

20.	What else do I need/want to know about this artifact to help me understand the group that I am serving?	
21.	What questions would I ask those who owned/made/used this artifact, if I could?	

CONNECTIONS

22.	What sources do I need to consult to find out information about this artifact?	
23.	How does this artifact connect with other artifacts from this same group?	

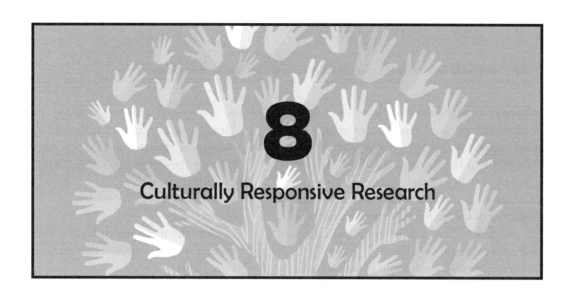

8

Culturally Responsive Research

Research is the systematic investigation of an issue, problem, or question, which is designed to produce generalizable knowledge. In this chapter, we examine the concept of knowledge and the type of knowledge (or epistemological frames) that has traditionally been the reference point in the United States. We examine the concept of research, and what it means to engage in culturally responsive research. Discussions of practice based on evidence have been prominent in the speech-language pathology literature since the late 1990s. As part of these discussions, levels of evidence have been identified, which suggests that not all evidence (i.e., research) is equal (American Speech-Language-Hearing Association [ASHA], 2017). These levels of evidence represent a "formal system of categorizing" research based on the study design, quality, and relevance (ASHA, 2017). The levels of evidence promoted by ASHA are presented in Table 8–1.

This focus on various levels of evidence, and the perception that research with higher levels of evidence (Level Ia or Ib) have more rigor and are therefore better, has failed to

TABLE 8–1. Levels of Evidence

Strongest Evidence	Ia	Well-designed meta-analysis of more than one randomized controlled trial
	Ib	Well-designed randomized controlled study
	IIa	Well-designed controlled study without randomization
	IIb	Well-designed quasi-experimental study
	III	Well-designed nonexperimental studies (i.e., correlational and case studies)
Weakest Evidence	IV	Expert committee report, consensus conference, clinical experience of respected authorities

Source: Adapted with permission from ASHA (1997–2017). *Assessing the evidence.* Retrieved from http://www.asha.org/Research/EBP/Assessing-the-Evidence/

include discussions about the extent to which these more "rigorous" research studies are culturally responsive (Bal & Trainor, 2016).

Some of the history regarding the role that research has played in communities of color, as well as research ethics, is reviewed. Examples of culturally responsive research in the professions of speech-language pathology and audiology will be addressed. We end the chapter with a discussion about potential barriers that diverse populations face with regard to participating in research projects and provide some suggestions of how culturally responsive research can be effectively implemented.

LEARNING OBJECTIVES

After reading, discussing and processing the information presented in this chapter, you will be able to demonstrate the following knowledge, skills, and attitudes:

1. Knowledge
   a. To explain micro, meso, and macro levels of analysis that can be used to engage in systematically examining language and hearing development and use
   b. To explain the importance of critical self-reflection for becoming a more culturally responsive researcher
   c. To discuss the role that scientific racism has had in the poor reputation of research within communities of color
   d. To describe the relationship between culture and epistemologies
2. Skills
   a. Construct a culturally responsive research project beginning with the conceptualization of the research question(s) to the dissemination of the research findings
   b. Review current research produced in the fields of speech-language

pathology and audiology, and identify: (a) elements of culturally responsive research, and (b) ways to increase these elements within that published research
   c. Construct a culturally responsive research project
   d. Identify the three principles of human subjects research that minimize harm
3. Attitudes
   a. Demonstrate through journaling an appreciation and respect for various types of knowledges/epistemologies
   b. Demonstrate an ability to value how culture mediates research practices
   c. Recognize the relevance of culturally responsive research
   d. Recognize the importance of research ethics

KEY CONCEPTS

Key concepts addressed in this chapter are presented in Table 8–2.

"WHOSE KNOWLEDGE IS IT ANYWAY?"

We start this section with a question that is part of a title for a recent publication, "*Rethinking education: Whose knowledge is it anyway?*" (Unwin & Yandell, 2016). This question sheds light on an important issue underlying research in terms of which epistemologies are valued, and which ones are not. Epistemology refers to a division of philosophy that focuses on the study of knowledge and truth (Bradley, 2015). Eurocentric ways of knowing or epistemologies primarily have been the focus of research (Ladson-Billings, 2003: Romm, 2015), particularly in the fields of speech-

TABLE 8–2. Key Concepts

Action research	Macro level of research analysis
Critical self-reflection	
Cultural institutions	Meso level of research analysis
Culturally responsive research (CRR)	Micro level of research analysis
	Participatory action research
Epistemology	Research
Levels of evidence	

language pathology and audiology. These ways of knowing privilege the ways Western males think (Grosfoguel, 2012, p. 83), while other ways of knowing—feminist epistemologies (Anderson, 2000), epistemologies from the perspective of members of lesbian, gay, bisexual, transgender, queer, intersexual, asexual (LGBTQIA) communities, and "indigenous" (Smith, 2005) or "ethnic" epistemologies (Ladson-Billings, 2003, p. 398) have not always been included in U.S. educational institutions. When these ways of thinking have been included in U.S. curricula, they are often included as fringe or marginal ideas (Grosfoguel, 2012). Ladson-Billings (2003) states that the differences between Eurocentric and "ethnic" epistemologies depend on whether the "individual mind is the source of knowledge and existence" (p. 398) or whether knowledge is "contingent on relationships with others" (p. 398)—that is, whether knowledge is created individually or within and among groups.

In Chapter 3 we mentioned some epistemologies that have been excluded in research, particularly in speech, language, and hearing sciences. The scholars associated with those ways of thinking focused on macro level units of analysis (policies, social structures, and global forces) and knowledge created among groups, rather than on meso level (groups and communities) or micro level (individual) units of analysis. Focusing on macro level factors is important in providing services in the current global context in which we exist.

The macro level involves larger systems of interaction, such as those at the global level or interactions between local and global actors. These interactions include systems of relations locally (within one country) and globally (among countries), but are distant and external to those engaged in research (Blackstone, 2012; Wylie et al., 2013). When we use macro level structures, we are referring to the social structures, at the local and global level, that affect the daily lives of everyone, including those with communication disabilities. Note that social structures, the system of social arrangements and relations within a society, can also occur at the micro level (norms of individual behavior for example) and meso level (relationships between individuals and organizations as an example).

At the macro level, researchers examine social structures (i.e., politics, culture and cultural institutions,[1] economics, and state violence) that affect populations and/or people in a country, and/or global processes that affect international relations among countries (Blackstone, 2012). An audiologist conducting

---

[1]Cultural institutions serve the function of maintaining the culture (i.e., values, beliefs, assumptions) of those with power in a society, and they include schools, the media, the family, churches, and the legal system (Gramsci, 1971).

macro level research may engage in a comparative study of the consequences of globalization on hearing aid availability and accessibility in several different countries. A speech-language pathologist (SLP) working at the macro level may investigate the way cultural institutions in the world affect help-seeking behaviors of persons with communication disabilities in various countries in the world. Macro level inquires may also include examination or review of global documents, such as the World Health Organization International Classification of Functioning, Disability, and Health (WHO-ICF), World Report on Disability, or SLP and audiologist practices in various country contexts (Wylie et al., 2013), and the way these global documents inform services.

The meso level refers to a focus on groups, interactions among group members or between different groups (Blackstone, 2012), such as the interactions among male preschoolers or between male and female preschoolers; or among different-aged children with autism or between children with autism and their typically developing same-aged peers. Meso level is composed of phenomena that are external to the researchers, but close in proximity, such as national government policies, community needs, and national organizations such as ASHA or the American Academy of Audiology (AAA) (Wylie et al., 2013). For example, a SLP researcher conducting a meso level analysis may compare the development of pragmatics between children with autism and those with histories of maltreatment who are being schooled in the same city district. In an article by Wylie et al. (2013), examples of meso level processes based on World Report on Disability recommendations included government policy promoting service equity, and the role of national organizations (ASHA) in government decision making about programs and services (p. 10). At the meso level, researchers examine interactions within a community or region of a coun-

try—that is, interactions within and between groups (Blackstone, 2012).

The micro level can be conceptualized in a variety of ways, but we are using it to refer to the smallest circle of influence that a SLP or audiologist may have in the life of an individual. Micro level practice focuses on individuals and families. At the micro level, a SLP or audiologist will approach his or her role as one whose primary responsibility is to facilitate language, speech, communication, swallowing, or hearing for an individual to be successful in the various contexts in which that individual exists. Examples of SLP or audiologist practice at the micro level include collecting case histories from individuals and their family members; assessing individuals in various contexts, while focusing on the behavior, language, speech, or communication or hearing of the individual, and intervening with an individual in the context of clinic, hospital, school, academic classroom, or home. The micro level can even be reduced into smaller components such as focusing on assessment or intervention at the sound (phonological), word (morphological), or sentence level (Nelson, 2010; Nelson, Bahr & Van Meter, 2004), or considering the use of communication skills while interacting with others on a day-to-day basis (Nelson, 2010; Simmons-Mackie, 2014).

All living beings interact at all three levels simultaneously (Van Wormer & Besthorn, 2017), but focusing on and incorporating the macro level concerns into the work of SLPs and audiologists is grossly underrepresented in the speech-language pathology and audiology literature and curricula (Wickenden, 2013). SLPs and audiologists currently have a strong focus and robust skills focused on micro level changes through individual or small group assessments or interventions. To affect a true change in the lives of people with communication disabilities, it is important to also address macro level issues (Centers for Disease Control, 2017; Wickenden, 2013). This step of learning about, understanding, thinking about, and managing macro level issues is unavoidable, particularly if you want to be a culturally responsive researcher and service provider.

Utilizing or understanding and analyzing an issue at various levels helps us have a holistic interpretation of an issue (or practice), and can be useful in guiding future action, or policy development (Caldwell & Mays, 2012). The world is a complex organism. Thinking about micro, meso, and macro levels provides a framework for understanding how the individuals, organizations, communities, policies, as well as local and global social structures affect each other (WHO, 2002). Figure 8–1 is a simplified visual representation of the interaction between these different levels.

Research occurring at each of the levels mentioned above would lead to more culturally responsive practices. Epistemologies (ways of knowing) drive which research questions are asked, the theoretical frameworks used, which research methods are implemented, the nature of evidence, and how research results are interpreted. For SLPs and audiologists engaged in developing and implementing culturally responsive practices, being able to employ culturally responsive research is essential, which means thinking in a new way about research (Romm, 2003). This new way of thinking about research includes advancing epistemologies and methodologies that will be more consistent with the values, beliefs, assumptions, and worldview of those being served by the professions of speech-language pathology and audiology (Chilisa, 2012). Next is a discussion regarding conducting research with communities of color.

HISTORY OF RESEARCH WITH COMMUNITIES OF COLOR AND SCIENTIFIC RACISM

First Nations, African American, and Latin@/Hispanic communities have had a difficult history with being the subjects of research. These groups in particular in the United States have been victims of "scientific racism" (Schanche Hodge, 2012, p. 431). Research within these communities, historically, has been linked to

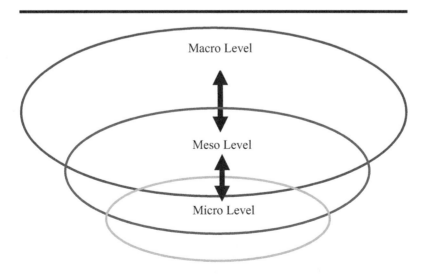

FIGURE 8–1. Interconnectedness of micro, meso, and macro levels.

colonialism, capitalism, imperialism, racialization, and demonization of groups thought about as being "different" (Gans, 2017; Smith, 1999). (Refer to Table 8–3 for definitions of these terms.)

This past research resulted in members of these communities being described as deficient, which served to justify their exploitation and to maintain the existing social order (Castagna & Sefa Dei, 2000). This justification has been prevalent throughout the history of the United States. One of the founding fathers of the United States, Thomas Jefferson, wrote that "all men were created equal," but believed otherwise. When speaking of the persons he himself enslaved, he stated, "Negro inferiority was obvious, [and] the criteria by which it might be established would have to be determined by science" (Graves, 2001, p. 42).

It is important to keep this history in mind so that it is not repeated. Currently, during this period of globalization, there is increased movement among people from disparate parts of the world. This means that refugees, migrants, and people of diverse cultural (including religious) practices and worldviews come into contact with each other. These groups are often presented as "dangers to national identity, well-being, safety and security" (Gans, 2017, p. 341). In the United States, for example, this very discussion is occurring from the current federal administration (2017) with regard to migrants, people who are of Arab descent, and people who practice religions other than Christianity. It seems that some of the ideas that support scientific racism are "creeping back" into the thinking in the United States (Byrd & Hughey, 2015).

In addition to people from communities of color in the United States being labeled as deficient when compared to White middle-class populations, there is a history of limited trust for researchers among communities of color. This lack of trust, or mistrust, stems from the ways that communities of color have been used, misused, and represented (or misrepresented) by researchers. The following are only a few of the thousands of examples available to make this point:

- Smallpox-infected blankets were distributed among First Nations communities by the British (1756–1763) to deliberately exterminate this group (Schange Hodge, 2012).
- In the early 1900s to treat trachoma, an eye disease, First Nations groups were

TABLE 8–3. Definitions of Colonialism, Capitalism, Imperialism, and Racialization

Concept	Definition
Imperialism	The expansion of one country's control over another.
Colonialism	Colonialism is a process that is part of imperialism, where one country gains control over another country and occupies that country with settlers from the country doing the colonizing.
Capitalism	An economic system that is based on private property, private ownership of profit-making apparatuses, and profit.
Racialization	Negative characteristics (behaviors, values, and worldviews) are attributed to groups considered to be outside of what a society may consider as normal (Gans, 2017).

Note. Colonialism, capitalism, and imperialism are discussed in the literature as being inseparable because capitalism is the driver of colonialism and imperialism (Amin, 2006).

subjected to the removal of eyelids, when with other groups eye washes and blood-letting were the typical treatment (Schange Hodge, 2012).

- In the 1920s and 1930s approximately 1/3 of all the women in Puerto Rico had been sterilized without their knowledge or through coercion (Denis, 2015).
- In the 1970s thousands of First Nations women and girls were sterilized without their knowledge or consent (Schange Hodge, 2012).
- For 40 years the United States funded researchers who studied the progression of syphilis in black male sharecroppers in Alabama. The men were told they were receiving a drug for their illness—they were not. They were also not given the appropriate drug to cure their illness when it became available (Tuskegee Study of Untreated Syphillis).
- In 1951 cells were taken from an impoverished female African American tobacco farmer without her knowledge or consent. These cells became the most important material for developing advances in medicine including the development of the polio vaccine, cloning, gene mapping, in vitro fertilization, and cures for certain cancers (Skloot, 2010). Although these cells were used to make these significant medical advancements, and others have profited from them, Henrietta Lacks' family has not, as of today.
- The United States Navy conducted tests with bombs and chemical weapons on the island of Vieques, which is part of Puerto Rico. People living on the island suffer 30% higher cancer rates than other Puerto Ricans, 381% higher rates of hypertension, 95% higher rates of cirrhosis, and 41% high rates of diabetes (Wheeler, 2010).
- Many English language learners have been immersed in English-only classrooms although research suggests that is not the

best way to acquire another language. It is important to build on the language in which the child is most proficient since language and literacy skills in one language transfer to the other (Mahendra & Namazi, 2014).

We have come a long way from research abuses occurring so frequently, although they still occur, particularly with respect to groups from cultural and linguistic, religious, and national backgrounds different from the researcher. The history of these and other abuses, however, remains strong in the historical memories of cultural groups, which facilitates the mistrust of some cultural groups of "research." These abuses can be minimized by engaging in culturally responsive research (CRR). In the next section, we explore the meaning of CRR.

CULTURALLY RESPONSIVE RESEARCH (CRR)

Culturally responsive research (CRR) "attempts to equalize the power between researchers and participants as they work collaboratively throughout the research process" (Berryman, SooHoo, & Nevin, 2013, p. 17). An essential component of CRR is to learn *from* research participants, how to best support the participants (Berryman et al., 2013).

In speech-language and hearing sciences, randomized controlled trials (RCTs) are considered one of the highest levels of evidence, which provoke perceptions that these types of trials produce "the most valid, reliable, and thus generalizable" knowledge (ASHA, 2017; Burns, Rohrich, & Chung, 2011; Trainor & Bal, 2014, p. 203) for every group. Trainor and Bal (2014) raise questions about RCTs and their relationship to culturally responsive research (CRR). They state that "the extant scholarship in special education has yet to amass robust knowledge that addresses the strengths and needs of the racial/ethnic, linguistic, and economic diversity present in U.S. classrooms and society" (p. 204). This same argument can be declared about scholarship in speech, language, and hearing sciences. All aspects of research are culturally mediated and situated beginning with the theoretical approach used to develop the question through to the dissemination of the results (Arzubiaga, Artiles, King, & Harris-Murri, 2008; Ford, 2010; Ford, Moore, Whiting, & Grantham, 2008). Surprisingly, few researchers explicitly mention engaging in CRR (Ford, 2010; Ford, Moore, Whiting, & Granthan, 2008).

CRR requires attending to the contextual factors (such as those outlined in the WHO-ICF, as well as social structures, policies, cultural practices) and how persons involved in the research negotiate these contexts (Trainor & Bal, 2014). It requires the use of theory and multiple methods that can manage the complexity of conducting research at the macro, meso, and micro levels (Trainor & Bal, 2014). CRR is conducted from multiple theoretical perspectives, not just from a medical model or from European or Western epistemological traditions (Berryman et al., 2013). It can include theories that value multiple ways of knowing, relational or collective ways of knowing such as feminism (Berryman et al., 2013), Queer theory (Browne & Nash, 2016), decolonizing (Smith, 1999) or ethnic (Ladson-Billings, 2003) methodologies, or African humanism (Collins, 2000)—which would be categorized as excluded intellectual traditions (see Chapter 3), particularly in the field of communication sciences and disorders. One basic commonality between these excluded traditions is that they use a critical approach, which means that researchers deconstruct the status quo, and acknowledge the role that social structures, unequal relations of power, and cultural practices play in behaviors and developmental processes. For CRR to be carried out and effective, it is important for researchers to understand how social structures affect the communities in which the research is taking place so that the research results can be applied broadly. This means understanding how macro and meso level factors affect communities and people with disabilities. Trainor and Bal (2014) identify several characteristics of CRR:

1. It requires a focus on personal experiences, cultural practices, and assumptions that researchers bring to study, in addition to the principle of combining research practice to applicable theory (Trainor & Bal, 2014); in other words, researchers approach projects recognizing that "knowledge is subjective, and value-laden" (Ford, 2010, p. 26; Hyter, 2014).

2. It utilizes theories and methodologies that have been developed for diverse cultural and linguistic groups, and have been shown to be relevant for the population being investigated (Ford, 2010, p. 26). For SLPs and audiologists, this means identifying theories that are beyond the ones usually relied upon (those that emerge from positivism), to theories that come from interpretivism, critical frameworks, or social theories of transformation (Santiago-Valles, 2005), utilizing methods such as participatory action research, ethnomethodology, ethnography, and conversational analysis.

3. It focuses on research questions that go beyond the interests of the researchers, to include the interests of the participating community members (Ladson-Billings & Tate, 2006), and includes members of the participating

community from the inception of the research—from conceptualization of the study to interpretation of the results.

4. It focuses on social structures and their influence on diverse cultural and linguistic groups (Ford, 2010), such as going beyond micro levels of research and focusing on human rights. In SLP research and audiology, a focus on human rights will engage more with the WHO-ICF (WHO, 2001), and the UN Convention on the Rights of People with Disabilities (UN, 2006) (Wickenden, 2013). The WHO-ICF (WHO, 2001) connects all aspects of disabilities, and how disabilities affect all aspects of a peoples' lives at the macro, meso, and micro levels (Wickenden, 2013).

5. It approaches research from an emic position (insider perspectives from inside the cultural group), not just an etic one (outsider perspectives from outside of the cultural group) (DeJarnette, Rivers, & Hyter, 2015), and utilizes the language of the participants (Ford, 2010). For example, a SLP conducting research to identify types of speech acts produced by young African American English–speaking children would examine the children's communication for speech acts reported in the literature as being produced in the African American English–speaking community. Such speech acts include those identified, for example, by DeJarnette (2009), Hyter (2000), Kochman (1972), Mitchell-Kernan (1972, 1973, 1989), Morgan (2002), Percelay, Monteria, and Dweck (1994), Rickford and Rickford (2000), Smitherman (1977, 2000), and Stockman et al. (2008), rather than only those identified by Dore (1974, 1975, 1977, 1978), Halliday (1975), and Tough (1977).

6. It includes sufficient numbers of participants from a range of cultural and linguistic backgrounds.

7. It includes instruments, assessments, data collection procedures, and interventions that have been demonstrated to be culturally responsive, which is connected to approaching research from an emic perspective.

8. It includes practices and behaviors on the part of the researchers that are transparent, such as being open about the histories that the researchers bring to the interpretation of the research results (Berryman et al., 2013), which allows trust to be developed between the researchers and the members of the community participating in the research endeavor.

9. It results in meso and macro level outcomes in addition to micro level outcomes, which are more likely to affect outcomes at the societal level, not just the individual level, such as changes in policies and practices. At the meso level it might include SLPs and audiologists urging their professional associations to provide input at the national level regarding insurance provisions for people with disabilities. At the macro level, international research agendas sponsored by a collaboration of professional organizations could contribute powerful data and tools to ensure communication disability is recognized. This process could drive change in practice and research (Wylie, 2013, p. 11).

10. It considers multiple worldviews and explanations for results (Ford et al., 2008, p. 89). Being able to make this consideration is dependent on the theoretical frames that guide the research endeavor. The theories that

lend themselves to being able to be used for considering multiple worldviews and explanations are those associated with interpretivism, the critical theories, and many of those that are considered as excluded intellectual traditions, as discussed in Chapter 3.

THE NECESSITY OF CRR

There has been a long history of discriminatory practices in research. These practices can be traced back to the 1800s, many of which occurred at the hands of persons who were doctors. Spitz (2005, p. xvi) outlines several heinous experiments that took place in the United States during the 1800s:

- Thomas Hamilton, a doctor in Georgia, put an enslaved person in a pit oven to study heat stroke.
- A doctor in Virginia (Walter Jones) poured scalding hot water over enslaved persons who were sick in order to determine if that would cure typhoid fever (Spitz, 2005).
- J. Marion Sims practiced an operation on enslaved women in Alabama, resulting in a cure for a birth-related condition that caused a continuous flow of urine from the vagina.
- Ephraim McDowell from Kentucky practiced removing ovaries from enslaved women.
- Crawford Long of Georgia, examining the way anesthesia worked, cut off two fingers of a young child. One finger was cut off with the use of ether, and the other was cut off without any anesthesia.

In 1924 German researchers were scolded in the literature by F. Lenz for "falling so far behind America in exploiting genetic knowledge in the interest of racial hygiene" (p. xix). Racial hygiene is a gentle name for eugenics, the science of trying to modify human genetic outcomes. There was a eugenics movement in the United States that was funded by Andrew Carnegie, the Rockefeller Foundation, and heavily supported by John H. Kellogg (of the cereal company) (Samaan, 2012). The foundation of the Nazi's ideas about a "master race" was based on the research occurring in the United States around eugenics. When Hitler became chancellor of Germany in 1933, he enacted a required sterilization law for persons with cognitive impairments, mental illnesses, epilepsy and alcoholism, and persons who were "coloured[2]" (Spitz, 2005). Between 1933 and 1945, Germany committed atrocities under the guise of experimentation. Table 8–4 includes a limited list of harm committed through research before and after federal law was enacted in 1974 to regulate research development and implementation, and to protect research participants.

As you can see from the list above, discrimination in research has occurred throughout history, and across fields of study including in speech, language, and hearing sciences. One of the most well-known cases in the field of SLP was that of Wendell Johnson. Johnson was a psychologist and SLP with a special interest in semantics and stuttering. One of Johnson's master's thesis students conducted a study to determine if labeling a person a stutterer would cause the person to become disfluent (Manning, 2010). In this study, the 22 participants were members of an orphanage in Iowa. Half of this group of children was praised for their fluent speech, but the other

---

[2]Victims of Nazi Germany's concentration camps do not only include people who were Jewish but also those who were LGBTQIA, mentally ill, Sinti, Roma, and Black. Black Germans have never been publically memorialized and are rarely recognized as victims of the Holocaust (Carr, 2003).

TABLE 8–4. Research Harms Committee Throughout the Decades

Decade	Events
1930s	Tuskegee syphilis study; 600 Black men in Alabama who had syphilis but did not receive adequate treatment even when the cure became available; continued for 40 years The Monster Study by Wendell Johnson (see below)
1940s	German experimentation on Jewish, men, women, and children included, but was not limited to: • conducting bone transplants; • conducting head injury experiments where a child was hit on the head with a hammer repeatedly; • immersing people in cold water to study hypothermia; • studying malaria by infecting prisoners with malaria and then treating them with different drugs to test whether the drugs were effective or not; and • deliberately exposing prisoners to mustard gas, which left severe chemical burns. Infecting prisoners and persons with mental illnesses in Guatemala with syphilis. In Guatemala from 1946 to 1948, some research involved intentionally infecting over 1300 subjects with venereal diseases to test the effectiveness of penicillin. Only 700 subjects were given penicillin and 83 died as a result of the study. The subjects were not informed that they were participating in an experiment. Injected experimental flu vaccine into male patients at a state mental hospital in Ypsilanti, MI, then exposed them to flu later. Development of the Nuremberg Code outlining what one could and could not do legally when conducting experiments with human subjects.
1950s	When the Asian flu pandemic was spreading, federal researchers sprayed the virus in the noses of 23 inmates at a prison in Maryland to compare their reactions to those of 32 virus-exposed inmates who had been given a new vaccine. Government researchers attempted to infect 24 volunteering prison inmates with gonorrhea using two different methods in Atlanta. Many illiterate Puerto Rican women who did not speak English were used to test contraceptives before the drugs were determined to be safe by the U.S. Federal Drug Agency. CIA conducts mind control research studies using LSD in subjects who were not informed.
1960s	The Willowbrook Study took place at a state school for children with cognitive impairments. The children were intentionally given hepatitis C orally by feeding them the feces of infected children, and by injection to see if they could be cured. Researchers injected cancer cells into 19 debilitated patients at a Jewish Chronic Disease Hospital in New York. The goal was to determine if the bodies would reject the cancer cells. Helsinki Declaration published ethical principles for research on human subjects.
1970s	Milgram study—at Yale, where Stanley Milgram conducted experiments on administering electric shocks to others. The results of this study revealed that people are willing to do things that they consider wrong when given an order by an authority figure. Congress passes the National Research Act, authorizing federal agencies to develop human research regulations. The Belmont Report on ethical research using human subjects was released.

continues

179

TABLE 8–4. *continued*

Decade	Events
1980s	NASA was warned about possible O-ring failure, due to cold weather in the space shuttle Challenger. NASA decides to go ahead with the launch, and the Challenger explodes and kills the crew.
	Two agencies are formed, the Office of Scientific Integrity and the Office of Scientific Integrity Review for the purpose of investigating scientific misconduct.
	The National Institutes of Health require all graduate students on training grants to receive education in conducting responsible research.
1990s	U.S. funded doctors did not give AIDS drug (AZT) to all of the HIV-infected pregnant women in a study in Uganda, although the drug would have protected their newborn babies.
	Pfizer gave an antibiotic (Trovan) to children with meningitis in Nigeria, although there were doubts about this drug's effectiveness for that disease. It is thought that the experiment caused the deaths of 11 children and disabled many others.
2000s	High-profile researchers were accused of plagiarism or were found to fabricate and falsify data.
	The Environmental Protection Agency revised human subject rules in response to a congressional mandate to strengthen protections for children and pregnant or nursing women.
2010s	A fraudulent paper was published in 1998 by Andrew Wakefield and colleagues, linking autism to the measles vaccine. It was retracted in 2010.
	Researchers were able to genetically modify an H5N1 avian flu virus, so that it can be transmitted between mammals. This virus is lethal with a mortality rate of 60%.

Source: Based on Spitz (2005), Stobbe (2011), and Resnik (2017).

half was berated for their speech and called stutterers. The results were that typical speaking children who received the negative input experienced psychological stress and speech problems that occurred throughout their lives. The University of Iowa apologized to the victims' families in 2001 when the thesis was made public.

The case of Wendell Johnson and his student is clearly a problem; however, there are subtle problems in speech-language and hearing sciences. Most notably, there have been long-standing concerns about overrepresentation and underrepresentation of students of color and those who are English language learners on the caseloads of SLPs and on special education roster. Studies concerned about overrepresentation of children of color in special education have prompted federal legislation and policies focused on reducing "minority disproportionate representation" in special education (Fread Albrecht, Skiba, Losen, Choong-Geun, & Middleberg, 2011; Morgan et al., 2015; U.S. Department of Education, Office of Civil Rights, 2011). The literature on the reasons why children of color have been reported to be overrepresented in special education services includes institutionalized racism resulting in typical behaviors being characterized as disordered or deficient; schools' use of academic standards that are more in sync with middle-class White families' experiences, values, and worldviews; many children of color receive a lower quality education based on underfunding of schools in impoverished neighborhoods; or children of color have more exposure to biological and environmental toxins placing them at higher risk for cognitive impairments and academic challenges (Morgan et al., 2015). Explanations of underrepresentation of children of color in special education have included the limited access of families to special education services due to socioeconomic, linguistic, or cultural mismatches between family values and the educational institutions; and families preferring to receive support from extended family members rather than professionals. A recent study examining early childhood longitudinal data of 20,100 children who started school in 1998–1999, and who had data analyzed from their kindergarten, first, third, fifth, and eighth grades found that for this cohort, children of color were underrepresented in special education rather than overrepresented (Morgan et al., 2015). Whether children from diverse cultural and linguistic backgrounds are over- or underrepresented in special education services, including speech-language pathology and audiology, is inconsistently reported. We believe, however, that engaging in CRR and culturally responsive practices will help to mitigate the over- and underrepresentation of diverse populations in special education.

Research Compliance

When engaging in research, it is essential that research ethics are followed. The Human Subjects Institutional Review Board (HSIRB) review of research proposals is based on three principles: (a) respect for persons, (b) beneficence, and (c) justice (U.S. Department of Health and Human Services, 1979). Respect for persons is based on the assumption that people are autonomous, and vulnerable populations have a right to protection. For those who can make their own decisions, they should be provided with sufficient information about the research study for them to make an informed decision about whether to participate in the research study. For vulnerable populations, such as children, prisoners, or persons with diminished intellectual capacities, an advocate representing their best interest decides whether people from vulnerable groups will participate in the research study. This principle is applied through informed consent and assent protocols. Informed consent is when the person invited to participate in a research study, who is able to make his or her own decisions or who has a representative who makes decisions for him or her, voluntarily accepts the invitation. This acceptance occurs without coercion. Assent is what one who is too young to give consent (because they are not yet an adult) gives to demonstrate her or his willingness to participate in an activity.

Beneficence means that research participants will be treated ethically and will be treated in a manner that maximizes benefits and minimized harms. This principle is enacted when decisions of research participants are respected, and when researchers demonstrate concerns about the participants' safety through the implementation of a cost–risk analysis. The rule of thumb is that the research study should not cause harm, but if it does, only minimal harm. If the research study has the potential to result in some minimal harm to the participants, then the benefits of the research should be high. Beneficence extends beyond the research participants but to society at large; that is, the research outcomes should result in benefits for society, or a field of study, but not just an individual or small group of people.

Justice refers to the principle of equal distribution of benefits from the research study across socioeconomic, racial, cultural, gender, linguistic, and national boundaries. Research injustice occurs when some groups benefit from the research and other groups are excluded or when research is conducted only on one group (White middle-class men) resulting in limited information about typical development of members of other racial, cultural, and socioeconomic groups. This principle of justice also refers to when one group shoulders the burden of the research risks and this burden is not placed on others (a trial of a new high-risk medicine is studied in prisoners only rather than in various segments of the population).

ENGAGING IN CULTURALLY RESPONSIVE RESEARCH

Culturally responsive research is all-encompassing in that CRR methods run through each stage of a research project, from the theory that guides the research questions and methodologies, to the interpretation and dissemination of the results. Following, we discuss steps for how to engage in CRR. Then we review a research study published in 2009 by researchers who used CRR. We present this study as only one example of how CRR was infused into each stage of the research process.

Skills of CRR Researchers

To be a CRR investigator, it is important to first be willing to become more culturally responsive, which means participating in learning *throughout your lifetime* that results in knowledge, skills, behaviors, and dispositions that facilitate effective engagement across cultures, inclusion of diversity, and improved services and changed policies that are more effective in an intercultural context (Campinha-Bacote, 2002; Hyter, 2014). As discussed in Chapter 2, a significant aspect of

becoming more culturally responsive is engaging in critical self-reflection on a consistent basis over a lifetime (Ford, 2008). To be "critical," as it is used here, means to think beyond current reality to reevaluate one's knowledge, and to seek alternative ways of thinking, knowing, and meaning (Subedi, 2010). Self-reflection is the activity of assessing one's thoughts, knowledge, skills, behaviors, and perspectives, and it leads to self-awareness. When engaged in critical self-reflection, the researcher meticulously questions her or his own assumptions, challenging himself or herself to examine those assumptions from alternative viewpoints (Conner, Gallagher, & Ferri, 2011). Critical self-reflection is a powerful learning tool, as a person questions himself or herself with the ultimate goal of improving self-awareness as mentioned earlier, but also one's own knowledge, behaviors, and practice, and disposition toward social justice (Ford, 2008; Zeichner & Liu, 2010). Critical self-reflection is a skill that is fostered in the professions of speech-language pathology and education, for example, as it is a core component of developing and monitoring clinical competence and classroom teaching. Engaging in critical self-reflection will lead to the researcher being more aware of the assumptions that each party (researchers and participants), brings to the research experience (Trainor & Bal, 2014), and an awareness that assumptions and knowledge are culturally mediated and may differ among groups.

We are all cultural beings, even those of us engaged in research. All people have culture, which in this text is defined as the underlying assumptions, beliefs, and values that guide daily behaviors or practices. Culture permeates everything, including the conceptualization, methodologies, analysis, and interpretations of research. In short, the creation of knowledge—research—is "subjective, and value-laden" (Ford, 2010, p. 26; Hyter, 2014). Engaging in culturally responsive research is an acknowledgment "that the decisions we (researchers) make have power" (Ong, 2017). Following is a list of some of the questions that Ford et al. (2008) suggest researchers ask themselves before engaging in research that includes participants from cultural backgrounds different than the researcher:

1. How do I feel about working with individuals or groups that are different from me? What stereotypes, biases, and fears do I hold of other groups? How do these views affect my work including research questions hypotheses, literature review, instrument development or selection, data interpretation, and data use?

2. How are the expectations that I hold of diverse individuals/groups different from those of individuals in my own group?

3. How much time and effort am I willing to devote to learning about alternative theories and models associated with diverse groups? (p. 88)

In addition to being consistently engaged in critical self-reflection, developing cultural awareness is important for engaging in CRR. Researchers engaged in CRR make an effort to understand the perspective of the diverse groups being included in the research. If researchers engaged in the communities that they were involving in their research, some cultural awareness would develop. Some of the questions that researchers can ask themselves when being aware of the cultural groups with whom they are working include the following:

1. What is "race/culture," and how does it affect teaching and learning self-concept and racial identity (and the construct under investigation)?

2. What are the cultural beliefs, values, norms, and traditions of the diverse participants represented in my sample?

What cultural beliefs, values, norms, and traditions of the diverse participants are not represented in my sample? What are the socioeconomic (access to resources) and political (ability to exercise power in their own interests) characteristics of the participants represented in the research sample?

3. What data collection strategies/procedures are culturally compatible with the participants in the study? For example, do participants feel more comfortable with surveys or interviews? (Ford et al., 2008, p. 88)

Another characteristic of researchers engaged in CRR is that their experiments are approached from a disposition of social justice; that is, they make sure to include individuals from diverse cultural and linguistic backgrounds in their research projects, and make a conscious effort to promote social justice (Ford et al., 2008). In the "further reading" section of this chapter, we provide the title of a text that presents definitions of social justice based on theoretical frameworks.

Begin With a Theoretical Framework

As you continually operate from a posture of critical self-reflection, begin the conceptualization of the culturally responsive research project from a theoretical perspective. Remember that one goal of CRR is to produce knowledge *with* the research participants, which creates an equitable distribution of power between the researcher and those being researched (Berryman et al., 2013). (See Chapter 4 for a discussion on culture and power.) Theories that lend well to being utilized as a framework that guides culturally responsive research include those within the interpretivism (ethnomethodology and ethnography) and critical frames (Marxism, critical social theory). Although interpretivist theories are now more frequently incorporated into research in speech, language, and hearing sciences more than before, theories within the critical frames are seldom employed in these fields. We discussed the premises of the interpretivism and critical frameworks in Chapter 3. Here, we discuss some of the frameworks that were developed, adopted, or suggested by SLPs and audiologists living and working in majority world countries, or working with diverse communities in their home countries. These frameworks are critical consciousness (Freire, 1990; Hyter, 2008, 2014), political consciousness (Kathard & Pallay, 2013), sociocultural theory (Daniels, 2008; Rogoff, 2003), the biopsychosocial model (Engel, 1980), and a social theory of transformation or praxis (Santiago-Valles, 2005).

Critical Consciousness

Critical consciousness (or conscientização) is a concept popularized by Paulo Freire (1990), a Brazilian educator, theorist, and writer, who based it on Frantz Fanon's[3] (1952) concept of conscienciser. Critical consciousness is based in critical social theory (discussed in Chapter 3), and is the ability to question one's social, cultural, political, economic, and environmental situation. In other words, it includes understanding what macro level forces are, how these forces act in the world, and how they affect daily life, and includes the ability to take action against structures that exploit, dominate, or exclude (Freire, 1990). Hyter (2008, 2014) speaks of critical consciousness as imperative knowledge and skills needed to be culturally and globally responsive service providers. SLPs and audiologists approaching research endeavors using critical consciousness will be interested in examining all of the social structures that may affect (facilitate or hinder) communication processes.

Political Consciousness

Political consciousness is an aspect of critical consciousness. It is similar in that it facilitates examination of "how selected forces at the macro-level (policies), meso-level (professional knowledge) and microlevel (individual services) may enable or limit services to underserved majority" (Kathard & Pillay, 2013, p. 84) in order to provide more equitable services to underserved populations. It is different than critical consciousness in that it can be used to focus on political issues (i.e., unequal relations of power) rather than the broader social structures, which in addition to politics includes economics, culture (cultural institutions), and state-sanctioned violence (Hyter, 2014). Kathard and Pillay urge SLPs and audiologists to become political actors to effect change using an "equity driven population-based approach" (p. 88). SLPs and audiologists approaching research from a political consciousness perspective will be concerned about equity of research at all levels of interactions.

Sociocultural Approach

A sociocultural approach comes out of the work of Vygotsky and focuses on the human experience (Daniels, 2008). The primary premises of this approach are that: (a) human beings are "born into culturally organized worlds" (Daniels, 2008; Rogoff, 2003); (b) the meanings of experiences are derived from interactions with other people (Daniels, 2008); and (c) these social interactions take place within the context of cultural meanings (Daniels, 2008; Rogoff, 2003; Vygotsky, 1978). SLPs and audiologists using the sociocultural approach to concep-

---

[3] Frantz Fanon was born in Martinique and was an Afro-Caribbean psychiatrist.

tualize a research project will take into consideration the cultural meanings adopted by research participants, and the ways that those meanings were derived from interactions with other cultural actors within the participants' social communities.

Biopsychosocial Model

The biopsychosocial model (Engel, 1980; Harris, Fleming, & Harris, 2012; Penn, 2002) acknowledges contextual factors as included in the WHO-ICF. Specifically, people who use this model recognize the relationship between social factors (relationships, socioeconomic issues, cultural practices) and health outcomes including access to health care and health disparities (Harris et al., 2012), which can be extended to speech, language, and hearing outcomes. The biopsychosocial model can be used to validate "the knowledge, experiences and values of individuals regarding their own wellbeing and health" (Harris et al., 2012, p. 42). SLPs and audiologists approaching research from a biopsychosocial model will be interested in questions focused on the relationship between social determinants of health and speech, language, and hearing outcomes.

Social Theory of Transformation (Praxis)

Santiago-Valles (2005) defines the social theory of transformation as praxis. *Praxis* is a term that emerges from Marxism and Critical Social Theory, and was used by Paulo Freire (1970) to refer to the collective reflection and action on the world (i.e., social structures that exploit, dominate, or exclude) in order to transform the world (Freire, 1970, p. 36). It is important to note that reflection without action is not praxis; similarly, activism without critical reflection is not praxis. Both critical reflection and action are required for praxis to exist (Freire, 1970, p. 52). One is engaged in praxis when a theory (or idea or skill) is tried out collectively (i.e., not individually), then reflected on critically, changed based on the collective critical reflection, and then reenacted taking into consideration the changes made as a result of the critical reflection (Freire, 1970; Santiago-Valles, 2005). Researchers approaching problems using praxis focus on critically evaluating social structures affecting daily life, raising the consciousness of others about unequal relations of power (exposing unequal relations of power), and then engaging in activities with others to transform those unequal relations of power. In this vein, SLPs and audiologists approaching research from the perspective of a social theory of transformation will focus on the unequal relations of power resulting from communication disabilities, and ways to help others realize those inequities, and then working with others such as community members, to transform the structures causing the inequities or inequalities.

Researcher Team

To engage in CRR, ideally, we would put together a research team of people from diverse cultural and linguistic backgrounds, but also various disciplinary backgrounds. These co-researchers, including those who are members of the community where the project takes place, will be able to bring a range of viewpoints to the assumptions that undergird the research methods, research analyses, and interpretation of results (Ashing-Giwa, & Kagawa-Singer, 2006; Bal & Trainor, 2016).

Criteria for Inclusion/Exclusion of Research Participants

When devising criteria for inclusion and/or exclusion from a research project, to be more culturally responsive is to include details about the rationale for the inclusion or exclusion of individuals from diverse cultural and linguistic backgrounds. When these inclusion criteria have been presented, they include information that goes beyond racial and language characteristics. There should be some discussion of differences among participants regarding such factors as living conditions (socioeconomic status and social interactions), access to resources (economics), and abilities to take decisions in their own interest (politics or power). Thinking about these characteristics will help "maximize" the incorporation of people from diverse cultural and linguistic groups as participants in research endeavors (Bal & Trainor, 2016).

Research Purpose and Research Questions

In CRR the purpose of the research should go beyond the personal or professional interests of the researchers and the researchers' fields of study. The research purpose should include the strengths, interests, and needs of the participants and their communities (Bal & Trainor, 2016). A concern for the community and the issues in which the community members are interested, can facilitate research studies that are conceptually and methodologically responsive to the participating populations, resulting in more effective collaborations between the researchers and communities (Ashing-Giwa & Kagawa-Singer, 2006). SLPs and audiologists engaged in CRR will develop research projects that directly address concerns of those participating in the research project, and produce deliverable benefits to the participants' communities (Ashing-Giwa & Kagawa-Singer, 2005, 2006).

As an example, Dr. Hyter and some colleagues (Veeck, Veeck, Hyter, & Santiago-Valles, 2004) conducted three focus groups and over 10 hours of interviews with Latin@s/

Hispanics living in Southwest Michigan. They talked about the concerns of participants regarding economic problems, and issues associated with the maintenance of their cultural practices, racism, racial profiling, minimal representation at levels of the government, and lack of social services appropriate for their families (Veeck et al., 2004, p. 30). Once data were analyzed, the researchers reported the data to the community during a community meeting, where study participants, community members, government officials, public school administrators, and faculty from the local universities were present, resulting in the City Council expanding policy decisions regarding the Latin@/Hispanic population. The overall outcomes were less than hoped for, but it was a start to continuing conversations and negotiations between the community and the government officials charged with meeting the needs of all of the community members. This example utilizes participatory action research (PAR), which is one of the more prominent methods used in CRR in addition to ethnographic methods (which was discussed in Chapter 7). PAR has a particular history of being more sensitive to cultural diversity and is already part of the history of activist scholarship in countries around the world including those in Africa and Latin America (Fals-Borda, 2006; Zavala, 2013). In PAR, the research participants become the co-researchers in that they have active roles in the conceptualization of the study and the development of the research question, and the collection, analysis, and interpretation of data (Becvar & Srinivasan, 2009; Berryman et al., 2013; Gallagher et al., 2011).

Other aspects of the research project presented in Table 8–5 have been adapted from Bal and Trainor's (2016) rubric for CRR as well as other literature focused on the components of CRR (Ashing-Giwa & Kagawa-Singer, 2006; Bal & Trainor, 2016; Trainor & Bal, 2014).

TABLE 8–5. Components of Culturally Responsive Research

Review of the literature	It is important for the literature review to discuss alternative conceptualization of the research problem and the corresponding concepts being investigated.
Collecting research data	To collect research data, a relationship among the researchers and the communities in which the research is taking place is important (Bal & Trainor, 2016). This relationship will help to develop trust among community members and researchers.
Data collection instruments	Instruments for data collection should be valid and reliable for diverse populations. The constructs measured should be relevant for the participating groups. Instruments that are translated should meet specifications for linguistic equivalence (the translation and backtranslation to ensure accurate translation of items), functional equivalence (similar meanings across translations allowing analysis of the same construct in both languages), cultural equivalence (similar interpretations of items across languages), and metric equivalence (same level of item difficulty across measures) (Peña, 2007).
Data collection methodologies	Multiple data collection and analysis procedures can be used within the same study—that is, conduct qualitative and quantitative methods. Qualitative research methods are used to examine and analyze expository information that does not include numbers. For example, analyzing data from interviews, focus group data, artifacts and documents, diaries, observations, and conversation groups would be considered qualitative analyses. Quantitative research methods use numerical data that are changed into statistics. Quantitative methods include test scores and surveys with Likert scales. Additionally, engaging in participant action research is important for equalizing the role of the researchers and co-researchers (also referred to as study participants). There are activities on the companion website that focus on participation action research.
Data analysis and interpretation	Ideally the participants and other stakeholders will be involved in the data analysis and interpretation and the decision making based on the outcome of the research study. For example, focus groups made up of the research participants can be helpful in clarifying findings, interpreting the meaning of the findings in the context of their communities, generating new hypotheses, and identifying ways that the outcomes can be realistically applied to their communities. The goal of the research outcomes should have translational utility to the communities participating in the research study (Ashing-Giwa & Kagawa-Singer, 2006).
Dissemination of study results	Dissemination of culturally responsive research will be made to the scientific/professional community of the researchers via publications and/ or presentations, but should also be disseminated to the community of the study participants in forms that are widely accessible. This community should include all stakeholders including government officials, educators, parents, participants, health care providers, and advocacy organizations. The dissemination of the research outcomes ideally will result in a benefit to the community. Data disseminated to the community can be constructed in several ways such as a community meeting (as in the example about Hyter's research reported earlier), or pamphlets being distributed in various community venues, via a community-wide conference, or to a community advisory board or neighborhood association.

Box 8–1 presents a summary of a study conducted in 2003 by Deborah Hwa Froe- lich and Carol Westby. This research study is a good example of CRR in action. As you review the summary in Box 8–1, identify the components of the study that match the aspects of CRR discussed in this chapter. After you finish reviewing and making notes about the summary, read the original study. What additional aspects of CRR as discussed in this chapter could be added? How might those pieces be added?

Box 8–1

Purpose: To gain information regarding how Southeast Asian parents, children, and Head Start staff make sense of early childhood education, their roles in child learning, and the identification of disabilities or learning problems (p. 299). The problem being addressed by this study was why Southeast Asian children are not readily referred for special education services.

Theory: Ethnomethodology

Data Collection Methods: Ethnographic methods include semistructured inter- views, observations, and document analysis[4] (of the literature given to parents by Head Start). (Ethnographic methods were introduced in Chapter 7.) Multiple methods of data collection and multiple sources of data were used. The researchers addressed reliability and validity of data by examining confirmability (through participant confirmation of the semantic content of interviews, for example); credibility (based on the expertise of the researchers, and rigorous data collection); transferability (based on the "quality meth- odological design," the use of "multiple methodologies and data sources to develop a "thick" description of . . . perspectives" [p. 305]); and dependability (based on the use of multiple methodologies, and fidelity of data analysis) (pp. 304–305).

Data Analysis: Examination of the data (interviews, observations, documents) resulted in the revelation of four domains regarding the way education, parenting, child learning and disability, and discipline were conceptualized among the parents of Southeast Asian children, and the Head Start staff.

Outcomes: The data and results of the analysis were interpreted through Hofstede's (2011) cultural dimensions of independence/interdependence and power/distance relationships, resulting in a summary of assumptions that revealed possible reasons why the children were not being referred for special education services. Based on the assumptions identified through this study, the researchers stated that "Because of the Head Start organizational underlying assumptions about parents as equal partners and the contrasting cultural values of independence/interdependence and power/distance relationships, Southeast Asian children were not identified as having learning problems and consequently, did not receive special education services."

---

[4]Note that the authors referred to the Head Start documents as "artifacts."

IMAGINE

The Beatles were a famous singing group that existed in the 1960s and early 1970s. One of the singers, the late John Lennon, wrote a song called "Imagine." It is a song about thinking beyond what already exists, to imagine a better future. (You can hear the song and watch the video associated with the song here, https://www.youtube.com/watch?v=VOgFZfRVaww) That is what we want you to do now. Imagine for a moment that you could transform your profession in any possible manner. What would CRR look like in your profession?

Activity 8–1

Working with two or three others, think about and read about your own profession. Discuss the following questions.

1. What are some of the CRR examples that have been taught throughout the curriculum?
2. Are there barriers that prevent CRR from being used more widely in speech, language, and hearing sciences?

CHAPTER SUMMARY

In this chapter we focused on culturally responsive research. The chapter began by defining CRR and discussing the relationship between CRR and levels of evidence as outlined by ASHA. We reviewed the importance of considering diverse epistemologies when engaged in CRR rather than only those ways of thinking based on Western, White, middle-class males. It is also important to approach research across levels of interactions; that is, rather than focusing only on the micro level (individual development and disorders) to conduct CRR, the researcher needs to consider social forces at all of the levels in which a person interacts, such as at the meso level (organization of professional knowledge) and macro level (economic and political contexts; policies). The chapter ended with an example of CRR in action.

FURTHER READING

Austin, M. J., Branom, C., & King, B. (2014). Searching for the meaning of social justice. In M. Austin (Ed.), *Social justice and social work: Rediscovering a core value of the profession* (pp. 1–18). Los Angeles, CA: Sage

Vining, C. B., & Allison, S. R. (2000). *Navajo perceptions of developmental disabilities: Project Na'nitin institute manual.* Albuquerque, NM: University of New Mexico.

Westby, C. E., & Vining, C. B. (2004). Cultural variables affecting research with Native American populations. *SIG 14, Communication Disorders and Sciences in Culturally and Linguistically Diverse Populations, 11,* 3–17.

REFERENCES

American Speech-Language-Hearing Association (ASHA). (2017). *Steps in the process of evidence-based practice.* Retrieved from http://www.asha.org/Research/EBP/Assessing-the-Evidence/

Amin, S. (2006). Colonialism is inseparable from capitalism. *L'Humanite.* Retrieved from http://www.humaniteinenglish.com/spip.php?article70

Anderson, E. (2017, Spring). Feminist epistemology and philosophy of science. *The Stanford encyclopedia of philosophy.* E. N. Zalta (Ed.). Retrieved from https://plato.stanford.edu/archives/spr2017/entries/feminism-epistemology

Arzubiaga, A. E., Artiles, A. J., King, K. A., & Harris-Murri, N. (2008). Beyond research on cultural minorities: Challenges and implications of research as situated cultural practice. *Exceptional Children, 74*, 309–327.

Ashing-Giwa, K., & Kagawa-Singer, M. (2005). Can a culturally responsive model for research design bring us closer to addressing participation disparities? Lessons learned from cancer survivorship studies. *Ethnicity and Disease, 15*, 130–137.

Ashing-Giwa, K., & Kagawa-Singer, M. (2006). Infusing culture into oncology research on quality of life. *Oncology Nursing Forum, 33*(1), 31–36.

Bal, A., & Trainor, A. A. (2016). Culturally responsive experimental intervention studies: The development of a rubric for paradigm expansion. *Review of Educational Research, 86*(2), 319–359.

Bankert, E. A., & Amdur, R. J. (2006). *Institutional review board: Management and function* (2nd ed.). Boston, MA: Jones and Bartlett.

Becvar, K., & Srinivasan, R. (2009). Indigenous knowledge and culturally responsive methods in information research. *The Library Quarterly: Information, Community, Policy, 79*(4), 421–441.

Berryman, M., SooHoo, S., & Nevin, A. (2013). Culturally responsive methodologies from the margins. In M. Berryman, S. SooHoo, & A. Nevin (Eds.), *Culturally responsive methodologies* (pp, 1–32). Bingley, UK: Emerald Group Publishing Limited.

Berryman, M., SooHoo, S., Nevin, A., Barrett, T. A., Ford, T., Nodelman, D. J., . . . Wilson, A. (2013). Culturally responsive methodologies at work in education settings. *International Journal for Researcher Development, 4*(2), 102–116.

Blackstone, A. (2012). Sociological inquiry principles: Qualitative and quantitative methods v. 1.0. Retrieved from https://open.umn.edu/opentextbooks/BookDetail.aspx?bookId=139

Bradley, D. (2015). *A critical introduction to formal epistemology.* London, UK: Bloomsbury Academic.

Browne, K., & Nash, C. J. (2016). Queer methods and methodologies: An introduction. In C. J. Nash & K. Browne (Eds.), *Queer methods and methodologies: Intersecting queer theories and social science research* (pp. 1–24). New York, NY: Routledge.

Burns, P. B., Rohrich, R. J., & Chung, K. C. (2011). The levels of evidence and their role in evidence-based medicine. *Plastic Reconstructive Surgery, 128*(1), 305–310.

Byrd, W. C., & Hughey, M. W. (2015, September 28). Born that way? "Scientific" racism is creeping back into our thinking. Here's what to watch out for. *The Washington Post.* Retrieved from https://www.washingtonpost.com/news/monkey-cage/wp/2015/09/28/born-that-way-scientific-racism-is-creeping-back-into-our-thinking-heres-what-to-watch-out-for/

Caldwell, S. E. M., & Mays, N. (2012). Studying policy implementation using a macro, meso and micro frame analysis: The case of the Collaboration for Leadership in Applied Health Research and Care programme nationally and in North West London. *Health Research Policies and Systems, 10*(32). doi:10.1186/1478-4505-10-32

Campinha-Bacote, J. (2002). The process of cultural competence in the delivery of healthcare services: A model of care. *Journal of Transcultural Nursing, 13*(3), 181–184.

Carr, F. W. (2003). *Germany's Black holocaust, 1890–1945: The untold truth.* Lakewood, CA: Scholar Technological Institute of Research.

Castagna, M., & Sefa Dei, G. J. (2000). An historical overview of the application of the race concept in social practice. In A. Calliste & G. J. Sefa Dei (Eds.), *Anti-racist feminism: Critical race and gender studies* (pp. 19–37). Halifax, Nova Scotia: Fernwood.

Centers for Disease Control (CDC). (2017, July 28). *Social determinants of health.* Retrieved from https://www.cdc.gov/socialdeterminants/

Champion, T. (1998). "Tell me somethin' good": A description of narrative structures among African American children. *Linguistics and Education, 9*(3), 251–286.

Champion, T., Seymour, H., & Camarata, S. (1995). Narrative discourses among African American children. *Journal of Narrative Life History, 5*(4), 333–352.

Chilisa, B. (2012). *Indigenous research methodologies.* Los Angeles, CA: Sage.

Collins, P. H. (2000). *Black feminist thought: Knowledge, consciousness and the politics of empowerments* (2nd ed.). London, UK: Harper Collins.

Conner, D. J., Gallagher, D., & Ferri, B. A. (2011). Broadening out horizons: Toward a plurality of methodologies in learning disability research. *Learning Disability Quarterly, 34*(2), 107–121.

Daniels, D. (2008). Working with people who stutter of diverse backgrounds: Some ideas to consider. *ASHA SIG 4 Perspectives on Fluency and Fluency Disorders, 18*, 95–100.

Degoy, L. (2006). [Patrick Bolland, Trans]. Samir Amin: Colonialism is inseparable from capitalism. *L'Humanité in English*. Retrieved from http://www.humaniteinenglish.com/spip.php?article70

DeJarnette, G. (2009, April). *Developing a culture sensitive taxonomic classification of discourse in African American English*. Presentation given to the Annual Convention of the National Black Association for Speech-Language and Hearing, Atlanta, GA.

DeJarnette, G., Rivers, K. O., & Hyter, Y. D. (2015). Ways of examining speech acts in young African American children: Considering inside-out and outside-in approaches. *Topics in Language Disorders, 35*(1), 61–75.

Denis, N. A. (2015). *War against all Puerto Ricans: Revolution and terror in America's colony*. New York, NY: Nation Books.

Dore, J. (1974). A pragmatic description of early language development. *Journal of Psycholinguistic Research, 4*, 343 – 350.

Dore, J. (1975). Holophrases, speech acts, and language universals. *Journal of Child Language, 2*, 21–40.

Dore, J. (1977). "Oh them sheriff": A pragmatic analysis of children's responses to questions. In S. Ervin-Tripp & C. Mitchell-Kernan (Eds.), *Child discourse* (pp. 139–164). New York, NY: Academic Press.

Dore, J. (1978). Variation in preschool children's conversational performances. In K. Nelson (Ed.), *Children's language* (Vol. 1, pp. 397–444). New York, NY: Gardner Press.

Engel, G. L. (1980). Clinical application of the biopsychosocial model. *American Journal of Psychiatry, 137*, 535–544.

Fals-Borda, O. (2006). Participatory (action) research in social theory: Origins and challenges. In P. Reason & H. Bradbury (Eds.), Handbook of action research: Concise paperback edition (pp. 27–37). Thousand Oaks, CA: Sage.

Ford, D. Y. (2010). Conducting research that is culturally responsive. *Gifted Child Today, 34*(3), 25–27.

Ford, D. Y., Moore, J. L., Whiting, G. W., & Grantham, T. C. (2008). Conducting cross-cultural research: Controversy, cautions, concerns, and considerations. *Roeper Review, 30*(2), 82–92.

Fread Albreacht, S., Skiba, R. J., Losen, D. J., Chung, C.G., & Middelberg, L. (2012). Federal policy on disproportionality in special education: Is it moving us forward? *Journal of Disability Policy Studies, 23*(1), 14–25.

Freire, P. (1970). *Pedagogy of the oppressed*. New York, NY: Continuum.

Freire, P. (1990). *Education for critical consciousness*. New York, NY: Continuum.

Gallagher, D. J., Conner, D. J., & Ferri, B. A. (2011). Broadening our horizons: Toward a plurality of methodologies in learning disability research. *Learning Disability Quarterly, 34*(2), 107–121.

Gans, H. J. (2017). Racialization and racialization research. *Ethnic and Racial Studies, 40*(3), 341–352.

Garrod, J. Z. (2006). A brave old world: An analysis of scientific racism and BiDil. *McGill Journal of Medicine, 9*(1), 54–60.

Gramsci, A. (1971). *Selections from the prison notebooks*. New York, NY: International.

Graves, J. L. (2002). *The emperor's new clothes: Biological theories of race at the millennium*. Piscataway, NJ: Rutgers University Press.

Green, J. (1985). The narrativization of experience in the oral style. *Journal of Education, 167*(1), 9–35.

Grosfoguel, R. (2012). The dilemmas of ethnic studies in the United States: Between liberal multiculturalism, identity politics, disciplinary colonization, and decolonial epistemologies. *Human Architecture: Journal of the Sociology of Self-Knowledge, X*(1), 81–90.

Halliday, M. A. K. (1975). *Learning how to mean: Explorations in the development of language*. London, UK: Edward Arnold.

Harris, J. L., Fleming, V. B., & Harris, C. L. (2012). A focus on health beliefs: What culturally competence clinicians need to know. *SIG 14 Perspectives on Communication Disorders and Sciences in Culturally and Linguistically Diverse (CLD) Populations, 19*, 40–48.

Hofstede, G. (2011). Dimensionalizing cultures: The Hofstede model in context. *Online Readings in Psychology and Culture, 2*(1), https://doi.org/10.9707/2307-0919.1014

Hyter, Y. D. (2000). *"Play wit'cho (with you) no more": Ignoring as a potential communicative function by female speakers of African American English* (Unpublished raw data). Western Michigan University, Kalamazoo, MI.

Hyter, Y. D. (2008). Considering conceptual frameworks in communication sciences and disorders. *ASHA Leader, 13*, 30–31.

Hyter, Y. D. (2014). A conceptual framework for responsive global engagement in communication sciences and disorders. *Topics in Language Disorders, 34*(2), 103–120.

Hyter, Y. D., Rivers, K. O., & DeJarnette, G. (2015). Pragmatic language of African American children and adolescents: A systematic synthesis of literature. *Topics in Language Disorders, 35*(1), 8–45.

Kathard, H., & Pallay, M. (2013). Promoting change through political consciousness: A South African speech-language pathology response to the World Report on Disability. *International Journal of Speech Language Pathology, 15*(1), 84–89.

Kochman, T. (1972). *Rappin' and stylin' out: Communication in urban Black America*. Urbana, IL: University of Illinois Press.

Kumagai, A. K., & Lypson, M. L. (2009). Beyond cultural competence: Critical consciousness, social justice, and multicultural education. *Academic Medicine, 86*(6), 782–787.

Labov, W. (1972). *Language in the inner city*. Philadelphia, PA: University of Pennsylvania Press.

Labov, W., & Waletsky, J. (1967). Narrative analysis. In J. Helm (Ed.), *Essays on the Verbal and Visual Arts* (pp. 12–44). Seattle, WA: University of Washington Press. Reprinted in 1997, *Journal of Narrative and Life History, 7*, 3–38.

Ladson-Billings, G. (2003). Racialized discourses and ethnic epistemologies. In N. K. Denzin & Y. S. Lincoln (Eds.), *The landscape of qualitative research: Theories and issues* (2nd ed., pp. 398–432). London, UK: Sage.

Ladson-Billings, G., & Tate, W. F. (2006). *Research in the public interest: Social justice, action, and policy*. New York: Teachers College Press.

Lindsay-Dennis, L. (2015). Black feminist-womanist research paradigm: Toward a culturally relevant research model focused on African American girls. *Journal of Black Studies, 46*(5), 506–520.

Mahendra, N., & Namazi, M. (2014). Becomoing bilingual: When children learn a second language, what's the best way to support them and their families? Hint: It's not about sacrificing the language they already know for the one they're seeking to learn. *ASHA Leader, 19*, 40–44.

Mainess, K. J., Champion, T. B., & McCabe, A. (2002). Telling the unknown story complex and explicit narration of African American preadolescents: Preliminary examination of gender and socioeconomic issues. *Linguistics and Education, 13*(2), 151–173.

Manning, W. H. (2010). *Clinical decision making in fluency disorders* (3rd ed.). Clifton Park, NY: Delmar Cengage Learning.

Mitchell-Kernan, C. (1972). Signifying, loud-talking and marking. In T. Kochman (Ed.), *Rappin and stylin out: Communication in urban Black America* (pp. 315–335). Urbana, IL: University of Illinois Press.

Mitchell-Kernan, C. (1973). Signifying. In A. Dundes (Ed.), *Mother wit from the laughing barrel* (pp. 210–328). New York, NY: Garland Publishing.

Mitchell-Kernan, C. (1989). Signifying and marking: Two Afro-American speech acts. In J. J. Gumperz & D. Hymes (Eds.), *Directions in sociolinguistics: The ethnography of communication* (pp. 161–179). New York, NY: Basil Blackwell.

Molina Azorin, J. M., & Cameron, R. (2010). The application of mixed methods in organizational research: A literature review. *The Electronic Journal of Business Research Methods, 8*(2), 95–105.

Morgan, M. (2002). *Language, discourse and power in African American culture*. Cambridge, UK: Cambridge University Press.

Morgan, P., Farkas, G., Hillemeier, M., Mattison, R., Maczuga, S., Li, H., & Cook, M. (2015). Minorities are disproportionately underrepresented in special education: Longitudinal evidence across five disability conditions. *Educational Researcher, 44*(5), 278 – 292.

Nelson, N. W. (2010). *Language and literacy disorders: Infancy through adolescence.* Boston, MA: Allyn & Bacon.

Nelson, N. W., Bahr, C. M., & Van Meter, A. M. (2004). *The writing lab approach to language instruction and intervention.* Baltimore, MD: Paul H. Brookes.

Ong, A. (2017, January 21). *Embracing culturally responsive research and evaluation practice.* Retrieved from https://www.washington.edu/museology/2017/01/21/embracing-culturally-responsive-research-evaluation-practice/

Peña, E. D. (2007). Lost in translation: Methodological considerations for cross-cultural research. *Child Development, 78*(4), 1255–1264.

Penn, C. (2002). Cultural narratives: Bridging the gap. *Folia Phoniatrica et Logopaedica, 54*(2), 95–99.

Percelay, J., Monteria, I., & Dweck, S. (1994). *Snaps.* New York, NY: Quill Morrow.

Petersen, C., & McCabe, A. (1983). *Developmental psycholinguistics: Three ways of looking at a child's narrative.* New York, NY: Plenum.

Resnik, D. B. (2017). Research ethics timeline (1932–present). *National Institutes of Environmental Health Sciences.* Retrieved from https://www.niehs.nih.gov/research/resources/bioethics/timeline/

Rickford, J. R., & Rickford, R. J. (2000). *Spoken soul.* New York, NY: Wiley.

Rodriguez, K. L., Schwartz, J. L., Lahman, M. K. E., & Geist, M. R. (2011). Culturally responsive focus groups: Reframing the research experience to focus on participants. *International Institute for Qualitative Methodology, 10*(4), 400–417.

Rogoff, B. (2003). *The culture nature of human development.* New York, NY: Oxford University Press.

Romm, N. R. A. (2015). Conducting focus groups in terms of an appreciation of indigenous ways of knowing: Some examples from South Africa. *Qualitative Social Research, 16*(1), Art 2.

Samaan, A. E. (2012). *From a "race of masters" to a "master race": 1948 to 1848.* Createspace.com.

Santiago-Valles, W. F. (2005). Producing knowledge for social transformation: Precedents from the Diaspora for twenty-first century research and pedagogy. *The Black Scholar, 35*(2), 50–60.

Schanche Hodge, F. (2012). No meaningful apology for American Indian unethical research abuses. *Ethics and Behavior, 22*(6), 431–444.

Simmons-Mackie, N. (2014). Micro and macro traditions in qualitative research. In M. J. Ball, N. Muller, & R. L. Nelson (Eds.). *Handbook of qualitative research in communication disorders* (pp. 17–38). New York, NY: Psychology Press.

Skloot, R. (2010). *The immortal life of Henrietta Lacks.* New York, NY: Random House.

Smith, L. T. (1999). *Decolonizing methodologies: Research and indigenous peoples.* London, UK: Zed Books.

Smith, L. T. (2005). Building a research agenda for indigenous epistemologies and education. *Anthropology and Education Quarterly, 36*(1), 93–95.

Smitherman, G. (1977). *Talkin and testifyin: The language of Black America.* Detroit, MI: Wayne State University Press.

Smitherman, G. (2000). *Talkin that talk.* New York, NY: Routledge.

Spitz, V. (2005). *Doctors from hell: The horrific account of Nazi experiments on humans.* Boulder, CO: First Sentient.

Stobbe, M. (2011, February 27). Ugly past of U.S. human experiments uncovered: Tests included exposing mental patients, prisoners to infectious diseases. *NBCNEWS.com.* Retrieved from http://www.nbcnews.com/id/41811750/ns/health-health_care/t/ugly-past-us-human-experiments-uncovered/#.WS28yYczVYc

Stockman, I. J., Karasinski, L., & Guillory, B. (2008). The use of conversational repairs by African American preschoolers. *Language, Speech, and Hearing Services in Schools, 39,* 461–474.

Subedi, B. (2010). *Critical global perspectives: Rethinking knowledge about global societies.* Charlotte, NC: Information Age.

Tough, J. (1977). *The development of meaning.* New York, NY: Halsted Press.

Trainor, A. A., & Bal, A. (2014). Development and preliminary analysis of a rubric for culturally responsive research. *Journal of Special Education, 47*(4), 203–216.

Unwin, A., & Yandell, J. (2016). *Rethinking education: Whose knowledge is it anyway?* (no-nonsense guides). Oxford, UK: New Internationalist.

U.S. Department of Education (2011). *New data from the U.S. Department 2009–10 Civil Rights data collection show continuing disparities in educational opportunities and resources.* Retrieved from https://www.ed.gov/news/press-releases/new-data-us-department-education-2009-10-civil-rights-data-collection-show-conti

U.S. Department of Health and Human Services. (1979, April 18). *The Belmont report: Office of the secretary ethical principles and guidelines for the protection of human subjects of research: The National Commission for the Protection of Human Subjects of Biomedical and Behavioral Research.* Retrieved from https://www.hhs.gov/ohrp/regulations-and-policy/belmont-report/index.html#xethical

Valentijn, P. P., Schepman, S. M., & Bruijnzeels, M. A. (2013). Understanding integrated care: A comprehensive conceptual framework based on the integrative functions of primary care. *International Journal of Integrated Care, 13,* 1–12.

Van Wormer, K., & Besthorn, F. (2017). *Human behavior and the social environment, macro level: Groups, communities and organizations* (3rd ed.). Oxford, UK: Oxford University Press.

Vazquez-Montilla, E., Reyer-Blanes, M. E., Hyun, E., & Brovellim E. (2000). Practices for culturally responsive interviews and research with Hispanic families. *Multicultural Perspectives, 2*(3), 3–7.

Veeck, G., Veeck, A., Hyter, Y. D., & Santiago-Valles, W. (2004). Changing times: A case study of Hispanic-Americans in Southwest Michigan. *The Great Lakes Geographer, 11*(1), 28–44.

Vygotsky, L. S. (1978). *Mind in society: The development of higher mental processes.* Cambridge, MA: Harvard University Press.

Wane, N. (2013). [Re]Claiming my indigenous knowledge: Challenges, resistance, and opportunities. *Decolonization: Indigeneity, Education & Society, 2*(1), 93–107.

Wheeler, J. (2010, May 3). The poisoning of Puerto Rico: The U.S. Navy left Vieques, but for many the cancer remains. *In These Times.* Retrieved from http://inthesetimes.com/article/5869/the_poisoning_of_puerto_rico

Wickenden, M. (2013). Widening the SLP lens: How can we improve the well-being of people with communication disabilities globally. *International Journal of Speech-Language Pathology, 15*(1), 14–20.

World Health Organization (WHO). (2002). *Innovative care for chronic conditions: Building blocks for action, global report.* Geneva, Switzerland: Author.

Wylie, K., McAllister, L., Davidson, B., & Marshall, J. (2013). Changing practice: Implications of the World Report on Disability for responding to communication disability in underserved populations. *International Journal of Speech-Language Pathology, 15*(1), 1–13.

Zavala, M. (2013). What do we mean by decolonizing research strategies? Lessons from decolonizing, indigenous research projects in New Zealand and Latin America. *Decolonization: Indigeneity, Education & Society, 2*(1), 55–71.

Zeichner, K., & Liu, K. Y. (2010). A critical analysis of reflection as a goal for teacher education. In N. Lyons (Ed.), *Handbook of reflection and reflective inquiry: Mapping a way of knowing for professional reflective inquiry* (pp. 67–84). New York, NY: Springer.

9

Working With Interpreters

This chapter focuses on the development of skills for working with an interpreter. There are over 350 languages spoken in this country with Spanish being the most often used second language. Thus, it is likely that you have already provided services to an individual who speaks a language other than English. There are ethical issues and legal ramifications and mandates that have propelled the wide use of interpreters in medical, educational, and business practices. It is no longer an option, but a necessity and a culturally responsive practice to know how to access and work with interpreters appropriately. After reading this chapter and engaging in the learning activities, you will achieve the learning objectives listed below.

LEARNING OBJECTIVES

After reading, discussing and processing the information presented in this chapter, you will be able to demonstrate the following knowledge, skills, and attitudes:

1. Knowledge
   a. Identify why culture is an important part of the interpreting process
   b. Describe why the use of a child to interpret is strictly prohibited and

the use of other family members to interpret is a poor choice
   c. Distinguish between consecutive interpreting and simultaneous interpreting
   d. Identify the roles and responsibilities of an interpreter in the interpreting process
2. Skills
   a. Recognize the skills of a "trained" interpreter compared to an "untrained" interpreter
   b. Use the three parts of the interpretation process called BID (briefing, interaction, debriefing)
   c. Use an interpreter successfully during assessment and intervention in the practice of speech, language, and hearing science
   d. Recognize the potential for medical errors and educational errors when an interpreter is not used with second language speakers
3. Attitudes
   a. Advocate for the use of a "trained" versus "untrained" interpreter as a valued member of the health care and educational team
   b. Accept the role you may need to play in the training of your own interpreter

c. Facilitate the use of interpreters by acting as a resource of information in this area

d. Be a lifelong learner by using policies such as CLAS Standards, the Joint Commission Patient-Centered Standards, and the National Standards for Interpreters in Healthcare in your work

KEY CONCEPTS

Key concepts addressed in this chapter are presented in Table 9–1.

DEFINING INTERPRETER

The words *translator* and *interpreter* are often used interchangeably, and a translator may be requested, when in fact, an interpreter is needed. The two terms are similar in that they are both associated with language but one is the written word (translate) and the other is the spoken word (interpret) (NLSC, 2014). Each of these skills is highly specialized. We focus on interpreting. Interpreting is a broad process and goes beyond simply taking information from the *source* language (SL) of the first speaker to the *target* language (TL) of the second-party listener. There is a large cultural

component in the interpreting process, which is frequently not taken into consideration. In Chapter 1, we discussed the many facets of culture. It is important to be cognizant of how our understanding of culture influences our skill as interpreters. Consider the following scenario. In this interview the interpreter is directing questions to the mother rather than to the son. The son abruptly stops the session, and the family walks out of the appointment.

Box 9–1
Interpreting Interaction

Individuals in the interpreting event: Doctor (English), Interpreter (English and Vietnamese), Son Jason (English and Vietnamese), Mr. and Mrs. Wu (Vietnamese).

Doctor: Good morning Mrs. Wu. How are you doing this morning?

Interpreter: Chào buổi sáng Bà Wu. Bà có khỏe không?

Mrs. Wu: Tôi khỏe. Chồng tôi đang mắc chứng đau nửa đầu.

Interpreter: I am doing well. It is my husband that is having migraine headaches.

Doctor: Mr. Wu, you are not feeling well?

Interpreter: Ông Wu, ông cảm thấy không khỏe à?

TABLE 9–1. Key Concepts

Source Language	CLAS Standards
Target Language	BICs
Interpreter	CALPs
Translator	BID
Consecutive Interpreting	Paralanguage
Simultaneous Interpreting	

No response from Mr. Wu.

Son: I am Jason, my dad is not feeling well.

Interpreter: Tôi là Jason, bố tôi không được khỏe.

Doctor: Good to meet you, Jason.

Interpreter: Rất vui được gặp anh, Jason

Doctor: Mrs. Wu, can you tell me how long the headaches have been occurring?

Interpreter: Bà Wu, hãy cho tôi biết chứng đau đầu này đã kéo dài bao lâu rồi?

Mr. Wu: Tôi mệt.

Interpreter: I'm tired.

Mrs. Wu: Nhưng chúng ta đã đến gặp bác sĩ rồi đây.

Interpreter: But we came so far to see the doctor.

Doctor: Mrs. Wu, what medications is he on?

Interpreter: Bà Wu, chồng bà đã dùng những loại thuốc nào?

No response from family members.

Son: We are leaving now, my dad is not well.

Interpreter: Chúng tôi sẽ rời đi bây giờ, bố tôi không được khỏe.

Family leaves.

Doctor and Interpreter are left a little stunned.

Pause and think for a moment about what may have been the cause of this family walking out of the doctor's appointment. Could the interpreter and/or doctor have committed a cultural violation? If so, what might

it have been? In some cultures, as depicted in the example above, it is the oldest son who is the decision maker and the person addressed when the family is present. If the interpreter is not aware of this aspect of the culture, there may be negative consequences for the family dynamic. The mother may be punished later for not redirecting the conversation or the son may end the session prematurely without reason, as he did in this scenario. Although the interpretation exchange was excellent in the scenario, it was the cultural misunderstanding that resulted in the breakdown of communication.

The type of interpreting that occurred in the scenario with Mr. and Mrs. Wu is called *consecutive interpreting*. But there are two types of interpreting—consecutive interpreting and simultaneous interpreting—which will be discussed later in the chapter. In this scenario, the doctor was the *source* language (English) speaker. The interpreter took the doctor's message and relayed it in the *target* language, Vietnamese. The second speaker, Mrs. Wu, using the *target* language, reverses this event with the interpreter. This type of communication takes time, and it cannot be rushed. Allowing sufficient time is critical to the success of consecutive interpreting. Box 9–2 presents other examples of consecutive interpreting. An additional consecutive interpreting scenario is provided in the PluralPlus companion website which can be used to practice as a group.

Box 9–2

First Exchange

DOCTOR: Do you have headaches?

INTERPRETER: ¿Tiene Ud. dolores de cabeza?

PATIENT: Tengo migrañas.

INTERPRETER: I have migraines.

Second Exchange

DOCTOR: Is this the first time you have such a severe pain?

INTERPRETER: ¿ Es la primera vez que tiene dolor de cabeza tan furte como éste?

PATIENT: Sí, tengo mareos, y dolor constante en mis oido, los dientes y las sienes.

INTERPRETER: Yes, I am dizzy, and I have constant pain in my ear, my teeth, and my temples.

Third Exchange

DOCTOR: It could be your tonsils or your external auditory canal.

INTERPRETER: Puede ser sus amígdalas o su conducto auditivo externo.

PATIENT: La pupila de mí ojo no está clára.

INTERPRETER: The pupil of my eye is not clear.

DOCTOR: Open and close your eyes.

INTERPRETER: Abre y cierra los ojos.

Figure 9–1 illustrates how the interpreter is the conduit between the two (or more) speakers as noted by the parallel arrows. There is an extensive amount of active listening involved for all parties in consecutive interpreting. The burden is on the interpreter to hold the words from each speaker in memory and present them accurately in another language. Thus, speech is broken into small segments as a facilitating technique for the interpreter. This can result in a more stilted mode of communication among the speakers. It is unnatural to control the length and number of the speaking segments, then stop to wait up to 30 seconds or more for a reply (during which time the interpreter is communicating with the other person). Naturally occurring conversation moves rapidly at a rate of about 150 to 170 words per minute, which is much too fast for the interpreting sequence (Yuan, Liberman, & Cieri, 2006). Figure 9–2 shows one arrangement of seating in a consecutive interpreting scenario. The two women in the forefront represent the two speakers, and the interpreter sits to the side. In consecutive interpreting, the conversation takes place between the two main speakers. Although the interpreter is also speaking, his or her only role is to serve as a facilitator of the communication. The interpreter clarifies, but does not contribute otherwise to the conversation.

Another type of interpreting is called *simultaneous interpreting* and is used in diverse contexts, such as meetings or conferences where the interpreter almost simultaneously relays the message to an audience or an individual. The interpreter can be sitting next to one person and whispering or speaking quietly into his or her ear, or they may be sitting in a soundproof booth away from the meeting wearing a headset passing on the message immediately to a group of individuals also wearing headsets (Figure 9–3). The United Nations uses this latter type of service. Figure 9–4 shows a simultaneous interpreter system.

The information in this chapter describes only the process of consecutive interpreting, which is more commonly used in the clinical context. We begin by presenting a scenario that depicts a situation where there has been a breakdown in communication. The health care provider knows a "little" Spanish, but could also be French, Vietnamese, German, Chinese, or any language. She is friendly, communicating at a basic level in the second language, but in her own words, "I am not an interpreter, but I know enough to get by."

Consecutive Interpreting

Speaker1 talks
to interpreter.

Speaker1
finishes talking.

Interpreter talks
to Speaker2.

FIGURE 9–1. Interpreter communication between speakers. Illustrated by Severin Provance.

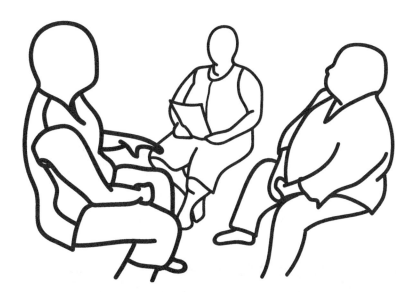

FIGURE 9–2. Consecutive interpreting seating arrangements. Illustrated by Severin Provance.

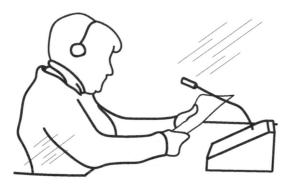

FIGURE 9–3. Interpreter in booth for simultaneous interpreting. Illustrated by Severin Provance.

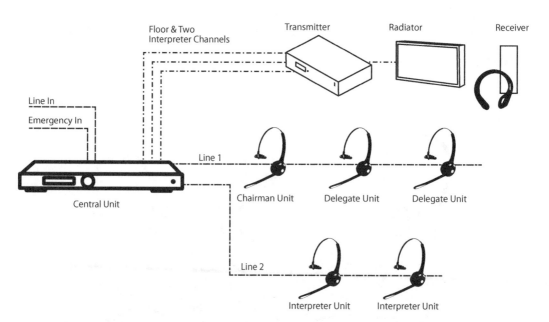

FIGURE 9–4. Simultaneous interpretation system. Illustrated by Severin Provance.

Box 9–3

In the clinic waiting room sits a family including a young father and mother and their 5-year-old son who is not feeling well. Their primary language is Spanish, but they do speak a few words in English and understand a little English. The parents are being ushered to the back exam room by an office assistant whose directions they did not understand. She only speaks English and is speaking quite fast. She led them down the hall from the waiting room, and they followed her lead but were a little afraid. The office assistant was friendly; however, she did not notice that the family was afraid. The family was compliant, so nothing seemed out of order. She assumed that they understood English because they said a few words in English. They also were very good at detecting body language and nonverbal cues. The office assistant said something in English which the family did not understand. When she said goodbye, they understood. She left them in the back exam room where they turned and looked at each other, confused. They did not know how long they would be in the cold room, whom they would see, or how they would communicate with their limited English skills. The doctor finally enters the room to take the child's temperature and takes note, from the medical chart, that the family is Spanish speaking. The doctor has learned a little about communicating with individuals whose primary language is not English, so she is somewhat confident. She took Spanish in high school and speaks a little Spanish like many of her friends. She smiles, introduces herself with her words in Spanish coming out slowly and deliberately. She examines the child. The parents ask her a question in Spanish, which she understands. However, she has difficulty formulating an appropriate sentence in Spanish to answer their question. She is doing her best. She smiles again and says, "la intérprete viene" (the [female] interpreter comes) and is relieved when the interpreter arrives.

The family has now interacted with two health care providers, and their needs have not been met. Each situation resulted in inadequate communication and has left the family more and more confused and afraid. This scenario happens daily in clinics, classrooms, hospital rooms, offices, and workplaces. How would you feel if you were the doctor? Would you do anything different? If you were the mother or father, would you feel confident that your child's medical care was addressed well? It is critical to be well equipped to communicate with individuals who speak languages other than English. Sometimes English language skills are not at a level necessary to communicate in an educational or health care environment where decisions that affect the lives of individuals will be made. Although we may be bilingual English/Spanish (after English, Spanish is the most often spoken language in the United States and Spanish is the second most spoken language in the world after Chinese [Shin, 2018]), there are at least 350[1] other languages spoken in the United States, and we may hear many of them throughout our workday (USCB, 2015). It is important to be informed ahead of time of the language skills needed for our clinical encounters of the day. In order to be assured of a positive communicative outcome for all individuals, we must realistically assess our personal skill set for communicating in the language needed. If we are unable to use the language adequately, we need to prepare in advance by locating an interpreter who can help us successfully communicate in the professional setting.

---

[1]It is important to note that several sources report the number of languages in the United States differently (Tamasi & Antieau, 2015). Also, language groups that might be considered different languages by researchers may be counted as the same language by the U. S. Census. The point here is that there are probably more the 350 languages in the United States (Tamasi & Antieau, 2015).

THE NEED FOR AN INTERPRETER

We have identified that there is a need for a skilled and **trained** interpreter. But how do you find such an interpreter? How do you access an interpreter every time you need one? For example, in the school setting, there may be an individual who has been trained as an interpreter for schoolwide or districtwide use. You may be able to locate an interpreter by contacting the English as a Second Language (ESL) Department or Special Education office in your school or district. Some of the best contacts may come from your colleagues at work. They may have had an interpreter who was assigned to them or to a group of them. Frequently, your employer will have a list of companies from which to hire trained interpreters through an hourly contract. If you are unable to identify an interpreter through any of these resources, you may need to resort to contacting your state professional organization or a national interpreters association, such as the ones listed at http://www.ncihc.org/interpreter-associations. This same process can be followed in any workplace setting when an interpreter is needed. Generally, the Human Resources office or the Title IX personnel in your organization should have some information on interpreters or be able to refer you to a source. Often, however, it is up to you as the professional to identify an interpreter because your organization may not offer that resource directly. The use of telephonic interpreter services should be limited to unique situations where other options are not possible in order to stay in compliance with Standard 4 of the National Standards for Culturally and Linguistically Appropriate Services (CLAS) in Health and Health Care (USDHHS, 2001a, 2001b, 2013).

CLAS Standard 4

- Title VI of the Civil Rights Act of 1964 entitles all individuals receiving federal assistance access to language assistance services (Chen, Youdelman, & Brooks, 2007)
- Title VI of the Civil Rights Act of 1964 requires that all health care organizations receiving federal funding provide individuals access to language assistance services
- The language assistance services must be available without regard to the size of this language group in the community
- Language assistance should be ideally provided by bilingual staff, but trained, contract, or volunteer interpreters are also acceptable

The CLAS standards were instituted in 2000 and enhanced in 2013. The Joint Commission (JACO) followed their lead (NCIHC, 2014) by publishing an important monograph in 2009 called *Advancing Effective Communication, Cultural Competence, and Patient- and Family-Centered Care: A Roadmap for Hospitals.* JACO recognized the importance of patient-centered communication and the need for trained interpreters by making it an accreditation requirement. At the admissions stage of care, the health care provider must identify the patient's preferred language for discussing health care. Both of these documents address the need to use the first language or strongest language of the person.

It also is important to discuss the ways in which an interpreter should *not* be selected. First, using the bilingual person down the hall, who speaks the language of the patient or student, is not the answer. This person may know the basics of the language, *Basic Interpersonal Communication Skills* (BICs), and be capable of speaking the language in a personal setting face-to-face. However, their ability to use the language at a level appropriate for gathering professional information in a medical or educational exchange may be minimal. A higher level of language use is called *Cognitive Academic Language Proficiency* (CALPs) (Cummins, 1979, 2008). Even if the individual is at a CALPs level of language skill, the use of professional vocabulary may be limited. In addition, there are strict Health Insurance Portability and Accountability Act (HIPAA) regulations in place to protect the confidentiality of health information (USDHH, 2003). The person you "pull in" to interpret may recognize the patient or student, and later may unknowingly discuss privileged information outside of the facility. Unfortunately, this happens more than it should. They would not be aware of the strict ethical standards by which a trained interpreter must abide.

It is important to re-emphasize that simply speaking a language, does not assure that the individual can use appropriate educational or medical vocabulary in the language as would be expected from a professional interpreter. For example, a bilingual employee who works in the office down the hall and speaks Mandarin Chinese may be called in on an emergency basis to interpret information about a laryngeal cancer diagnosis. You may think that, surely, this would never happen. But yet, it does. The individual does not understand the severity of the situation and is not familiar with the medical terminology related to cancer. Unfortunately, in an effort to be helpful, they are placed in a situation where they may make up words, omit parts of the discussion they do not agree with, are uncomfortable with, or do not understand. To ease their anxiety, they may depict a "false fluency" by interjecting irrelevant personal information or oversimplifying the information (Flores, 2005). They could ultimately provide incomplete or even incorrect information to the patient, family, or organization. This could place the individual

in great danger at many levels and may cause harm to the person. Bilingual employees are more than willing to help, although they may not understand the situation they are entering. Table 9–2 provides a list of 10 errors made in interpreting as described in this scenario. Examples of interpreter breakdowns can be found in the World's Apart videos (Grainger-Monsen & Haslett, 2003; Green, Betancourt, & Carrillo, 2003). Additional examples of interpreter breakdowns will be found in the PluralPlus companion website.

There are situations in which employees are given additional duties to serve as an interpreter, apart from their regular position. They are not trained interpreters but are simply bilingual speakers. Many times they are called "ad hoc" interpreters. In this instance, the employee is taken away from his or her primary job to serve as an interpreter. In some states, employees are paid an additional 10 cents per hour above their regular pay to serve as interpreters. Using bilingual speakers in this manner may negatively affect their primary job performance because of the regular interruptions. This can set them up for fail-

TABLE 9–2. Errors Made in Interpreting

1.	Misunderstand severity of situation
2.	Make up words
3.	Avoid parts they do not agree with
4.	Avoid parts they are uncomfortable with
5.	Avoid parts they do not understand
6.	Add irrelevant personal information
7.	Oversimplify information
8.	Provide incomplete information
9.	Provide incorrect information
10.	Cause danger or harm as a result of errors

ure in the interpreter scenario as well, because they have not received the training necessary to be a skilled interpreter. Sometimes, bilingual employees receive specialized training in order to also serve as interpreters as part of their job. In this situation, they would be serving dual roles for their employer. It is critical for the employee to understand that when serving as an interpreter, he or she must adhere to a strict code of ethics for interpreters that may not be required in regular employment. Compliance with a code of ethics could make it difficult for some individuals to serve as interpreters in their work setting. Langdon and Cheng (2002) describe a code of ethics for interpreters working with speech-language pathology and audiology and also for professionals who use an interpreter. There are many important skills necessary to provide ethical services as an interpreter. Table 9–3 provides a summary of these points. This information is also reviewed later in this chapter when discussing the responsibilities and skills of the interpreter.

Dr. Salas-Provance has trained medical interpreters who were adding the interpreting role to their primary position in the organization. This situation occurs quite often. The employment of a full-time interpreter is rare, and many organizations have limited funding to hire contract interpreters. The individuals encountered by Dr. Salas-Provance were interested in receiving formal training and improving their skills for interpreting. They wanted to accept interpreting work only when they felt linguistically and culturally competent. For many, prior to their formal training, they were required to interpret as part of their job, no matter their comfort level. They prepared as well as they could ahead of time, but many of the assignments were given at the last minute. They were fearful that they would not understand the message and give incorrect information. However, they knew to ask for clarification as needed. Although they did

not intend to offer advice while interpreting, many reported that they quickly aligned with the Spanish speakers and were easily swayed into a more casual conversation than dictated by their professional role. They felt that the advice they offered was harmless and did not cross professional boundaries. This is an area that is important to review regularly with the interpreter. In fact, if the professional feels that this is occurring, he or she is advised to stop the interpreter and ask questions. The professional may "feel" that not all information from the second language speaker has been relayed back. It is impossible to know for sure if the professional is receiving all the information being communicated. For that reason, a high level of trust must develop between the interpreter and the professional. As mentioned earlier, it is acceptable to stop the interpreter and have him or her explain what was communicated with the patient or student at that moment. It has been found that the highest errors of untrained interpreters were the omission of information and answering for both the professional and the second language speaker (Napels et al., 2015). Remember, it is not acceptable for the interpreter to cross boundaries by taking on your role or talking for you. The crossing of boundaries by the interpreter is an ethical problem that may have serious negative consequences for the patient, client, or student. Many of the employees who were also interpreters appreciated the opportunity to learn a new skill and to have new professional development goals. Interpreters who begin in this manner may look for full-time work in this area as a result of this initial exposure to the field of interpreting.

The use of family members or adult friends as interpreters is inappropriate, and the use of children is strictly prohibited per Standard 6 of the CLAS Standards. Children should not be used to interpret for their parents and they should not serve, under any circumstances, as the interpreter when they

TABLE 9–3. Summary of Points of Importance for Interpreters: From A to Z

A	**A**void any bias or stereotyping
B	**Be** sure to include all information and do not omit information
C	**C**onsider the importance of your role on the team
D	**D**o not editorialize or offer advice
E	**E**xamine and improve your skills on a regular basis
F	**F**ormal training in the dynamics of interpreting is essential
G	**G**o to professionals when information is unclear
H	**H**old all information in strict confidence
I	**I**nterpret exact message spoken and be true to interpreting
J	**J**oin professional organizations
K	**K**now the HIPAA rules for maintaining privacy of information
L	**L**anguage skills at native or near native levels are needed
M	**M**anage pacing of the three-way communication appropriately
N	**N**ote-taking can improve retention and accuracy
O	**O**ffering personal opinion is inappropriate
P	**P**rofessional development should remain a lifelong priority
Q	**Q**uestion both the professional and client for clarity
R	**R**emember to use the BID process for interpreting
S	**S**end the correct nonverbal messages
T	**T**reat everyone with respect regardless of their role
U	**U**nderstand the role of each person in BID
V	**V**alue and maintain the integrity of the process
W	Prepare **W**ell and in a timely manner for each event
X	**EX**pand your knowledge of cultural and linguistic diversity
Y	**Y**ield control to the professional and do not speak for him or her
Z	Listen with ra**Z**or focus

are the student or patient. Use of adult family members or friends may be an option under extreme situations, but this is not ideal. This arrangement can occur only after the family has been notified of the availability of a free interpreter (see CLAS Standard 5 below).

CLAS Standard 6 (Mandate)

- Health care organizations must ensure the competence of language assistance provided to limited English proficient patients/consumers by interpreters and bilingual staff. Family and friends should not be used to provide interpretation services (except on request by the patient/consumer).
  - Minor children should never be used as interpreters or be allowed to interpret for their parents when they are the patients/consumers.

CLAS Standard 5 (Mandate)

- Health care organizations must provide to patients/consumers in their preferred language both verbal offers and written notices informing them of their right to receive language assistance services.
  - Families have a right under Title VI to receive language assistance services. According to the CLAS Standards, families must first be notified that a free interpreter is available.

CLAS Standard 4 (Mandate)

- Health care organizations must offer and provide language assistance services, including bilingual staff and interpreter services, at no cost to each patient/consumer with limited English proficiency at all points of contact, in a timely manner during all hours of operation.
  - Based on Title VI of the Civil Rights Act of 1964

To use an adult family member as the interpreter, a specific request must be made for that person, and it must be acceptable to the professional. The amount and accuracy of information exchanged can be seriously compromised when a trained interpreter is not used. No matter the level of training, it is important for the interpreter to be a neutral party; a family member as an interpreter is a questionable choice. The use of anyone except a trained interpreter may put the professional and an organization at personal and legal risk (Chen et al., 2007). The individual may receive subpar care that may result in danger or harm.

Care that was delivered in an inadequate manner is shown through one story from the World's Apart video (Grainger-Monsen & Haslett, 2003). Mr. Mohammad Kochi is a 63-year-old man who came to the United States from Afghanistan many years ago. In his country, he was identified as an elder and leader. Following the surgical removal of a cancerous tumor, the family was assured of the success of the surgery. At a later point, it was reported that parts of the cancerous tumor still remained. Unfortunately, the youngest daughter, who served as the interpreter during that appointment, was uncomfortable relaying this information, choosing rather to allow her father to remain hopeful. The father understood some of the information during this appointment, but the remainder of the family was not told of his cancer diagnosis. When advised at a subsequent appointment that it was time to begin chemotherapy, Mr. Kochi refused. His eldest daughter was very confused with this recommendation as she thought there had been a complete remission of the cancer. There are many cross-cultural events occurring in this scenario, which are a source of good discussion. But, the most important point here is that the use of the young child as an interpreter set off a succession of communication breakdowns that affected the delivery of adequate health care for Mr. Kochi and may eventually cost him his life.

Provision of services in a culturally responsive manner has been directed at the federal level through the CLAS Standards and the JACO Cultural Competence Standards.

The Individuals with Disabilities Education Improvement Act (IDEA 2004) mandates that assessments occur in the language of the individual. Tests must be administered in a manner devoid of racial or cultural discrimination. The tests must be administered in the child's native language or other mode of communication. The child should be able to perform to the best of his or her abilities. When you are unable to find a bilingual professional who can test in the individual's language, then a "trained" interpreter must be used. When a trained interpreter is not used, the results may be invalid. Some professionals may not use interpreters because they feel confident in their linguistic skills but are not fully aware of their linguistic limitations. The top three causes of interpreter errors are (a) unqualified interpreter, (b) professional with inadequate basic skills, and (c) lack of understanding of cultural beliefs and traditions (Nápoles et al., 2015). It has been observed that in an attempt to compensate for lack of language proficiency, the professional slows his or her speech, speaks louder, and overarticulates speech. The hope is that the person can be put at ease so that some basic level of information is communicated, affirming that "at least they got the 'gist' of it." Most likely, however, the person and his or her family are more confused than ever, frightened, and probably will never return to that professional again. This mistake is also costly. The individual seeking services must reschedule appointments elsewhere. Money is spent or insurance is billed unnecessarily for an unsuccessful appointment or session, and everyone has wasted their time. The educational and/or medical consequences for communication breakdowns can include (a) giving permission for unneeded testing, examinations or surgeries; (b) misunderstanding of a medication schedule resulting in being over- or undermedicated; (c) delay in receiving health services that could have stopped a disease; (d) delay in provision of services that could have

improved communication at an early stage; (e) poor compliance or underuse of services due to the inability to understand the treatment plan; and most importantly, (f) poor patient/client satisfaction. In addition, parents who do not speak English cannot advocate for their child if they do not understand the child's problems. Beyond the needs of the child with a disability, parents may miss opportunities for their intellectually advanced child when they are reluctant or unsure of how to use services offered to them in the school or how to access after-school services. Children who are not assessed in the appropriate language may be misdiagnosed as having a speech and language delay or some other type of communication disorder. This may lead to an inappropriate recommendation for therapeutic services or special education placement. In the long term, they may be denied an appropriate education and its social and economic advantages.

RESPONSIBILITIES OF THE INTERPRETER

The professional can expect the interpreter to conduct the interpreting scenario in a responsible manner. Ten core responsibilities of the interpreter that will improve the interpreting process are identified in Table 9–4. Interpreters have specific roles and responsibilities in the variety of settings in which they will be needed, such as in a routine medical or clinical visit, legal proceedings, a teacher-parent conference, a hearing aid evaluation, a bedside swallow exam, a treatment session, or a comprehensive speech and language assessment. In addition, interpreters will have a range of experience from those who have served as an interpreter in an organization for many years, those who are interpreting for a single individual on a regular basis, those who accept an occasional contract on a case-by-case basis, or those who

TABLE 9–4. Responsibilities of the Interpreter

1. Say "NO" if necessary
2. Keep all information confidential
3. Respect privacy of the individuals
4. Remain neutral
5. Do not give independent advice
6. Do not interject own ideas
7. Remain true to interpreting
8. Interpret exact messages spoken
9. Do not stereotype
10. Do not allow personal bias

may be called on to interpret as a last resort or in an emergency. Again, the expectation is that in all these situations, the interpreter will be prepared to provide excellent and ethical service. In the latter situation, the interpreter needs to quickly evaluate her preparation and ability to interpret successfully. If necessary, the interpreter must say "no" to that interpreting request. This is an important ethical decision, and interpreters, just like all professionals, must maintain a high degree of ethical standards. The consequences of accepting an interpreter role beyond their skill level are serious and may result in long-term damage to an individual and their family from educational or medical misinformation. There may also be legal ramifications if serious errors occur as a result of the poor interpreting.

Another responsibility of the interpreter is to keep all information confidential and respect the privacy of the individual. The interpreter should not discuss any information he or she hears in the interpreting event outside of the event or with individuals who are not associated with the case. This can be a challenge when interpreters are in small communities where individuals have known each other for generations. This is the same problem faced by all professionals in these small communities. However, many educators and health care professionals are bound by their professional code of ethics, and the importance of privacy and confidentiality is ingrained throughout their education. An interpreter may not be certified, and many times their training occurs quickly. This same urgency of the importance of privacy and confidentiality may not be as evident and must be discussed regularly with the interpreter.

The interpreter must also remain neutral and unbiased. This may be difficult initially. Interpreters are not sole representatives of any of the parties, either the patient, client, or student. Their role is to facilitate the conversation that occurs between the individuals present so that the involved persons can achieve the purpose of the event. The interpreter must not "take sides" and interpret in a way that favors one party over the other. For example, while assisting in the testing of a child, in their desire to have the child perform well, the interpreter may unknowingly give the child additional cues. Although the interpreter should remain neutral, one of the nine Standards of Practice for the National Council on Interpreting in Health Care is advocacy. This organization acknowledges the role that an interpreter may play in protecting individuals from harm and from any mistreatment. The interpreter should follow the policies and procedures of their organization in this regard.

Interpreters may feel they know a patient well because they share a language and culture. Thus, they may be tempted to give independent advice to the patient or their family that is contrary to the professional's advice. Interpreters must refrain from interjecting their own thoughts and ideas (editorializing) and remain true to the interpretation by relaying only the exact messages being spoken. The interpreting must be accurate, complete, and void of personal bias. It is important to ensure that stereotyping does not influence the interpreter's words or actions. Self-evaluation of unconscious bias should be assessed regularly. The American Speech-Language-Hearing Association (ASHA, 2010) offers a cultural competence checklist called Personal Reflection that is very helpful.

Activity 9–1

Take the list of responsibilities from Table 9–4 and identify a situation whereby each one of those responsibilities is abandoned and a second situation where the interpreter abides by the responsibilities. We model this activity with the first responsibility. In the first scenario we have a patient with TBI in a skilled nursing facility (SNF) who we are seeing for the first time. The extended family is waiting for us, and we call in the interpreter to assist in the interview. The interpreter is comfortable with this type of case as she has worked in the SNF for several years. She says, "Yes," and the interview is a success.

- Why do you think the interpreter said "Yes" in this situation?
- Is there any reason why she should reconsider?
- What kind of information should she have requested before making a decision?

In the next scenario, we are again in the SNF, and there has been an emergency situation with a patient with whom you are working and a family member is upset. A meeting has been set up with the chief executive officer of the SNF, the family member, the family's lawyer, and you. The interpreter feels very uncomfortable with this level of executive interpreting, and although she works in the facility, she says that being in an office with this many professionals makes her very nervous, and she says "No." Fortunately, she has done so with enough time, so that you can identify another interpreter. If the interpreter were to say "Yes" despite her fears, she may not be able to process words correctly, inter-

pret quickly enough for the advanced level of communication, and the "legal jargon" may be well outside her knowledge base. This very intense and important meeting could be easily undermined by an interpreter who is not well-prepared for the job and who should have said "No."

- Why do you think the interpreter said "No" in this situation?
- Is there any reason why she should reconsider?
- What kind of information should she have requested before making a decision?
- What would have happened if it was not possible to bring in an alternative interpreter?

The interpreter and the professional both have a responsibility to make the interpreting event successful for the patient, client, or student. There is a certain level of vulnerability for all parties, but especially for those who do not understand or speak the language; the professional and the person being served. They must rely on the interpreter to provide information that is factual, unbiased, and correct. For example, if the interpreter has an unconscious bias toward children who misbehave, she may dismiss the concerns of the parent, blaming the parent and the parent's poor parenting skills for the child's behavior problems. This opinion may be communicated to the professional with a tone of voice that portrays disagreement. Both the professional and the child (through the parent) are vulnerable in this situation and have taken on a great deal of risk. In another example, if the interpreter feels uneasy about the lifestyle of transgender individuals, she may sabotage the care the patient receives by not relaying information to the professional correctly or may choose to omit pieces of information with which she does not agree that, in fact, could be helpful to the professional. This situation would be unacceptable at all levels. A conversation between the professional and the interpreter ahead of time may alert the professional to any potential biases or problems in this area.

It is important for the interpreter to meet with the professional ahead of time to review the case. At this time, the professional should provide the important background information of the case and describe the critical information that the professional will need from the meeting. The interpreter also has an important role to play, and he or she should use this time to talk about cultural aspects that may impact the communication with the individual. This is a good time to bring up "housekeeping" items such as where to sit and the technical aspects of the interpreting process. This "briefing" period will be discussed later in the chapter. Depending on the setting, there may be little time for the briefing, especially if the interpreter is called in quickly. But, the professional and the interpreter may have developed a long-standing relationship of mutual trust and understanding and be able to communicate easily and quickly about each patient, client, or student prior to the interpreting event.

SKILLS OF THE INTERPRETER

The ideal interpreter will be a "trained" interpreter. This training can range from continuing education courses, to a one-day seminar or weeklong workshop in the area of interpreting. The interpreter also may be trained over time, "on the job." Most states do not have a certification process for interpreters; however, there is excellent direction offered by the National Council on Interpreting in Health Care (NCIHC, 2005) through the development of their 32 National Standards of Practice in nine areas. In addition, the NCIHC offers standards for training programs with an accompanying self-assessment tool to analyze the level of your training (NCIHC, 2011). Table 9–5 shows a sample of the 32 standards across nine areas. The nine headings correspond to the nine principles in the NCIHC National Code of Ethics. The standards of practice can be used to confirm that the work of the interpreter is at the highest levels. This information can serve as a set of

TABLE 9–5. Code of Ethics for Interpreters

Code of Ethics	Standards of Practice	
Accuracy	No part of the message is omitted	Ask speaker to pause or slow down
Confidentiality	Do not discuss case with family	Do not leave notes in public view
Impartiality	Do not reveal personal feelings	Do not interpret for family member
Respect	Use culturally appropriate ways	Encourage patient/provider eye contact
Cultural awareness	Learn traditional remedies	Identify cultural misunderstandings
Role boundaries	Limit personal questions	Do not advise on health care matters
Professionalism	Be honest and ethical at all times	Support blameless culture
Professional development	Keep up to date with terminology	Attend professional workshops
Advocacy	Alert professional to appropriate levels of respect	Identify a cultural cure for hearing pain

Source: Adapted from National Council on Interpreting in Health Care (http://www.ncihc.org).

benchmarks from which to evaluate the skill set of interpreters in your school, practice, or organization.

The best interpreters demonstrate native or near native proficiency in both languages. They have superior knowledge of terminology and concepts relevant for clinical and nonclinical encounters, for educational work settings during assessment and treatment sessions, and for communication needed in a variety of other professional environments. In the earlier scenario of the family with the 5-year-old child in the clinic, we can imagine a different situation where the first health care provider is also serving as the interpreter for the case. She would be in tune with the family, knowing that they were nervous; thus, she would have patiently listened to their concerns. The family may have given her critical and private information as they walked down the hall, personally aligning with her because they speak the same language. When the doctor enters the room, she would have shown her professional integrity by sharing everything she has learned about the family and would have remained in the room placing the doctor and family at ease.

Now the interpreter exchange can begin in earnest. Some expectations for this encounter are that the interpreter will *have knowledge of the specific vocabulary* needed in the setting, and that she will be *true to the interpreting*. She must remain *patient in the process*, and maintain a *slower and regular pace*. Research in the aspect of pacing during the interpreting process reveals that using an interpreter should add very little time to the event when an interpreter with the appropriate skill sets is used (Flores, 2005). Much of the added time is due to additional questions that may be needed for clarification and understanding regarding the culture, and the interpreter needs extra time to reframe your concepts because there may be no conceptual equivalence in other languages. The interpreter must have *excellent*

listening skills and be able to focus intently on the speaker. She cannot become distracted by other people in the room or noises outside the room. All electronic devices should be turned off to avoid distraction. One of the areas that is not discussed enough is the interpreter's role in *expressing the emotion* of the individuals. This is a skill that must be developed, and the interpreter should not feel inhibited in expressing these emotions. If the mother says, "My baby woke up in the night screaming from pain in his ear!," the interpreter cannot relay this message with a flat tone, "My baby woke up in the night screaming from pain in his ear." The added emotion provides nonlinguistic information for the professional that is important in measuring this parent's level of anxiety, and possibly, the severity of the child's problem. In the example of the baby with ear pain, the mother may have expressed that she placed cotton with Mentholatum or Vicks VapoRub in the baby's ear canal to help with the pain. The interpreter should be aware of this *cultural variation* and *relay its significance to the professional* (Salas-Provance, Erickson, & Reed, 2002). The best possible outcomes are achieved when sufficient time is given to training the interpreter ahead of the session or event, in not only the technical aspects of interpreting, but also about the cultural history of the population the interpreter will serve. As a result of this training, the professional trusts that the interpreter will relay information accurately to the student or family and provide her with the same. Although maintaining *privacy and ethical behavior* are our final two skills, they are probably the two most important. The interpreter must respect the privacy of all individuals (HIPAA was discussed earlier) and adhere to all the ethical standards set forth in the interpreting profession. Tables 9–5 and 9–6 provide summaries of interpreter responsibilities and skills.

TABLE 9–6. Core Interpreter Skills

1. Be knowledgeable of specific vocabulary
2. Remain true to interpreting
3. Remain patient in process
4. Speak slowly
5. Be a good listener
6. Express emotions of the individual
7. Understand cultural variation
8. Relay pertinent information to professionals
9. Respect privacy
10. Be ethical

BID INTERPRETING PROCESS

Interpreting can occur in a variety of environments. It may be a teacher and parent standing at the door of a classroom with the teaching assistant suddenly asked to join them as the interpreter. It can be a speech-language pathologist working with a critical case calling for the interpreter to come immediately to facilitate communication between the person and the professional. Neither of these is an ideal scenario, but they happen often. If possible, it is best to be able to prepare for the interpreting event in advance and to set up the room so it is conducive to communication by three or more individuals for consecutive interpreting. During the interpretation, you and your interpreter will use a three-step process for consecutive interpreting, which includes a **b**riefing, **i**nteraction, and **d**ebriefing (BID). The BID process can be used to maximize the interpreting event (Langdon & Saenz, 2015).

The *briefing* should occur prior to entering the interpreting event and away from the patient, student, or client. During the briefing, the professional will review the facts of the case with the interpreter, as well as identify concerns or points that they may want clarified related to culture or language. The interpreter becomes a part of the health care team at this point and is allowed, per HIPAA regulation (DHHS, 2003), to receive private medical information. In the educational setting, the interpreter may be part of the team that is preparing the Individualized Education Plan (IEP) or part of a speech, language, hearing, or swallowing assessment. What is said during the briefing will vary by the health care or educational setting, whether it is a familiar or unfamiliar situation for the interpreter, the length of time available to complete the briefing, and the professional's understanding of the role of the interpreter. The interpreter has many points to make during the briefing. First, he or she must learn the names of the individuals for whom he or she will interpret and the purpose of the meeting. If possible, the correct pronunciation of the family name should be practiced by the professional. For example, the Spanish last name of "Jaramillo" would be pronounced as "Ha-ra-mee-yo" with a rolled "r" if possible, and not "Jara-mil-lo." The mispronunciation of the family surname may be offensive to the family members and start the professional off on the wrong foot. Following this, the interpreter should stress to the professional the importance of speaking directly to the family, student, or patient and not to hold the primary conversation or side conversations with the interpreter. It is important to be considerate of any cultural rules that may limit the amount of direct eye contact with a person. The professional should not make requests to the interpreter, such as, "Ask them why they came to see me today," rather the professional should be advised to look at the individual(s) and say, "Why did you come in to see me today?" When the individual responds, "I came because my son is having trouble speaking," the interpreter would be true to the interpreting and say the exact words from the target language, using the word "I" not "They said their son is having trouble speaking." The use of the first person when rendering the message from one party to the other makes the communication sound more natural as if they are truly "talking" to each other. This takes practice and is not easy to accomplish, because it feels unnatural for the interpreter.

During the briefing, the interpreter should also discuss some specifics of the interpreting process. One of these is identifying a system for controlling the pace of the interpreting or a signal when there is misunderstanding during the process. An unobtrusive hand signal or word could be used to slow down or stop the exchange. The interpreting process should proceed at a slow pace. Should the pace speed up, the use of this hand signal will be critical to controlling the flow of the interpreting. There is a rhythm created among the group when the interpreter is allowed sufficient time to move from one person to another seamlessly. Unfortunately, many times, the professional starts a thought and wants to complete it, ignoring or not noticing the cue to slow down or stop. The briefing is a good time for the interpreter to give the professional some communication strategies for successful interpreting. Avoid using idiomatic speech (it is difficult to interpret "It is raining cats and dogs"), simplify your sentences, but keep them complete. Fragmented sentence structures make it more difficult for the interpreter to follow the thought pattern. It is natural to ask several questions at a time, and maybe even change your mind in the middle of a sentence. However, this makes it impossible for the interpreter to retain the information and to select the important points. Working memory storage capacity is limited to three to five meaningful items (one to three sentences) in most instances, and technical jargon of five or six sentences at a time is not likely to be retained

in full (Cowan, 2010). The interpreter's task is very cognitively demanding, requiring him or her to attend to the message from the source language, concentrate on the task, remember the message, understand the message and analyze it, then reform the message into the target language. There is valuable, critical, and potentially, life-changing information being relayed through the interpreter, and it is not an option for the interpreter to forget bits and pieces and to paraphrase using only the information he or she feels is important or that he or she can recall. This is an important reason for the briefing to include information about pace of the communication. Poor pacing of the communication exchange (too rushed) can render the interpreting process useless and unproductive.

During the briefing, the interpreter should advise the professional to introduce themselves in the language of the individuals to establish a culturally sensitive environment from the beginning. This may be uncomfortable for the professional, but it is rarely too much of an inconvenience for the professional to say "good day" and "my name is" in a second language. This is appreciated by the individuals who are not English speakers. For example, the professional may say in Spanish, "Buenos dias, me llamo Sara, soy la doctora o la maestra." (Good day, my name is Sara, I am the doctor/teacher). Immediately, the conversation moves to the interpreter, who introduces himself or herself in the language of the individuals and also does a short briefing with them regarding the pace and the hand signal or words for slowing down or stopping the conversation. The interpreter encourages them to provide any type of information they feel may be helpful for the professional.

During the briefing of the professional, the interpreter can provide information on any cultural aspects that he or she feels may be important for understanding the individuals, or to make them more comfortable. For example, if the interpreter has been told that the reason they are meeting today is to tell the family that the grandmother has Alzheimer's disease, it may be tempting for the doctor to ignore the grandmother and speak directly to the sons or daughters in the room. This would be a significant cultural misstep, as the grandmother in many cultures is held in high esteem, and eye contact and communication are directed to her first, even if others in the family respond.

The briefing in an educational setting may look different from that in a medical setting, where the interpreter meets the professional shortly before the appointment. If the interpreter is part of an IEP meeting, he or she may meet with the speech-language pathologist in the therapy room or classroom the day of the meeting or earlier in the week to review the case file. The parent may join them there for the briefing before meeting the rest of the team, or the briefing could occur at the same time as the scheduled appointment or meeting.

The second step of the BID process is the *interaction* (I). There are a variety of ways that the interaction can take place, depending on the purpose of the interaction, the number and makeup of individuals involved, and the length of time for the interaction. For this example, consider a situation where there is a therapist, a parent, and an interpreter. The formal greeting takes place with the interpreter doing a short briefing with the parent in the manner described earlier. Everyone takes their seats, with the therapist and the parent facing each other. The interpreter sits next to the parent, but slightly to the side and back so the line of vision is directly between the professional and the parent (the sitting arrangement can vary greatly determined by the naturally occurring sitting or standing positions and size of the room). It is tempting for the parent and the professional to direct their attention to the interpreter, as that is the person who speaks their language. It can be a bit awkward

at first for two people who do not understand what the other is saying to hold a conversation and maintain eye contact. However, if done correctly, with a rhythm and flow, the other aspects of communication can frame and hold the conversation. It has been found that as little as 7% of communication is channeled through the spoken words, 38% is the tone of voice, and 55% is body language (Mehrabian, 1981; Mehrabian & Wiener, 1967). Although a formula cannot be strictly followed in an activity as fluid as verbal communication, it holds in most instances. Of course, the words must be understood, which is accomplished through the interpreter, but there is much more being communicated than words. If the therapist or the parent communicate only through the interpreter, these additional cues are lost. There are many nonlinguistic cues that can enhance the communication. Tai (2014) speaks of three characteristics of body language that can influence language: *intuitive*, *communicative*, and *suggestive* features of body language. For example, when the word "hurt" is used, this can be paired with a scowl across the forehead or a hand to the belly, which happen *intuitively* when you hurt in those areas. The *communication* feature allows for a holistic and approachable environment that sets the foundation for communication. You may have "felt" that in some groups you are more comfortable talking even before the first word is spoken. The *suggestive* feature may come in to play when there is hesitance in the communication; thus, you may hold your hands out to invite or accept more interaction or brighten your eyes to show interest and an invitation to speak. One of the responsibilities of the professional is to make a "connection" with the student, patient, or client. Clearly, this is more difficult when we do not know their language, but with an interpreter in the mix, we are now free to ease into that connection through our nonverbal communication.

Nonverbal communication has also been termed *paralanguage* (O'Neil, 2009). There are additional areas to consider in the use of paralanguage. Because the patient or student may already be feeling vulnerable or possibly afraid as a result of their limited language skills, paralanguage becomes an influencing factor in the interpreting interaction (Haviland et al., 2017). Most of the time we are unaware of paralanguage as the influences do not come from speaking. One example of this is our body language or kinesics. As soon as the professional enters the room, a hand is extended with a smile as part of the words of welcome. Remember that a handshake may not be appropriate in all cultures (Hall, 1990), and this would be an important cultural aspect to discuss with the interpreter during the briefing. Proxemics is another part of paralanguage and is related to the way we position ourselves during communication. We know that there are culturally defined uses of space to which we must adhere to avoid offending others (Hall, 1990). If the professional is a male and the patient or student is female, there may be gender roles related to space and interaction. The verbal message may be lost if the space aspect is not taken into consideration. Other messages carried through paralanguage are those of time, voice, and clothing, among others. Without a word, arriving late on a consistent basis, speaking with a shaky voice, or wearing solely black clothes may be understood and measured by others based on their own experiences. The nonverbal message we portray is left for others to interpret; thus, we must do everything possible to send the intended nonverbal message. The paralanguage communicated during the interaction process should be such that it is not offensive and supports the seriousness of the interaction taking place. There are also cultural aspects to consider. For example, in many cultures, a person with an advanced degree is held in higher esteem, especially those with the "doctor" title. It is incumbent on the professional to break this barrier with the patient or student as soon as possible. In some Buddhist and Muslim countries it may be considered rude to show the bottom of the foot. Should the professional cross his or her leg while sitting, placing one on top of the other so the bottom of the shoe is visible (the dirtiest part of the shoe), this can be taken as a sign of disrespect, and a breakdown in communication could occur. Some individuals from Latin America, may say "yes, yes, yes" (si, si, si) even if they do not understand, saying later to the interpreter "que pasó"/What happened? Be sure to take the time to know that the patient is understanding the communication exchange. The debriefing part of the interpreter scenario, which is discussed later in the chapter, will be helpful in this area. For the interpreter, it is important to understand the regional language of the individuals with whom you are communicating. The use of colloquialisms may be regionally and culturally determined. For example, the patient could say, "my foot hurts"/me duele la "pata." The interpreter would want to refrain from showing surprise at the use of the Spanish word for "pata" (the foot of an animal) rather than "pie" (foot for a human) in this exchange.

With everyone in their best sitting or standing position, the *interaction* part of BID continues. Communication through an interpreter takes additional time, and this must be taken into consideration when setting up the appointment. This aspect alone presents a significant challenge to successful interpreting. All professionals have tight schedules, and in the managed care system of today, with decreasing reimbursements, the average time spent with a physician is 15 to 16 minutes (National Center for Health Statistics, 2012). This makes the doctor–patient relationship difficult to establish. One study showed that patients are redirected after speaking for only 23 seconds (Marvel, Epstein, Flowers, &

Beckman, 1999). Another study revealed that even when the length of an office visit remains equal, when comparing exemplary and non-exemplary physicians, exemplary physicians offer more emotional support and more family involvement resulting in greater positive communication with their patients (Marvel, Doherty, & Weiner, 1988). The challenge of time in the interpreting process must be factored in and discussed with the professional beforehand. In order to meet the needs of the individuals in an interpreting event, a priority must be made to set aside additional time for this process to be a success.

The interaction part of BID is where the relationship is established. The information that is exchanged during this event either allows the patient or student to understand their situation thoroughly or results in a breakdown of communication. The goals of the event are not met either for the professional or the individual when there is a communication breakdown. The communication can be successful when the professional keeps his or her sentences short and concise, keeping in mind that the interpreter can retain less than 1 minute in immediate recall. When the professional becomes long-winded, he or she increases the probability that the interpreter will paraphrase and the message will be incomplete or incorrect. Another good strategy during the interaction is to pause frequently, even if it feels unnatural, which it is, but it is critical. Professionals tend to use a great deal of "field" terminology that is difficult to interpret. The interpreter should be made aware during the briefing, or earlier, of specific terminology that will be used. Simplify the verbal communication without risking the accuracy of the message the patient or student needs to hear. For example, if the interpreter needs to relay that the child has a neurological impairment with significant verbal apraxia, the interpreter must be able to get this information across in

a way that the parent can understand. This is not a time to use words that are close, or make up something that could result in the parent misunderstanding the severity of his or her child's condition. The interpreter and the professional may both take notes during the interaction on relevant behaviors noticed in the interaction, questions, or misunderstandings. Especially when an interpreter is used for assessment purposes, the notes may be valuable during the test analysis. An interpreter can ask for clarification during the interaction at any time in order to more correctly relay a message or provide cues or prompts as needed in an assessment. The National Council on Interpreting in Healthcare has information for the interpreter on the basics of note-taking for consecutive interpreting (NCIHC, 2016). There is an excellent training webinar that you can access on Baby Steps for Note-Taking by the NCIHC. This webinar includes information on strategies to recall information such as visualization, sound repetitions, and focusing on key words. The main point of note-taking is to capture ideas, and this can be done through words, shapes, or symbols. Successful note-taking includes both being able to write the note, but even more importantly, being able to read the note. We refer you to this webinar for further information in this area.

The final piece of the BID process is the *debriefing* (D). This is usually a short period of time in the medical appointment, but may be longer in a school or clinical setting. At this time, the interpreter can speak to any culturally relevant aspects of the interaction that he or she feels should be considered in the case. For example, the interpreter may have noticed that the patient was nodding in agreement with the doctor about the need to follow a certain diet to control her diabetes. Later, the patient may have expressed to the interpreter that she doesn't like the foods being recommended. In the ideal setting, the interpreter would have communicated that information to the professional immediately so the doctor and the patient could have had a conversation about options. But, it is still not too late, and a community liaison may be dispatched to the patient's home to discuss diet as a result of the interpreter's information. In a therapeutic or assessment debriefing, the clinician and the interpreter review their notes, discuss any difficulties in the session, discuss student responses, examine parts of the test together, and prepare for the next session. When the clinician reports the findings of an assessment they would describe how the interpreter was used.

CHAPTER SUMMARY

This chapter has provided an overview of the best culturally responsive practices for the use of an interpreter, including the roles and responsibilities of an interpreter and the BID (briefing, interaction, debriefing) process of interpreting. There is one final important point to consider. The use of an interpreter requires the professional to carefully think through the role the interpreter will play in the communication event and the level of risk that the professional is taking by using an interpreter. There is less risk of error as a result of poor interpreting in such situations as: (a) an introductory exchange such as is done when entering an office for an appointment, or (b) a situation where the information is consistent across patients and the responses are predictable, such as an examination protocol where you are expecting a certain answer. Some other examples of a low risk of error scenarios include the following:

■ testing when you are asking the child to "chose the blue ball" (from several colors of balls) or "point to the boy playing"

(where the boy is shown in several different activities);
■ in a doctor's office where you may say, "remove your hearing aid" or "raise your right hand"; and
■ taking background information, questions that the interpreter will have preferably had time to review ahead of time, and then be able to interpret easily and provide the responses uniformly.

There are numerous situations where the "stakes" are high and the interpreting errors can result in serious medical injury, misdiagnosis of a disorder, or misunderstanding of the plan of treatment or other recommendation. Some of these high risk of error settings include:

■ using an interpreter at the bedside for a swallow study;
■ serving as a representative for the IEP team and family;
■ interpreting for an assessment protocol; and
■ transmitting serious educational or medical information to the student, patient, or family.

Numerous medical errors are reported as a result of miscommunication across languages. It has been almost 20 years since the Institute of Medicine first reported that tens of thousands of Americans die each year as a result of medical errors (Institute of Medicine, 1999) in their report, To Err Is Human: Building a Safer Health System. The errors resulting from poor interpreting are considered knowledge-based errors, based on the delivery of incomplete or inaccurate information to the individual. These errors occur in both the medical and educational areas. The Agency for Healthcare Research and Policy reports that nearly 9% of the population (similar to the English language learning population in the

United States of 8.6%.) is at risk for an adverse event because of language barriers (AHRPR, 2012). In one seminal story, a young man named Willie Ramirez remains a quadriplegic today as a result of the misunderstanding of the Spanish word *intoxicado*. In Spanish the word can mean that a generalized illness is affecting the person. This is how this family was using the word. In English it can mean that the person has overdosed on drugs or alcohol or both. This is how the physician was using the word. He chose to treat the young man for a drug overdose and did not order brain tests. In reality, Willie was left for 2 days with an undiagnosed intracerebellar hemorrhage. Neither the doctor nor the family thought that the use of an interpreter was required, although there were severe communication breakdowns and confusion in the emergency room and days after. This was a medical error in language confusion that cost $71 million (Price-Wise, 2008). A trained interpreter may have allowed a successful outcome in this story. In fact, studies show that the medical error rate is cut in half when trained medical interpreters are used (Napoles et al., 2015). Medical errors are common with limited English speakers, and the frequency doubles when family members or untrained interpreters are used. Naples et al. (2015) found that the overall error rate was about 30% with untrained interpreters with errors of omission and answering for the patient or professional being the most common types. Significant errors were reduced by 75% with trained interpreters. Flores et al. (2003) reviewed pediatric encounters in a hospital outpatient clinic. The "ad hoc" interpreter encounters had higher numbers of significant medical errors, 77% versus 53% compared to the trained interpreters. Omissions were the most frequent types of errors. We have presented several interpreting secenarios in the PluralPlus companion website extended learning section for your review.

There is little information on errors in practices of speech-language pathology and audiology resulting from the use of untrained interpreters, or the lack of interpreters. ASHA along with other organizations offer continuing education opportunities to learn about the prevention of medical errors in general. Information on errors made as a result of a language communication breakdown would also be beneficial.

Finally, maintaining high ethical standards is critical in our work as speech, language, hearing, and swallowing professionals. The ability to make appropriate diagnostic and treatment decisions is paramount and at the core of an ethical practice. Thus, it would be inappropriate to relegate treatment or diagnostic decision making to an interpreter, either trained or untrained. It is not acceptable to ask an interpreter to make a decision, such as, "Do you think this therapy goal is relevant for this child?" or "would an informal or formal assessment be best?" There may be some situations where you have developed a long-standing relationship with your interpreter, and they are serving more as a paraprofessional, SLPA, or audiology technician. In this situation, there may be flexibility in these matters on a case-by-case basis. However, great caution must be taken before the information provided by an interpreter is used solely to make professional decisions. It takes great effort to use an interpreter correctly, and it will take time and commitment to use an interpreter successfully in your workplace.

In the end, it is the professional's ultimate responsibility to decide whether the interpreting is reliable and accurate. If you have any concern in this area, it is best to terminate the communication exchange until you feel assured that the interpreter is capable of providing accurate information. There must be a high level of trust and respect between the interpreter and the professional. The final outcome of the consultation, evaluation, therapy, or meeting always remains the ethical responsibility of the professional. The interpreter has no professional responsibility for the outcome. The interpreter must, however, provide the most accurate interpreting possible and abide by the interpreter codes of ethics as mentioned earlier in the chapter.

Schyve (2007) provides an excellent overview of how language differences can be a barrier to quality and safety for medical and other health professionals. The integration of evidence-based practices in our work, or in our case, the culturally responsive practices throughout this book, is posited as a solution. He describes the "triple threat" for diverse individuals who do not speak English as a first language. The first threat is the language difference, the second threat is the cultural difference, and the third threat is low health literacy. Although the use of translation was not discussed in this chapter, an interpreter may be able to assist in translation materials. It is vital to translate materials into the language of choice in order for individuals to understand their educational and medical situation. However, the ability to understand and process oral communication also is a barrier to health literacy. Presenting a parent with a set of instructions for ways to assist their child at home with a language disorder, feed their baby with a cleft palate, or use the augmentative communication system for their child with autism, among others, can be overwhelming and taxing. Accurately processing that information may be impossible for an individual who speaks English as a second language. Using the interpreter is one tool to better communicate with second language speakers with communication and swallowing disorders. As we have learned, there are many threats to their recovery and using an interpreter appropriately may be the key to ease the burden significantly. The patient, client, or student has the right to be fully informed of his or her medical or educational status. The use of interpreting services can assure that this happens. The use of an interpreter can also help us provide successful educational and health care outcomes for our patients, clients, and students.

FURTHER READING

Flores, G., Laws, B., Mayo, S. J., Zuckerman, B., Abreru, M., Medina, L., & Hardt, E. J. (2003). Errors in medical interpretation and their potential clinical consequences in pediatric encounters. *Pediatrics, 111*, 6–14.

Grainger-Monsen, M., & Haslett, J. (2003). *Worlds apart: A four-part series on cross cultural healthcare, video modules.* Boston, MA: Fanlight Productions. Retrieved from http://www.fanlight.com/downloads/Worlds_Apart.pdf

Green, A., Betancourt, J., & Carrillo, E. J. (2003). Worlds apart: Facilitator's guide. *Commonwealth Fund.* Retrieved from http://www.cmwf.org/usr_doc/worlds_apart_guide2.pdf

Mohammad Kochi's Story. https://www.youtube.com/watch?v=K5d_iPaUrWw

REFERENCES

Agency for Healthcare Research and Quality (AHRQ). (2012). *Improving patient safety systems for patients with limited english proficiency.* Retrieved from http://www.ahrq.gov/professionals/systems/hopital/lepguide/index.html

American Speech-Language-Hearing Association (ASHA). (2010). *Cultural Competence Checklist: Personal reflection.* Retrieved from http://www.asha.org/uploadedFiles/Cultural-Competence-Checklist-Personal-Reflection.pdf

Chen, A. H., Youdelman, M. K., & Brooks, J. D. (2007). The legal framework for language access in healthcare settings: Title VI and beyond. *Journal of General Internal Medicine, 22*(2), 362–367.

Cowan, N. (2010). The magical mystery four: How is working capacity limited and why? *Current Directions in Psychological Science, 19*(1), 51–57.

Cummins, J. (1979). Cognitive/academic language proficiency, linguistic interdependence, the optimum age questions and some other matters. *Working Papers on Bilingualism, 19,* 121–129.

Cummins, J. (2008). BICS and CALP: Empirical and theoretical status of the distinction. In B. Street & N. H. Hornberger (Eds.), *Encyclopedia of language and education, Volume 2: Literacy* (2nd ed., pp. 71–83). New York, NY: Springer Science + Business Media.

Department of Health and Human Services (DHHS). (2003). Use and disclosures to carry out treatment, payment or health care operations. *Code of Federal Regulations*, Vol. 1, Section 164-506, Title 45.

Flores, G. (2005). The Impact of medical interpreter services on the quality of health care: A systematic review. *Medical Care Research and Review, 62*(3), 255–299.

Flores, G., Laws, B., Mayo, S. J., Zuckerman, B., Abreru, M., Medina, L., & Hardt, E. J. (2003). Errors in medical interpretation and their potential clinical consequences in pediatric encounters. *Pediatrics, 111,* 6–14.

Grainger-Monsen, M., & Haslett, J. (2003). *Worlds apart: A four-part series on cross cultural healthcare, video modules.* Boston, MA: Fanlight Productions. Retrieved from http://www.fanlight.com/downloads/Worlds_Apart.pdf

Green, A., Betancourt, J., & Carrillo, E. J. (2003). Worlds apart: Facilitator's guide. *Commonwealth Fund.* Retrieved from http://www.cmwf.org/usr_doc/worlds_apart_guide2.pdf

Hall, E. T. (1990). *Understanding cultural differences, Germans, French and Americans*, Yarmouth, ME: Intercultural Press.

Haviland, W. A., Prins, H. E. L., McBride, B., & Walrath, D. (2017). *Cultural anthropology: The human challenge* (15th ed.). Boston, MA: Cengage Learning.

Individuals with Disability Education Improvement Act (IDEA: 2004). *Subchapter II: Assistance for education of all children with disabilities.* Retrieved from http://uscode.house.gov/view.xhtml?path=/prelim@title20/chapter33/subchapter2&edition=prelim

Institute of Medicine. (1999). *To err is human: Building a safer health system.* Retrieved from http://www.nationalacademies.org/hmd/~/media/Files/Report%20Files/1999/To-Err-is-Human/To%20Err%20is%20Human%20 1999%20%20report%20brief.pdf

Langdon, H. W., & Cheng, L. L. (2002). *Collaborating with interpreters and translators.* Eau Claire, WI: Thinking Publications.

Langdon, H. W., & Saenz, T. I. (2015). *Working with interpreters and translators: A guide for speech-language pathologists and audiologists.* San Diego, CA: Plural.

Marvel, M. K., Doherty, W. J., & Weiner, E. (1988). Medical interviewing by exemplar family physicians. *Journal of Family Practice, 47*(5), 343–348.

Marvel, M. K., Epstein, R. M., Flowers, K., & Beckman, H. B. (1999). Soliciting the patient's agenda: Have we improved? *Journal of American Medical Association, 281*(3), 287.

Mehrabian, A. (1981). *Silent messages: Implicit communication of emotions and attitudes* (2nd ed.). Belmont, CA: Wadsworth.

Mehrabian, A., & Wiener, M. (1967). Decoding of inconsistent communications, *Journal of Personality and Social Psychology, 6,* 109–114.

Nápoles, A. M., Santoyo-Olsson, J., Karliner, L. S., Gregorich, S. E., & Pérez-Stable, E. J. (2015). Inaccurate language interpretation and its clinical significance in the medical encounters of Spanish-speaking Latinos. *Medical Care, 53*(11), 940.

National Center for Health Statistics. (2012). *National Ambulatory Medical Care Survey: State and National Summary Tables: Time spent with physician: United States, Table 29.* Retrieved from http://www.cdc.gov/nchs/data/ahcd/namcs_summary/2012_namcs_web_tables.pdf

National Council on Interpreting in Healthcare (NCIHC). (2005). *National standards of practice for interpreters in healthcare.* Retrieved from http://www.ncihc.org/assets/documents/publications/NCIHC%20National%20Standards %20of%20Practice.pdf

National Council on Interpreting in Healthcare (NCIHC). (2011). *Healthcare Interpreter Train-*

ing Program self-assessment based on the National Standards for Healthcare Interpreter Training Programs. Retrieved from https://ncihc.mem berclicks.net/assets/documents/Interpreter%20 Training%20Program%20Self-assessment% 2006-22-2011%20(2).pdf

National Council on Interpreting in Healthcare (NCIHC). (2014). *A crosswalk of the National Standards for Culturally and Linguistically Appropriate Services (CLAS) in health and healthcare to the Joint Commission hospital accreditation standards* (pp. 1–16). Retrieved from https:// www.jointcommission.org/assets/1/6/Cross walk-_CLAS_-20140718.pdf

National Council on Interpreting in Healthcare (NCIHC). (2016). *Baby steps to note-taking for consecutive interpreting.* Retrieved from https:// www.slideshare.net/NCIHC/baby-steps-to-notetaking-for-consecutive-interpreting

National Language Service Corps (NLSC). (2024). *Understanding interpretation and translation.* Retrieved from http://www.nlscorps.org/images/ Translation_and_Interpretation_Tutorial.pdf

O'Neil, D. (2009). *Hidden aspects of communication.* Retrieved from http://anthro.palomar.edu/ language/language_6.htm

Price-Wise, G. (2008). Language, culture, and medical tragedy: The case of Willie Ramirez. *HealthAffairsBlog.* Retrieved from http://health affairs.org/blog/2008/11/19/language-culture-and-medical-tragedy-the-case-of-willie-ramirez/

Salas-Provance, M. B., Erickson, J. G., & Reed, J. (2002). Disabilities as viewed by four generations of one Hispanic family. *American Journal of Speech Language Pathology, 11*(2), 151–162.

Schyve, P. M. (2007). Language differences as a barrier to quality and safety in healthcare: The Joint Commission perspective. *Journal of General Internal Medicine, 2*, 360–361.

Shin, S. J. (2018). *Bilingualism in schools and society: Language, identity, and policy* (2nd ed.). New York, NY: Routledge.

Tai, Y. (2014). The application of body language in English teaching. *Journal of Language Teaching and Research, 5*(5), 1205–1209.

Tamasi, S. & Antieau, L. (2015). *Language and linguistic diversity in the U. S.: An introduction.* New York, NY: Routledge.

The Joint Commission. (n.d.). *Advancing effective communication, cultural competence, and patient- and family-centered care: A roadmap for hospitals.* Retrieved from http://www.jointcom mission.org/assets/1/6/ARoadmapforHospitals finalversion727.pdf

U.S. Census Bureau (USCB). (2015). Census bureau reports at least 350 languages spoken in U.S. homes. *American Home Community Survey.* Retrieved from https://www.census.gov/ newsroom/press-releases/2015/cb15-185.html

U.S. Department of Education (USDE). (n.d.a). IDEAs that work. *Office of Special Education and Rehabilitative Services.* Retrieved from https://www.osepideasthatwork.org/

U.S. Department of Education (USDE). (n.d.b). Individuals with Disabilities Education Act (IDEA). *Office of Special Education and Rehabilitative Services.* Retrieved from https://www2 .ed.gov/about/offices/list/osers/osep/osep-idea .html

U.S. Department of Health and Human Services (USDHHS). (2001a). National standards for culturally and linguistically appropriate services in healthcare: Executive summary. *Office of Minority Health.* Retrieved from https:// minorityhealth.hhs.gov/assets/pdf/checked/ executive.pdf

U.S. Department of Health and Human Services (USDHHS). (2001b). National standards for culturally and linguistically appropriate services in healthcare: FINAL REPORT. *Office of Minority Health.* Retrieved from https:// minorityhealth.hhs.gov/assets/pdf/checked/ finalreport.pdf

U.S. Department of Health and Human Services (USDHHS). (2003). *Summary of the HIPAA privacy rule.* Retrieved from https://www.hhs .gov/sites/default/files/privacysummary.pdf?lan guage=es

U.S. Department of Health and Human Services (USDHHS). (2013). National standards for culturally and linguistically appropriate services in healthcare: A blueprint for advancing and sustaining CLAS policy and practice. *Office of Minority Health.* Retrieved from https://www .thinkculturalhealth.hhs.gov/pdfs/Enhanced CLASStandardsBlueprint.pdf

Yuan, J., Liberman, M., & Cieri, C. (2006). Towards an integrated understanding of speaking rate in conversation. *Proceedings of Interspeech* (pp. 541–544).

10

Culturally Responsive Assessment

The purpose of this chapter is to describe culturally responsive assessment practices in the field of speech-language pathology and audiology. The importance of assessment from a multicultural perspective has been discussed broadly (Battle, 2002, 2012; Langdon, 2008; Roseberry-McKibbin, 2014). The assessment of bilingual children and adults requires clinical skills specific to this population and their needs (Goldstein, 2012; Kohnert, 2008). In-depth assessment strategies for speech, language, hearing, and swallowing disorders are documented well, and many of these sources also include important information for the assessment of culturally and linguistically diverse populations (Hegde & Freed, 2016; Hegde & Pomaville, 2016). Information on the assessment of bilingual language will be found in Chapter 5, Culture and Language, and assessment of audiology will be found in Chapter 6, Culture and Hearing Health.

LEARNING OBJECTIVES

After reading, discussing, and processing the information presented in this chapter, you will be able to demonstrate the following knowledge, skills, and attitudes:

1. Knowledge
   a. Explain the Hierarchy of Cultural Knowledge.
   b. Explain the effect of the cultural context on the development of speech and language.
   c. Explain the structure of a least-biased and culturally responsive assessment.
   d. Differentiate a language difference from a language disorder.
   e. Identify sound system differences in the Spanish and English languages.
   f. Identify the effects of culture in the assessment of fluency, cleft lip and palate, and voice disorders.
   g. Identify the consequences of using inappropriate assessment tools.
2. Skills
   a. Select an appropriate alternative assessment procedure for assessment of culturally and linguistically diverse populations.
   b. Use culturally and linguistically appropriate strategies during a bedside swallow examination.
   c. Use dynamic assessment to distinguish a difference versus a disorder.
   d. Use counseling strategies appropriate for multicultural populations.

3. Attitudes
   a. Show how the Hierarchy of Cultural Knowledge can help prepare you for an assessment.
   b. Demonstrate the ability to incorporate alternative strategies into an assessment.
   c. Acknowledge the value of using an interpreter in the assessment.
   d. Identify the importance of using emic approach in the assessment decision-making process.

KEY CONCEPTS

Key concepts addressed in this chapter are presented in Table 10–1.

CULTURALLY RESPONSIVE ASSESSMENT PRACTICES

Culturally responsive assessment practices accommodate variability found among people from a variety of cultural and linguistic groups. These practices assure that tests used in the assessments are fair and as unbiased as possible, and that the unique capabilities found in diverse groups are identified and validated.

Before you begin the assessment for a child or adult with a linguistic or cultural background different than your own, it is important to take a few minutes to first assess your own level of understanding of the culture of others and any bias you may hold regarding this culture. This moment of reflection will set the tone for your assessment and ensure that you will provide culturally responsive care. Use the Hierarchy of Cultural Knowledge (HCK) framework described in Chapter 3 as a barometer (Figure 10–1). Is your understanding of this culture at the lowest rung where your knowledge is based on stereotypes with potential inherent biases? Are you at risk for having misperceptions and incorrect expectations of this family dynamic? Or are you at the highest rung where you communicate with individuals from this cultural group and understand, value, and respect the influence of the culture on their everyday lives?

Additionally, think about your conceptual framework (Hyter, 2014) for providing culturally responsive care, also discussed in Chapter 3. What theoretical perspective undergirds the way you approach services? Will you focus only on the formal results of assessments (posivitism) or incorporate the client's perspective (interpretivism) or also be concerned with the contextual factors, such as policies and social structures, that may affect the person's ability to engage fully in his or her daily life (critical perspectives)? Where are you on the pathway to responsive "global" and cultural engagement (PRGCE) (Hyter, 2014, p. 116)? Have you acquired cultural humility—the ability to acknowledge that there are cultural values and practices just as valid as

TABLE 10–1. Key Concepts

Least-biased assessment	Alternative assessments
Dynamic assessment	Ethnographic interview
High-context culture	Low-context culture
Criterion referenced testing	Difference versus disorder
African American English as a rule-governed language system	Linguistic profiling

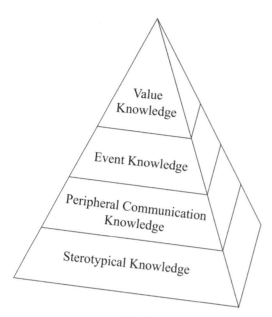

FIGURE 10–1. Hierarchy of cultural knowledge. Republished with permission of Delmar Learning, a division of Cengage Learning, from Salas-Provance, M. B. (2010). Counseling in a multicultural society: Implications for the field of communication sciences and disorders. In L. Flasher and P. Fogel (Eds.), *Counseling Skills for Speech-Language Pathologists and Audiologists* (pp. 159–189). Clifton Park, NY: Delmar; permission conveyed through Copyright Clearance Center, Inc.

your own? Are you culturally self-aware, and have you gained cultural knowledge, as indicated by your location on the HCK (Salas-Provance, 2010) discussed in the previous paragraph? Are you ready to engage with others from a position of reciprocity (Hyter, 2014)?

Activity 10–1

1. Using your developing conceptual framework, identify which theoretical position will guide your practice with a new referral you are scheduled to see soon.
2. Using the steps on the HCK and your conceptual framework, discuss a new referral that you are scheduled to see soon.

3. Using the steps on the HCK and your conceptual framework, discuss a current patient, client, or student on your caseload from a racially or ethnically diverse group.
4. Discuss the steps of the HCK and the PRGCE with your colleagues and where each of you feels the most comfortable at this point in time.
5. Discuss ideas of how you would move from your current level to one or two levels above on the HCK and/or the PRGCE.

Once you have taken the time to prepare yourself for the assessment, the next step is to review the cultural context within which the patient, client, or student has lived and how it has contributed to or framed the behaviors that you will observe in the assessment. An assessment strategy that keeps culture at its core will maintain focus on delivering a culturally responsive assessment. Attention to culture is the third prong or leg that maintains the balance of the assessment. Without a cultural focus, an assessment is at the minimum incomplete, possibly invalid, or at worst biased. A clinician takes the risk of making an incorrect diagnosis when culturally responsive assessment practices are not used.

As you review the following case example of a speech-language pathologist (SLP) interacting with the family of a preschool-age child, take note of:

- the educational information that the family needs to make an appropriate decision for their son's schooling;
- the family background information that the professional needs to have to provide effective services to the child; and
- the cultural knowledge, skills, and attitudes that are important for the SLP to have to provide appropriate services to a child who speaks a language that is different from their own.

Box 10–1
Case: Seth

The story of little Seth shows the importance of having a cultural focus of assessment, in this case, speech, language, and *culture*. The cultural context in which Seth has developed over the past 3 years is having a major impact on his speech and language development. Most professionals would agree that to place a 3-year-old, whose primary language is not English, in the back of a room day after day to play alone is a blatantly unfair and discriminatory practice. Yet, there are many true stories of just this scenario. Such a 3-year-old was brought to Dr. Salas-Provance in a school setting for an evaluation. She introduced herself in Spanish to the parents and Seth. The parents were immediately put at ease when they realized they were communicating with a bilingual service provider. Seth's big brown eyes looked up at his parents, then at her, tracking their conversation. This interaction was the beginning of the assessment and included important information. It could readily be seen that Seth was alert and attentive, at the same time being shy and on the verge of

tears. He was being considered for special education placement due to the fact that he would not talk in his preschool classroom and played alone the entire day. Was he selectively mute? Was he intellectually impaired? The parents were cautious and confused about this referral, but immediately reported that Seth did fine at home, played with his older brothers and sisters (he was the youngest), and spoke in Spanish well. The predictive validity of parent report for 2- to 3-year-olds has been found to be reasonably good for expressive language (Feldman, Campbell, Kurs-Lasky, & Rockette, 2005). This parent information was recorded and considered with other assessment findings. In this instance, after observing Seth play with his parents and conducting a speech and language screening in Spanish with the parents in the room, it was clear that Seth's main "problem," with the limited information gathered at this time, was that he was a primary Spanish speaker, a little shy, and would rather be home than at school.

Activity 10–2

Take a few minutes to brainstorm with two others, a list of information that you can insert into the columns of Table 10–2. Information, knowledge, skills, and attitudes needed to provide culturally, linguistically, and globally responsive services to the children and families in Seth's preschool classroom. Keep this chart in mind as you read the remainder of this chapter. At the end of the chapter, once you

have processed the Key Concepts and their definitions, you may revise the chart using a different color of ink.

Of course, not all assessments that involve children and adults from culturally and linguistically diverse backgrounds are going to be completed as quickly as that for Seth. There may be serious communication disorders that may need to be addressed with additional testing. But Seth's story shows how important it is for professionals to be aware of the tools

TABLE 10–2. Brainstormed List of Information, Knowledge, Skills, and Attitudes Needed to Provide Culturally, Linguistically, and Globally Responsive Services to Children and Families

Information	Knowledge	Skills	Attitudes

needed to have a successful outcome in their assessment, including the use of an interpreter, appropriate bilingual assessment materials, and the knowledge and skills to carry out test adaptations as necessary. When considering the speech and language assessment of bilingual and bicultural children, one of the most important diagnostic decisions is to distinguish between a "language difference" and a "language disorder."

There are differences associated with learning a second language, which are distinct from communication disorders. The child learning English as a second language has had limited experiences in the use of the English language. Difficulties associated with learning English should not be considered speech or language disorders. By testing in the native language, the clinician is more likely to recognize a true disorder. To effectively separate second language difference from communication disorder requires a complex and multifactorial assessment process that includes assessment in both languages. Culturally responsive practices will ensure that the individual is diagnosed correctly. The diagnostic process begins with an interview of the patient, client, or student.

APPROPRIATE ASSESSMENT PRACTICES, MEASURES, AND TOOLS

Interview Protocol

Before the testing begins, an appropriate case history must be taken. Information can be gathered in many ways. As occurred with Seth earlier, observations can begin in a hallway while talking with the parents and then continue in the evaluation room with the parents and the child together or the child alone. It can occur at bedside with a patient, or in a formal setting with a set amount of time dedicated to taking the case history. This time can be used to complete forms or review information submitted earlier. The way in which the professional and the client engage can follow a traditional model where the professional frames direct questions to receive specific answers. Or the interview can take on a conversational style, with spontaneous and equal amounts of information provided by all parties. The latter way of interviewing is more suitable for a diverse population and typical of the ethnographic interview style. In Chapter 7, the use of ethnographic interviewing is discussed. This type of interview makes it more likely that you will receive culturally relevant information during the interview.

No matter the disorder presented, it is important to have knowledge of the cultural and linguistic background of the people we serve. In Chapter 5, Culture and Language, we discussed a set of questions that may be used to learn the cultural background of an individual who is an English language learner. The set of 10 questions in Table 10–3 can be beneficial as a part of your assessment process to succinctly gather background information.

Start the interview by discussing issues related to the family structure, beliefs, and traditions. You may want to ask questions about implicit cultural beliefs such as gender roles in the family, child-rearing practices, beliefs

TABLE 10–3. Questions on Cultural and Linguistic Background for English as a Second Language Speaker

1. How long has the family been in the country?

2. How long has the patient been in the United States?

3. What is the language(s) spoken at home?

4. What is the patient's level of exposure to English?

5. What is the language skill of other family members?

6. What is the patient's language development history in each language?

7. What is the education level of the family?

8. What has been the acculturation pattern of the family?

9. What is the economic level of the family?

10. What is the family's cultural dynamic?

on disability, or educational values. In terms of family traditions, be sure that you are interviewing the appropriate family member(s) for that family dynamic (Ortega, 2016). For example, in many traditional Latin@/Hispanic families, the role of the father as the breadwinner and caretaker of the family would dictate that he be the decision maker and, therefore, the key person in the interview. For many immigrant families, those roles may be reversed. Children may be taking on the role as breadwinner or caretaker; thus, they become the main decision makers for the parents. Although it is not recommended that family members serve as interpreters, the reality is that many do interpret for each other. In fact, consider that in many cases, the elder family members may place more trust in their own family member than in an interpreter who is a stranger to the family. The use of an interpreter could appear invasive to the family. Be sure to have a thoughtful discussion with the family to bridge this cultural gap and to stress the need for an interpreter from outside of the family. Consider also that a person may come into the interview with several family members. There may be certain family members who should be included or excluded from the interview, but this should be done with sensitivity and consideration of the desires of the family. The student or patient may need to be interviewed alone as well as with family members, depending on the information that needs to be gathered. In order to allow for an authentic conversation to occur, a specific interview environment may be necessary. You may need to conduct the interview out in the community, over several sessions, or with a variety of family members. Because there is so much cultural variation among individuals and groups, the use of cultural humility as discussed in Chapter 3 can be useful. Here the professional does not claim to know the cultural intricacies of the family dynamic, but is open to learning, which can allow the family to be more open with you during the interview.

In many cultures, there can be mistrust of the professional, especially if the professional sets himself or herself up as the expert (Benkert, Peters, Clark, & Keves-Foster, 2006). On the other hand, in many cultures a high value is placed on professionals (e.g., therapists, teachers, and doctors) who will be respected. Frequently, the family will follow requests of professionals without question. Passive acknowledgment from the family can limit the amount of important information the health care professional will receive during the interview. Although family members may nod in agreement, they may only do so to avoid having to divulge private information, or they may be uncomfortable expressing their disagreement with the professional. For example, the professional may say to a family, "Your father can choke on foods, therefore, he should only have food that is pureed." The family may agree, but may still bring in foods from home either because they do not understand the severity of the disorder, or do not agree with the recommendation, thinking "regular" food from home will help make their family member better sooner. The use of professional terminology during an interview can be disorienting for families who may already

be upset or confused with the examination. A natural and engaging interactive communication style will place the family at ease. Early in the interview process, try to learn the family's beliefs on the disability of their family member (see Chapter 6; Glanz, Rimer, & Lewis, 2002; Kleinman & Benson, 2006; Salas-Provance, Erickson, & Reed, 2002, Sanchez & Wood, 2016). They may be more hopeful or more desperate than you expect. It is important to "know" or learn their true state of belief or understanding through a sensitive conversation.

As professionals who have years of experience in assessment, we know our cultural expectation for how the assessment process will proceed. However, a patient or student has not had these same experiences, and his or her expectation may be quite different from the professional's experience. Let's consider just one cultural aspect of the assessment, *time factor,* and how the element of time may vary across cultures. One way to examine cultures is through the anthropological reference of low-context versus high-context cultures (Hall, 1976), as outlined in Table 10–4.

Individual behavior may vary on the continuum of low- to high-context cultures or be a mix of the two. However, it is important to be aware of the effect of these belief

TABLE 10–4. Example of Low- and High-Context Culture

	Low-Context Culture	High-Context Culture
Communication	More words, spell things out, explain more, explicit, direct	Few words, assume common knowledge, indirect
Family	Individual, loosely defined family structure	Small close-knit group, traditional
Learning	Individual orientation, focus on detail, speed not accuracy	Group learning, connectedness, accuracy
Territory	Compartmentalized, privacy, farther apart	Communal, share space, stand close

Source: Based on Hall (1976).

principles on established behaviors. In Box 10–2, the culture of this First Nations family may be considered high context temporally. In this context, time is not easily scheduled, everything has its own time, the needs of people come first, and time is slow and it belongs to others and nature (Hall, 1976). The story that follows shows how this family managed time for an assessment within their cultural framework.

Box 10–2
Case: Mariah

As a member of cleft palate teams for many years, Dr. Salas-Provance is familiar with the team process whereby the family members come to their appointment early in the morning and are seen by several professionals throughout the day. The day culminates with a team meeting to review the day's patients. On one occasion, while collecting speech data on the speech development of children with cleft lip and palate, Dr. Salas-Provance had hoped to interview a family from a First Nations culture during their scheduled team visit and to record the speech of their baby for the study. Dr. Salas-Provance arrived early for the team meeting and set up the equipment, and was hoping to receive family approval for the recording first thing that day. Patients arrived for their evaluations throughout the day, but not the family for whom she was waiting. Finally, when the team was ending for the day, the family arrived. In fact, team members were getting into their cars to leave when a truck with this family in it arrived in the parking lot. The father reported that there were some family and transportation issues that morning. Because they had traveled several hours from a faraway reservation, the team surgeon quickly examined the 18-month-old baby. It was not likely that the child would have another team visit for at least 6 months if she was not seen that day. Unfortunately, it was too late for Dr. Salas-Provance to do a recording, and she could see that the opportunity to have the speech of this baby in the database had been lost. However, she spoke with the family and mentioned what she was doing in terms of her research. They listened intently and said, "We want Mariah recorded." Dr. Salas-Provance was overjoyed, of course, but it was too late to record that day. It was explained to the family that the center would not be available for a recording at a later time. Not to be deterred, the family presented another option. They invited Dr. Salas-Provance to go to their home on the reservation to complete the recording. This was a surprising turn of events; this was not something that would have been expected. She returned to their home on the reservation the next day and completed the recording and interview with parents, grandparents, and a few brothers, sisters, and neighbors in the room. They invited her to stay for lunch, which she did. While eating a lunch of freshly prepared home cooking, they explained that that they would do anything that they could to help Mariah. They felt that because of the cleft palate, she was a very special child and they wanted to be sure she could learn to talk with the "hole in her mouth."

Take a few minutes to brainstorm with two others to answer the following questions:

1. What are some other factors besides *time* that can be a cultural factor in an assessment?
2. Why did the family allow the SLP to go to their home?
3. Why is going to the home of a First Nations family on a reservation of significance?
4. What was the purpose of all the people in the room during the recording?
5. Would you have been comfortable joining the family for lunch? What may have resulted if the SLP had not accepted the lunch invitation?
6. Does this situation fit into your knowledge of expected behavior for this cultural group?

This story is a reminder of what a rare and special opportunity it is when we are invited into the sanctuary of a First Nations family's home, or the home of any family. We may carry stereotypes about families who come late to appointments, as our general expectation is that the family being assessed should be respectful of the time allotted to them by the professionals. But a culturally responsive framework requires us to look deeper into the family's world and be flexible and understanding. In communicating with families from across many cultures, it has been found that all families, no matter the culture, want the best care available for their children, parents, and other family members despite their views on time management.

As an activity, consider the low- and high-context cultural attributes and answer the following questions:

1. Where do I fit in this continuum of low- to high-context cultures?

2. Have I been considering this aspect of culture in others?
3. Does the fact that a person is from a low-context culture or high-context culture directly affect my assessment strategies?
4. Which attributes of low- and high-context cultures are most important for me to understand?

We now look at specific assessment strategies for individuals from culturally and linguistically diverse groups.

ALTERNATIVE ASSESSMENT PROCEDURES

The first part of an assessment is to select the appropriate tools. A standardized assessment requires the test delivery protocol to be completed as specified in the test manual. Any change to the testing delivery invalidates the examination. Before selecting a test, it is important to check if the person's ethnic and/or language background is represented in the normative sample. If not, you may still have reasons to use the test. However, you need to make adjustments to the test delivery format to fit the client's needs. If you make changes, they need to be explained on your diagnostic report and the test scores cannot be used in an official capacity, for example, as a standardized test score to place a student in a special education class. There may be information from the test that can provide important direction for your follow-up intervention.

It is possible to provide a least-biased and culturally responsive assessment by using several methods. As noted earlier, you can complete a norm-referenced standardized assessment if the test has been normed on the target group. When it has not, you can still use the standardized test by using alternative assessment methods (Table 10–5). A review of these methods is provided by Erickson and Iglesias (1986); Goldtstein (2000); Laing and Khami (2003); and Tolliver-Weddington and Myerson (1983).

An alternative to norm-referenced tests is the use of a criterion-referenced test. A more in-depth description of criterion-referenced testing is given on the PluralPlus companion website. In essence, you set up the task and measure the outcome. For example, we want to know whether the person can use the grammatical concept of "–ing." The criterion is to use 10 episodes of "–ing" while describing a picture in a 10-minute period of time. If eight episodes of "–ing" are used within the 10 minutes, then the task was completed with 80% accuracy. This can be completed at any complexity level needed for the patient, client, or student.

Modifying Norm-Referenced Tests

Even if you chose an appropriate norm-refer-enced test, it may not give you all the infor-mation you need. It is suggested that a variety of measures be used to fully assess speech and language skills in culturally and linguistically diverse individuals. As noted in Table 10–5, the administration procedures of the norm-referenced test can be modified.

Let's consider that we are administering a language test to a 12-year-old child, Abdel, who just immigrated to the United States from a Middle Eastern country. The child has stud-ied English for many years but has not partici-pated in a schooling structure similar to what is found in the United States. You feel com-fortable that a standardized test with adapta-tions will be appropriate. The child is hesitant

TABLE 10–5. Alternative Methods of Assessment

1. Use of criterion-referenced tests

2. Modification of norm-referenced tests by
   - Varying prompting
   - Completing test over several sessions
   - Completing test under several conditions in different locations (office, classroom, playground, home, patient room)
   - Using more than the allotted practice items
   - Extending the time of the testing
   - Allowing credit for a variety of responses beyond those accepted in test protocol
   - Scoring test twice, once by examiner manual direction and one with nonstandard adjustments

3. Measure processing abilities rather than language knowledge

4. Use of portfolio assessment methods

5. Use of narrative assessment methods

6. Use of dynamic assessment methods

7. Include an interpreter in administration of test

8. Develop a new test

in giving responses, so you *provide more than the allotted two prompts* on certain parts of the test. This is a successful strategy as he gets the answers correct with the increased prompting. The test is long and Abdel is tired. He is now using English more than ever before, which is still difficult for him, settling into a new school and making new friends. You decide to have him *return the next day to complete the test*. This allows the child to rest, which will maximize his performance on the test. You sense that he was uncomfortable in the conference room where you were testing, so you decide to *continue the testing in a room next to his classroom*. Immediately you see that he is more relaxed as he is in a familiar environment. You get to one part of the test where he must provide a list of words in a selected period of time. He does not understand the request so you *practice the task several times* before providing the test items. This allows him to learn the procedure before having to complete the test item. You are now at the end of the test administration, and it is clear that the *time allotted for the test has been exceeded*. You complete the final item where Abdel must describe the function of certain objects. You note that the items in the test are not familiar to him and he has not had experience with those objects. Instead of using the objects in the picture book, *you ask him to describe the function of items in the room and items with which he is familiar*. Clearly, you have had to adapt the test so you want to be sure to provide Abdel with as much credit as you can for his answers. You first score the test as the scoring manual directs and then *score the test again with the nontraditional adjustments made*. In reviewing the administration of the test, it appears that Abdel's true abilities are reflected and that a good diagnostic decision can be made for a discharge, placement in English language learning (ELL) services, or speech and language therapy.

Beyond making adjustments to a standardized test, you can consider other options including using: (a) *criterion referenced tests* (McCauley, 1996) where you measure task performance by a set of criteria you have established; (b) *portfolio assessments* (Herrera, Murry & Cabral, 2012; Kratcoski, 1998) where you collect and review student work over time, such as story writing tasks, spelling quizzes, or projects; (c) *narrative assessments* (Bliss & McCabe, 2012; Hedberg & Westby, 1993) where a child progressively completes narratives with supports or with the assistance of dynamic assessment methods (Gutierrez-Clellen & Quinn, 1993); and (d) *ethnographic assessments* (Westby, 1990) where you gather information about the student or patient from several individuals or from documents, such as reports. In ethnographic assessment, you are looking for examples of correct task completion. You want to identify the settings, tasks, situations, and environments in which the child or patient performs well. Finally, *dynamic assessments* (Gutierrez-Clellan & Peña, 2001; Peña, 2000; Peña et al., 2014; Petersen, Chanthongthip, Ukrainetz, Spencer, & Steeve, 2017) occur when you measure a child's performance, such as narrative retelling, before and after a teaching (mediation) component. Because dynamic assessment has been shown to be a useful tool for identifying language impairment in English language learners (Kohnert, 2013; Peña, Gillam & Bedore, 2014), a more detailed description follows.

Dynamic Assessment

Dynamic assessment has been used for more than 40 years and was first identified through the work of Vygotsky (1978). Vygotsky identified the Zone of Proximal Development (ZPD), which depicts the distance between the level of task performance when teaching is provided and when teaching is not provided. This distance has been identified as the "potential" the student has to learn the task.

Reuven Feuerstein added mediated learning to Vygotsky's theory (Fuerstein, Fuerstein, Falik, & Rand, 2006). Mediation or the mediated learning experience is an important component of dynamic assessment. It is the way that learning is experienced as it is intentionally mediated by a parent, teacher, peer, sibling, or others, such as a speech-language pathologist. The "mediating agent, guided by intention, culture, and emotional investment, selects, enhances, focuses, and otherwise organizes the world of stimuli for the learner . . . for that learner's enhanced and effective functioning" (Feuerstein et al., 2006).

Dynamic assessment can distinguish a difference from a disorder, which will allow us to recommend appropriate services, either ELL services or speech-language therapy. When the child is successful during the mediated learning portion of dynamic assessment, this indicates that ELL services are appropriate. If we are using dynamic assessment to examine the English language skills of a student, and to identify the possibilities within their level of English, the child should have basic interpersonal communication skills (BICS) in English (Cummins, 2008). An individual with BICS can communicate in the language at a social level, face-to-face, for everyday social communication. This is not a deficit model of assessment where the focus would be on the English skills they "do not" have. Dynamic assessments also can be conducted in both languages, if needed.

Dynamic assessment can be used for a child who, for example, is inappropriately using past tense irregular verbs in English, such as, "I *eated* my food yesterday." In this case, after one or a few teaching sessions, the child is able to say, "I *ate* my food yesterday." Additional training on irregular verbs like *drank* and *flew* allowed the child to transfer skills to other irregular verbs and be able to say, "I drank water yesterday" and "The bird flew yesterday." This child has shown that with

training or mediation he can learn. For some children, the teaching sessions may be longer. This child has now had an experience that he did not have before. The therapist has provided a culturally responsive assessment and received a good outcome. The child has shown us his ability to learn, he has transferred the strategies he was taught, and he has responded positively to the teaching.

The final option on the list of alternative methods of assessment is to develop a new measure. This is not a decision to be made lightly, and may only happen under extreme circumstances. Yet, there may come a time when this is the *only* choice you have.

Developing a New Screening Measure

Dr. Salas-Provance had the opportunity to develop a new screening measure while working as a bilingual consultant. She received a request from the state department to assess a large number of school-age children whose parents were summer migrant workers. Approximately 500 children were in need of a speech and language screening to be completed over 3 summer months. The children were predominantly Spanish speakers. Because there were no readily available bilingual test materials in 1978 when this screening took place, another means for screening was required. Dr. Salas-Provance developed a screening tool in Spanish using the phoneme targets of the *Goldman Fristoe Test of Articulation* (Goldman & Fristoe, 2015) as appropriate for the Spanish phonemic system. Five receptive language and five expressive language questions were included. There were three syntax and three morphology items. For connected speech, the children counted from 1 to 10 and produced a 2-minute spontaneous speech sample. The entire screening took 8 to 10 minutes. A picture of children playing in a field was used to elicit the speech sample. The screening tool was used consistently across all 500 children who ranged from 5 to 12 years of age. The results revealed rates of speech and language disorder typical of those found in the general population.

The development of a new measurement protocol to meet the needs of this group of Mexican children is an example of an emic approach of addressing issues where the professional takes the view of the local community. Generally speaking, emic (insider point of view) and etic (objective view from a distance) perspectives were first used by anthropologists to process and understand the social aspects of their research field (Loustaunau & Soho, 1997). Professionals in the field of multicultural counseling (and other fields including nursing, communication studies, business) have been using the emic and etic approaches for many years in order to make their counseling more culturally specific (Sue & Sue, 2002). It is a useful strategy for SLPs to develop culturally responsive assessment processes (DeJarnette, Rivers, & Hyter, 2015). The current screening measure was conducted in a way that considered the cultural framework and the experiences of the participants rather than using a purely empirical perspective as would be common.

When developing the screening protocol, both linguistic and cultural aspects of the group were considered. The screening was conducted in Spanish and the dialectal variation found in this group of Mexican children was incorporated into the protocol and the children were not penalized for use of their dialect. The measurement items and materials were culturally responsive to reflect the students' real experiences. Another important adaptation was related to cultural expectations. Many of the children had established cultural norms for interacting with an adult; the first group of children remained nonverbal in the 10 minutes allotted to them for the screening. To address that cultural behavior, a cultural broker from the community was brought in to participate in the screenings and served as a bridge by talking with the families and the children prior to their screening. She set them at ease by giving them "permission" to speak freely with an adult stranger. By using culturally responsive practices we can provide best practice and be confident that people will not be over-identified for clinical or educational services or dismissed without receiving appropriate treatment (Laing & Kamhi, 2003; Mattes & Omark, 1991).

In the next section we provide an overview of the culturally responsive assessment practices for several speech disorders including phonological disorders, fluency disorders, resonance disorder in cleft lip and palate, voice disorders, and swallowing disorders. The chapter closes with a review of culturally responsive counseling practices that may be useful during the assessment.

SPEECH SOUND ASSESSMENT

When we are evaluating the speech sound production of individuals who speak English as a second language, we need to have excellent knowledge of the phonemic system of the person's first language. Our knowledge of the sound system is key in making the decision on whether the individual is presenting a difference or a disorder. A speech sample must be gathered in a specific way for bilingual children (Bedore, Peña, Gillam, & Ho, 2010), and it is important to have a clear understanding of unique cultural situations that will encourage ease of communication. For example, if the child has not had access to books, it would not be appropriate to request that the child turn pages in a book and describe the story for your speech sample. If the child is most comfortable sitting on his or her parent's lap and talking with the parent in two languages, then that may be where the best speech sample will be elicited. Be prepared with objects or pictures that are relevant and meaningful to that cultural group so that your speech sample will be a valid assessment. It is less effective to request that an adult with a speech disorder talk about a child playing soccer than to have that person describe a picture of a family preparing or eating a meal familiar to them. Family photos are usually a good way to elicit speech that is culturally relevant at all levels.

Stand-Alone Articulation and Phonological Assessments

The use of stand-alone articulation tests and phonology assessments in the second language are assessment tools for identifying articulation or phonological disorders in children who speak a second language. These tests and materials are available through many venues, such as the Multilingual Children's Speech lab and others (Mattes & Omark, 1991; McLeod & Verdon, 2014) (http://www.csu.edu.au/research/multilingual-speech/speech-assessments). It will take additional time to prepare for and deliver an assessment for the linguistically diverse student or patient. In addition, an interpreter will be necessary if your knowledge and skills in the language are not at a level of competency to administer the test. For example, there is not a set standard of Spanish. There are many variations of Spanish spoken across the country, including Cuban Spanish, Mexican Spanish, and Puerto Rican Spanish, among others. But, generally, it is found that there are five primary vowels in Spanish. This is compared to English, which has 14 or more vowels. There are 18 consonants in Spanish and 24 in English (Goldstein, 2000) (refer to Figures 10–2 and 10–3, and Table 10–6).

A similar side-by-side view of phonetic inventories in other languages will allow you to evaluate how the child's sound system is developing in each language separately as well as their influence on each other. This is the first step in identifying a difference versus a disorder. The American Speech-Language-Hearing Association (ASHA) provides a phonemic inventory in Spanish and other useful phonological information on their website (http://www.asha.org/uploadedFiles/practice/multicultural/SpanishPhonemicInventory.pdf). There are computerized software programs that can assist with the transcription and analysis, including the Computerized Profiling (Long, Fey, & Channell, 2004); Computerized Articulation and Phonology Evaluation System (CAPES; Masterson & Bernhardt, 2006); and the Logical International Phonetics Program (LIPP; Oller & Delgado, 2000).

There is extensive information on phonological development and disorders in bilingual children that is beyond the scope of this chapter (Goldsetin & Gildersleeve, 2012). Knowledge of this body of work will allow you to provide culturally responsive services to bilingual children. Fabiano (2007) presents an excellent overview of the assessment process for phonological disorders in bilingual children. According to Fabiano, an evidence-based assessment would include: (a) single word and connected speech evaluation in both languages, (b) percent input and output in both languages (the hours each week that a child hears and uses the language), (c) an analysis of the phonetic inventory, (d) evaluation of the accuracy of consonants and vowels, and (e) an analysis of the phonological patterns. For example, in analyzing the influence of Spanish on English, we know that both the /t/ and /d/ in English are produced as a dentalized [t̪] and a dentalized [d̪] in the Spanish speaker. This is an example of how the Spanish phonemic system influences the production of English.

ENGLISH VOWEL QUADRILATERAL

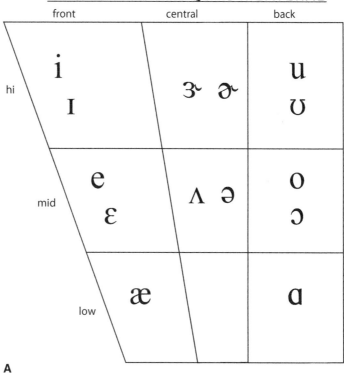

A

FIGURE 10–2. Vowel quadrilateral of English (**A**) and Spanish (**B**) vowels. Adapted from http://www.rose-medical .com/images/vowel-chart.jpg and https://qph.ec.quoracdn .net/main-qimg-3eb5e58b 5d426bf30a0cc7fec3e0d18d Illustrated by Severin Provance.

SPANISH VOWEL QUADRILATERAL

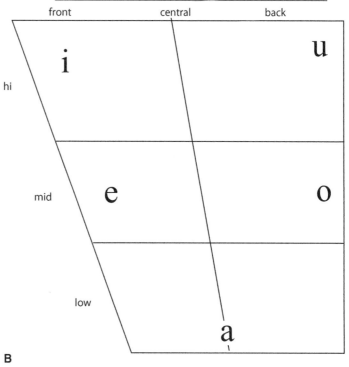

B

SPANISH & ENGLISH VOWELS

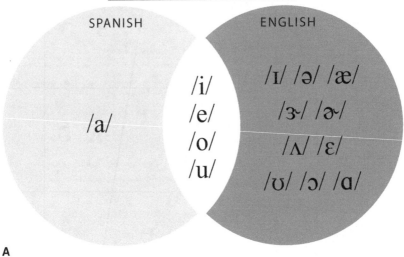

A

SPANISH & ENGLISH CONSONANTS

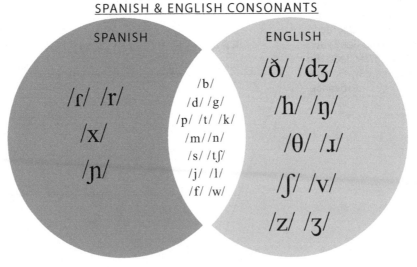

B

FIGURE 10–3. Spanish and English vowels (**A**) and consonants (**B**) White overlapping space includes those consonants and vowels shared by the two languages. Adapted from https://www.pinterest.com/doraliss/phonology. Illustrated by Severin Provance.

TABLE 10–6. Descriptions of the Unique Diacritic Symbols or Phonemes From Figure 10–3

Spanish Phonemes to English Word	English Phonemes to English Word	Spanish/English Phonemes to English Word
/ɲ/—ca*ny*on—ni*ñ*a/child	/ð/—*th*ose	/j/—*y*ellow
/ɾ/—r—to*r*tilla	/dʒ/—*j*udge	/tʃ/—*ch*air
/r/—*r*ayo/ray	/ŋ/—ri*ng*	
/x/—*h*amon/ham (scraping sound on the palate)	/θ/—*th*umb	
	/ɹ/ or /r/—*r*ed	
	/ʃ/—*sh*oe	
	/ʒ/—trea*s*ure	

Another example is the use of the vowel /ɛ/ prior to the blend /st/ so that the word "stamp" is now produced as "estamp" [ɛstamp]. This is a phonological processing pattern of "addition" in Spanish where the /ɛ/ is added before the /s/. An interpreter may be necessary to assist in conducting a complete and accurate analysis for Spanish and other languages. We now look at the use of African American English (AAE). Knowledge of this speech and language system will expand your skills when working with individuals who use AAE.

African American English

Assessing the language skills of AAE speakers remains challenging for SLPs; however, we know more now about this language variation than before. Some of the AAE features can seem similar to language impairments, and the reverse is also true. Features that may seem like AAE features could indeed be impairment (Seymour, Bland-Stewart, & Green, 1998). One strategy that has been used is to examine noncontrastive features of AAE—that is, features of AAE that do not contrast with general American English (GAE) (Pearson, Velleman, Bryant, & Charko, 2009; Seymour et al., 1998; Stockman, 1996). Sey-

mour et al. (1998) provide an instructive example highlighting the noncontrastive features of AAE. They presented three versions of a sentence:

1. John is a boy.
2. John __ a boy.
3. John is __ boy.

The main verb in the sentence above is the copula, which does not appear in sentence 2. The feature of AAE present in sentence 2 is called zero-copula, meaning that the use of the copula is optional—it can be present in this case but is not required. Therefore, statement 1 can be spoken by both an AAE speaker and a GAE speaker. Statement 2 is appropriate for an AAE speaker but not for a GAE speaker. Sentence 3 is not appropriate for either speaker. Deletion of the article "a" is not appropriate for either an AAE or a GAE speaker, which makes it a shared feature between both languages (Seymour et al., 1998, pp. 96–97).

When assessing the speech of children who use AAE, take into consideration that the use of phonemic and language structures is a well-established part of their communication system (Stockman, 1996). The speech of a child who uses AAE should be evaluated from the perspective of a difference, not a disorder, although there may be a speech or language disorder identified. One of the most commonly recognized characteristics of AAE phonology is final consonant deletion. Not every final consonant will be deleted, and this characteristic follows specific rules. For a consonant cluster (e.g., nd, sk, st) occurring at the end of words, the cluster is produced as a single consonant sound, but only in particular contexts. If the word with the cluster is followed by a word beginning with a vowel sound, all components of the cluster will be produced. The word "desk" will be produced

like "des" unless it is followed by a word beginning with a vowel, such as open. It is important for SLPs to understand the phonological features of AAE to provide culturally and linguistically responsive assessments (Horton-Ikard & Miller, 2004). Focusing assessment on noncontrastive features is a common practice when assessing phonological, morphological, and syntactic features of AAE.

Charity (2008) and Green (2002) present an overview of the research and linguistic characteristics of AAE. Some examples of consonant and vowel variation are included in Table 10–7.

TABLE 10–7. Examples of Consonant and Vowel Features of AAE

Consonant Variation		Vowel Variation	
Name	**Example**	**Name**	**Example**
Final consonant deletion (*Rule: occurs in front of words that begin with consonants*)	Desk → des Test → tes	pen-pin merger before nasal consonants	*pen* as *pin*, *ten* as *tin*
Devoicing occurs at the ends of words	b → p cab → cap	/iy/ /i/, /ey/ /e/ merge before /l/	*feel* and *fill*; *fail* and *fell* rhyme
/th/ produced as t, d, f, and v. /t/ and /f/ occur in medial and final positions. /d/ and /v/ may occur in the beginning, middle, or end of words	Bathroom → bafroom These → dese Smooth → smoov	oi	road → /roid/
/r/ and /l/ liquid vocalization or unstressed and not produced	/r/ and /l/ produced as a schwa vowel, e.g., court → [kot] or tore → *toe*		
–in' only for words with more than one syllable	He's runnin' fast		
skr associated with young AAE speakers or may be regional	str → skr street → skreet		
ask/aks alternation	I aks him a question		

Source: Based on Chasity (2008) and Green (2002).

It is essential to keep in mind that the phonological characteristics of AAE are produced according to rules (Green, 2002). There may also be variations across all language domains. Prosodic (Thomas & Carter, 2006; Thomas, 2015) variation should be considered in the assessment of the speaker of AAE, which should be part of a culturally responsive assessment protocol. The prosodic elements of AAE have been discussed in the literature since the 1960s (Baugh, 2003; Labov, 1968; Tarone, 1972, 1973; Wolfram & Fasold, 1974). Green (1990) found that yes/no questions asked by AAE speakers did not consistently end with a rising intonation. Hyter's (1994) dissertation data found that adolescents retelling the "Frog Goes to Dinner" story produced vowel elongations when introducing new characters, and these vowel elongations were accompanied by deictic gestures. In addition to prosodic and phonological elements, AAE includes syntactic, semantic, pragmatic rules, which were discussed in Chapter 5, Culture and Language.

John Baugh (2003) has quite extensively discussed "linguistic profiling"—the discrimination against (or in favor of) someone based on how he or she sounds, or more accurately, based on the ethnicity associated with the way he or she talks. To conduct culturally and linguistically responsive assessments with AAE speakers, it is important to use measures that are appropriate for this language variation. Table 10–8 lists several assessments that are appropriate for AAE. Let's turn our attention to fluency disorders next.

Fluency Disorders

Stuttering is the most common form of fluency disorder (Manning & DiLollo, 2017) and can be found in all languages and cultures (Van Riper, 1982). Stuttering occurs in both bilingual and monolingual children (Shenker, 2011), but there is evidence that it may occur more often in bilingual children (Borsel, Maes, & Foulon, 2001). It is known that in normal speech and language development, children go through a phase of speech disfluency, which may be common in second language speakers as well (Byrd, Bedore, & Ramos, 2015). Difficulty in speaking English as an additional language may be confused with stuttering. It may be that the individual who seems to be stuttering is actually pausing to search for the word in the second language or has hesitations because of the lack of confidence in speaking the second language. If a bilingual child is being assessed for a fluency disorder, he or she should be tested in both languages. Stuttering may in fact be a problem, but the degree of stuttering may vary depending on the language. The language of the SLP also may be a factor. It has been found that English-speaking SLPs may identify fewer and less severe stuttering in both languages compared to bilingual SLPs and may recognize the moments of stuttering more precisely for English speakers versus Spanish speakers (Lee, Robb, Ormond, & Blomgren, 2014).

There are cultural differences in attitudes toward stuttering that are important to consider (Ogundare, 2012). In the U.S. culture, stuttering is viewed as an abnormal speech production and often there are serious social consequences (Blood & Blood, 2016). However, it has been reported (Lemert, 1962) that in the Manganians, from the Mangaia Island of the Pacific Ocean, as well as in some countries in Africa, stuttering is accepted as an inborn characteristic, and in some First Nations/North American Indian societies stuttering is viewed as supernatural (Stewart, 1960). This information can be a critical piece to consider when speaking with the patient or family and when developing a plan of intervention. Because groups of people will range widely in their belief systems on stuttering, whether traditional or mainstream, it is critical to ask

TABLE 10–8. Assessment Measures and Processes Appropriate for Speakers of African American English

Use assessments that are primarily standardized on AAE speakers	• *Diagnostic Evaluation of Language Variation* (DELV) is the only test that falls into this category and is composed of
	   ○ *The DELV Screening Test* (Seymour, Roeper, & de Villiers, 2003) and
	   ○ *The DELV Norm-Referenced* (Seymour, Roeper, & de Villiers, 2005).

Use tests that accommodate language variations	• *Preschool Language Scale–5* (Zimmerman, Steiner, & Pond, 2011) • *The Structured Photographic Expressive Language Test:* Third edition (Dawson, Stout, & Eyer, 2003)
Use assessments developed with test bias review panel input	• As part of the test development process, review panels made up of professionals and scholars with expertise in assessment of children from diverse cultural and language backgrounds identify possible forms of test bias within preliminary test items for one or more populations (Wyatt, 2017, p. 531).
Be familiar with types of biases that can occur in standardized assessments	• Linguistic bias occurs when measures are used that assess speech and language processes that have variations without adjusting the scoring for those variations in production. • Situational bias is when the cultural communication style and expectations of the person being tested and that of the SLP or audiologist do not match. • Format bias refers to the use of assessment processes and formats that are not familiar (or less familiar) to the person being tested. • Value bias refers to when responses to a test question based on cultural or social norms of one group are considered correct, but those of another group are considered incorrect.
Modify existing assessment measures and procedures	• Use modified scoring or modified test administration procedures, e.g., adjusting scoring for dialect usage. Wyatt (2017) cautions that those who attempt to do modified test scoring need to be sufficiently familiar with the rules of AAE, and that any modifications need to be discussed in the diagnostic reports.
Dynamic assessment and other measures that focus on the process of learning	• Dynamic assessment is a method of assessment that identifies the person's potential for learning and modifiability rather than solely information about prior knowledge and skills (Pena, 2000). • Process-dependent measures (incidental word-learning tasks) (Brackenbury & Pye, 2005; Campbell, 1997) are useful for assessing vocabulary skills of children from diverse backgrounds (Wyatt, 2017, p. 533)
Supplemental assessment measures and procedures	• Language sampling (Stockman, 2010) • Narrative sampling and analysis (Champion, 1998; Hughes, McGillivray, & Schnmidek, 1997) • Curriculum-based and portfolio assessments (Nelson, 1989; Nelson, & Van Meter, 2002) • Parent and child interviews
Assessments focused on language universals and non-dialect-specific language abilities	• Minimum core competency (Stockman, 1996, 2008, 2013; Stockman, Newkirk, Swartzlander, & Morris, 2016). • Examination of subject-relative clauses (Burns, de Villiers, Pearson, & Champion, 2012; Oetting & Newkirk, 2011) • Noncontrastive features of AAE (Bland-Stewart, 2005; Seymour, Bland-Stewart, & Green, 1998)

Source: Adapted from Wyatt (2017, pp. 528–540).

the family for this information directly. This will allow you to clarify any misconceptions in their thinking or direct their understanding to commonly accepted information in the area of stuttering. Stuttering has affective, behavioral, and cognitive components (Bernstein Ratner, 2011) and all three aspects must be considered when working with a diverse population. The behavioral issues of dysfluent speech and secondary behaviors must be addressed separately from the issues related to belief systems and attitudes about stuttering.

Speech-language pathologists and audiologists may be familiar with culturally responsive practices pertaining to health beliefs and attitudes, but it is equally as important to be knowledgeable about culturally responsive practices regarding disability culture (Eddey & Robey, 2005). Boyle, Daniels, Hughes, and Buhr (2016) state that disability culture is composed of three components, "(a) shared history, (b) expressions of identity and meaning, and (c) pride" (p. 13). These authors share that certain sensitive practices should be incorporated into communicating and/or interacting with persons who stutter (PWS). These practices are listed in Table 10–9. We continue

our review of communication disorders with a look at the assessment of voice disorders in racially and culturally diverse persons.

Voice Disorders

The prevalence of voice disorders was found to be 1.7% in an adult U.S. population sampled (146.7 million people) from 2008 to 2012 (Benninger, Holy, Bryson, & Milstein, 2017) as identified through a review of the Commercial and Medicare MarketScan databases. A total of 17.9 million adults who sought medical services for voice disorders were identified through their insurance claims. The authors felt this was an underestimation of the prevalence of voice disorders as the representative pool was limited to those individuals seeking health care service. A prevalence rate of 6.6% for adults with voice disorders has been reported in other studies with 30% of adults reporting at least one vocal pathology event in their lifetime (Roy, 2005; Verdolini & Ramig, 2001).

Of the 17.9 million adults identified with voice disorder in the first study, those

TABLE 10–9. Sensitive Practices for Communicating With a Person Who Stutters

Practice	Description
Make eye contact	Maintaining eye contact facilitates communication, can provide information about the speaker's intentions, and provides positive social feedback to PWS, which can serve to facilitate positive change in PWS
Use person-first language	Such terms will be empowering for PWS
Demonstrate patience	Allow the speaker to take as much time as necessary to finish his or her conversational turn
Let the person who stutters, speak	Do not speak for PWS or attempt to complete his or her sentences or words
Focus on content	Focus on what is said rather than how it is said

Source: Based on Boyle et al. (2016, pp. 18–19).

in manufacturing jobs had the highest rate (35%) of voice disorders, followed by those in the service industry (24%). When compared to ethnically diverse populations in the workforce, with manufacturing jobs coded as "production" jobs, African Americans (15.6) and Latin@s/Hispanics (15.6) represent the majority of workers in this industry compared to Whites (5.5%) and Asians (9.3%). Similarly, African Americans (25.1%) and Latin@s/Hispanics (25.4%) are highly represented in the service industry, where Whites constitute 16.5% of the workers and Asians 16.1% of the workers (Current Population Survey [CPS], 2016). Although race and ethnicity were not extracted from the Commercial and Medicare MarketScan database, we can deduce from these two reports that a large number of individuals with voice disorders in this study may have been from racially and ethnically diverse groups. Employment in manufacturing jobs, where there may be higher exposure to carcinogenic chemicals and higher rates of smoking, makes individuals more vulnerable to voice disorders. Employees in the service industry, who often conduct their work in high noise environments where they are required to use a high voice volume and speak for long periods of time, are also at risk for voice disorders.

Ethnically and racially diverse individuals are more likely to live in impoverished areas compared to Whites and have negative health outcomes (Fiscella, Franks, Gold, & Clancy 2000; Musu-Gillette et al., 2016). Children living in impoverished areas and in Black neighborhoods (blocks) are more likely to be exposed to alcohol and tobacco advertisements (Widome, Brock, Noble, & Forster, 2013). Individuals in low SES groups have a higher rate of smoking (more cigarettes, more often, longer duration) (USDHHA, 2014). In terms of the use of tobacco (cigarettes, cigars, and smokeless tobacco), the lifetime use of tobacco is highest for First Nations groups (27.1%)

followed by Whites (21.6%), Latin@s/Hispanics (16.8%), Black/African Americans (12.7%), and Asians (6.9%) (AHA, 2017). High tobacco use is found in several groups including those living in low SES communities, First Nations, racialized groups, lesbian, gay, bisexual, transgender, queer, intersexual, asexual (LGBTQIA) individuals, those with disabilities, and those with mental illness. In fact, the lifetime tobacco use of people with psychiatric illness is extremely high at 56.1% of those with mood disorders, 55.6% of those with anxiety disorders, and 70.1% of those with schizophrenia (AHA, 2017). These statistics reflect a broader client population that may be affected with voice disorders due to smoking. Smoking not only affects the smoker's health, but there are harmful health consequences to those in the household who are exposed to secondary smoke. A long-term cigarette smoking habit in combination with high levels of alcohol consumption can lead to laryngeal cancer (Stewart & Semmler, 2002). It has also been reported that African Americans acquire laryngeal cancer at a younger age with a higher mortality rate compared to Whites (Steuer, Deiry, Parks, Higgins, & Saba, 2017). It is common for individuals in low SES environments to be diagnosed at the later stages of a disease process due to their poor access to health care. A late diagnosis of laryngeal cancer significantly reduces potential for recovery. African Americans were less likely to undergo laryngeal restoration (use of radiation therapy with concurrent chemotherapy) for locally advanced cancers, opting for a total laryngectomy instead (Hau, Daly, & Lee, 2012). The authors believed that a profound form of racial disparity was in effect, which may be associated with several factors such as: (a) physician's decision on patients' ability to complete extensive course of radiation; (b) lack of health care literacy whereby the patient did not understand the options; (c) lack of social or family support to complete treatment; (d) racial disparities in referral to oncology specialists; and (e) financial, health insurance, or transportation barriers. Laryngeal restoration could represent a significantly improved quality of life choice compared to a poorer quality of life following a total laryngectomy (Terrell, Fisher, & Wolf, 1998). The authors report that there appears to be a narrowing of this disparity gap. They further noted that the low SES of many of the patients may have been a large contributor to the disparity (unable to afford the surgery) beyond race. SES and health are associated at all levels, but most profoundly and negatively at the poverty level where diverse individuals are found in high numbers.

Few studies are available on the prevalence of voice disorders in racially and ethnically diverse children. In one study, Duff, Proctor, and Yairi (2004) analyzed the voices of 1,586 African American and 859 European American preschoolers ages 2 to 6. The protocol included teacher and parent identification and a screening by a SLP. Of the 3.8% found to have voice disorders, no statistical difference was found between races. In one unpublished study of 41 Black children and 79 White children ages 3 to 6, no differences were found in pitch on vowel prolongations (Steinsapir, Former, & Stempe, 1986). A commonly cited study by Haller and Thompson (1975) found that of 979 African American children from Harlem, ranging in age from 3 to 17, approximately 9% were found to have a speech disorder. The test protocol included conversational speech only. Of this group, 22% were identified with vocal hoarseness. They based this high prevalence rate on potential "conditions" in Harlem that caused the vocal symptoms. The association of impoverishment and voice pathology was noted earlier. In addition, the SLP rater was employed in an otolaryngology practice, and the authors felt that because of her heightened awareness of voice disorders, she may have overidentified children.

Standardized protocols for voice assessment should be used across all racial and ethnic groups (Roy et al., 2013). Detailed information on voice examination procedures has been well documented (Aronson & Bless, 2009; Boone, McFarlane, Von Berg, & Zraick, 2010; Stemple, Glaze, & Kelchner, 2004; Theis, 2010). Generally, the assessment begins with a comprehensive case history, which should include a history and etiology of the disorder, patient description of the problem, vocal use patterns, and other associated events and illnesses. The voice evaluation will continue with a peripheral examination of the vocal and oral musculature, viewing of the vocal folds through endoscopic imaging procedures (ASHA, 1998; Karnell,1994), measurement of aerodynamic function (Mehta & Hillman, 2007), perceptual assessment (ASHA, 2007; Kempster, Gerratt, Abbott, Barkmeier-Kraemer, & Hillman, 2009), and acoustic analysis (Colton, Casper, & Leonard, 2011). Following the assessment, recommendations should be made for intervention. As with any assessment, an interpreter should be available for people who speak a language different from the examiner.

One component of the voice evaluation is the measuring of the acoustic characteristics of the voice from which we will extrapolate voice function. Earlier in the chapter, we discussed the importance of normative data that reflect the diversity of groups of people for speech and language assessments. More often now, diverse individuals are included as part of the sampling population when developing assessment tools. This assures us that a test will be a valid and reliable measure to identify a "difference" from a "disorder." Unfortunately, there is very little normative data on the acoustic characteristics of the speech of racially and ethnically diverse groups to assist us in distinguishing a "voice" difference from a "voice" disorder. Interestingly, there have been arguments over the years on the appropriateness of anatomical and physiological measures that characterize individuals by race or ethnicity. It has been said that biological differences among and across racial/ethnic boundaries are so small that they may not exist at all (Barkan, 1992; Cavalli-Sforza & Cavalli-Sforza, 1995; Lieberman, Kirk & Littlefield, 2003; Lieberman & Reynolds, 1978). In one study, researchers used mitochondrial and Y-chromosomal data from two ethnic groups located in Central Asia. They concluded that instead of a "common genetic ancestry" (p. 49), ethnicity may actually be a socially constructed phenomenon (refer to Chapter 2 for further information on race as socially constructed), at least for these two groups (Heyer et al., 2009). If so, this would make the gathering of normative data across racial and ethnic boundaries unnecessary. There are others, however, that support the use of racial categories in scientific research (Hernstein & Murray, 1994; Pearson, 2002). It can be argued that in order to provide culturally responsive services, we should identify and use normative data for the entire population found in society, including those from racially and ethnically diverse backgrounds. The normative data could provide specific information that could be utilized to the group's benefit. It can be used as a baseline and a standard in assessment.

There are a limited number of studies that have attempted to provide normative data for culturally and linguistically diverse populations in the area of speech acoustics. One of the difficulties in conducting this research is assuring the results are truly a function of the biological characteristics of the race or ethnicity and not of the linguistic factors presented by language (dialectal) variations.

Early research in this area (Hudson & Holbrook, 1981, 1982; Lass, Almerino, Jordan, & Walsh, 1980; Lass, Tecca, Mancuso, & Black, 1979) focused on the comparison of the acoustic profiles of African American speakers versus White speakers. Findings show

that listeners were able to identify Black from White speakers from speech samples. They acknowledged that linguistic-phonetic features may have been one of the factors distinguishing the speakers. Studies analyzing vowel formants showed no differences between the groups. There did seem to be a trend toward greater fundamental frequency perturbation (jitter) in the vowels of Black children. Vowel prolongation studies found no difference among young children ages 3 to 6 in mean F_o (fundamental frequency) (Steinsapir, Forner, & Stemple, 1986). Walton and Orlikoff (1994) studied the vowel prolongations of 50 Black and 50 White males from 18 to 57 years of age. They identified several features present in the speech of the Black participants as compared to the White speakers, including: (a) increased frequency perturbation (jitter), (b) increased amplitude perturbation (shimmer), and (c) decreased harmonic-to-noise ratio. Listeners were able to detect the vocal perturbation difference. It was described as an additive noise difference. They concluded that the vocal quality rather than the vowel acoustic differences differentiated the voices of African American males from their White counterparts. A study conducted by Mayo and Grant (1995) that examined the fundamental frequency, vowel formant frequency, and jitter and shimmer in 30 Black and 30 White males did not find the differences that Walton and Orlikoff (1994) report. An early study (Boshoff, 1945) on 102 cadaver larynges of Bantu South African Blacks revealed anatomical differences when compared to 23 White South African larynges. The Black larynges were described as having "broader and stronger" muscles. This finding would suggest physiological differences as well (pp. 49–50).

Mayo (1990) investigated the fundamental frequency of African American speakers and found that male and female voices were lower and produced greater pitch variations than what had typically been reported in the literature for European American speakers. Mayo, Manning, and Hudson (1989) studied young African American males and found that their mean vowel formant patterns were lower than published norms for White males, but no statistically significant effect was found for fundamental frequency. In a study of 200 college-age African American students, Jones and Mayo (2001) identified reading fundamental frequency (RF_o). The data were compared to other studies (Study #2 and Study #3), with male subject RF_o found to be similar to Caucasian subjects in Study #2, but lower than that found in Study #3 with another group of African American males. The female subjects fell between the two groups in the comparative studies. It was found that the range in reading fundamental frequency was wider in all the African Americans studied compared to the Caucasian subjects. There appear to be within-subject and across-subject differences. Vargo (2012) measured the fundamental frequency of 30 African American and Caucasian males and females while sustaining vowels, during a speaking task and a reading task. There were no significant differences by race or by task. The African American females did have a higher F_o for the sustained vowel task compared to the Caucasian females. Refer to this study for a comprehensive review of the literature in this area.

Differences between the fundamental frequencies and formant frequencies of African American males and females were not always found to be statistically different for White speakers, but there appear to be perceptual differences (Alim, 2005; Baugh, 2000, 2003; Bullock, 2006; Gaither, Cohen-Goldberg, Gidney, & Maddox, 2016; Smalls, 2004; Wolfram, 2011). Acoustic pharyngometry (sound waves inside the vocal tract are analyzed by computer) was used to identify vocal tract variation across races. Vocal tract volume was found to contribute to acoustic differences in the voices of Chinese, White Ameri-

can, and African American speakers (Xue, Hao, & Mayo, 2006). There were extensive differences across and within gender and race. African American males were found to have the smallest vocal tract volume, followed by White American males then Chinese males. Oral volume was found to be the largest in Chinese men, and African American men had the largest pharyngeal length. This is a fruitful area of study that provides important information about vocal tract characteristics in racially and ethnically diverse individuals.

Andrianopoulos, Darrow, and Chen (2001a, 2001b) analyzed the vowels of three multicultural groups including African American, Hindi, and Chinese for fundamental frequency, spectral characteristics, and format structures. There were differences in vowel formats for [a], [i], and [u] across culture and race attributed to physiological differences. African American males and females exhibited lower F_3 for [i]. Chinese males produced more posterior positioning of the tongue for a lower F_2 and F_1. Significantly greater vowel and tongue height (lower F_1) were found for Hindi Indian male and female speakers. Compared to their cultural peers, Mandarin Chinese males and females produced significantly higher fundamental frequencies (that is the average of their highest and lowest F_o) with higher short-term and long-term vowel perturbation. The findings in these studies represent an important contribution to the body of evidence on normative acoustic data across cultures.

The studies reported here represent only a small sampling of the research in this area of study. The notion of identifying an individual by the acoustic characteristics of their voice remains a compelling and intriguing thought. However, there remain many limitations to the studies as noted by almost all the investigators in the review of literature presented. There are the confounding variables of race, age, health, gender, and their interplay with physiology that dictate the sound of our voices. To return to the words at the beginning of this section, it is important to identify a "voice difference" from a "voice disorder" for racial and ethnic groups if that information allows us to provide culturally responsive services. If we are able to use that normative data to provide appropriate assessments and interventions, that would represent an advancement in the field of communication disorders.

The voice assessment should include history on past illnesses and diseases. Diseases found in ethnic and racial groups could be associated with poverty, lifestyle, or geographic region as well as the genetics of the individual (Matthews & Gallow, 2011). However, low SES and poverty play a significant role in health outcomes. The large numbers of racial and ethnic emerging majority groups in low SES environments are more likely to suffer health consequences (Fiscella, Franks, Gold, & Clancy, 2008). Diseases that affect voice can include endocrine system diseases, like hyperthyroidism and hypothyroidism. They can result in a poor voice quality due to variations in fundamental frequency or dryness in the larynx (Mohammadzadeh, Heydari, Azuzu, Matos, & Hutfless, 2011). McLeod, Caturegli, Cooper, Matos, and Hutfless (2014) in a 15-year study of active duty military, found that endocrine disease such as Graves' disease, where the thyroid overproduces its hormone resulting in hyperthyroidism, was found more often in Blacks (women two times and men two and a half times as much) and Asians compared to Whites. Hashimoto's thyroiditis, where the immune system attacks the thyroid causing hypothyroidism, was found more often in Whites. Respiratory diseases have been known to effect voice quality as well. Tuberculosis (TB) remains a global health problem. TB is higher among racially and ethnically diverse populations and lower in Whites. The Centers for Disease Control and Prevention (CDC, 2016a) report that Asian Americans and Native Hawaiians/ Pacific Islanders present with the highest incidence of tuberculosis per 100,000 population (18.3) for both groups, followed by First Nations (6.1), African Americans (5.0), Latin@s/Hispanics (4.8), and Whites (0.6). Although genetic factors play a role, social and economic factors may also contribute to this high rate of TB in Asian Americans. Coussens et al. (2013) showed that individuals with African ancestry appear to have less immunity to the TB infection. Additionally, many prescription drugs have a negative effect on the voice. The New York Voice Academy provides a thorough list of these medications and their impact on voice quality (http://www.newyorkvoiceacademy.com/pdf/effects-drugs-on-voice.pdf). Adults with lower socioeconomic status are likely to have an increased risk for serious mental illness, and poverty has been linked to mental illness for decades (Adler et al., 1994). For individuals suffering from symptoms of mental illness, the long-term use of antipsychotic drugs may result in laryngeal dystonias, and the use of antidepressants can have a drying effect on the vocal folds. Latin@s/Hispanics are at high risk for cardiovascular disease because of high blood pressure, obesity, and diabetes found in these communities (American Heart Association, 2017). Diuretics, used to control high blood pressure, will increase fluid output and may cause dryness of mucous membranes. Some heart medications to reduce angina, as a result of the high blood pressure, may cause coughing and irritation to the vocal folds. Another disease that may affect the voice is asthma. It occurs over twice as often in African American children compared to White children. African American children are 10 times more likely to die of the disease (Jenson & Fraser, 2015). The prevalence of asthma in *adults* is overall 7.6%, Puerto Rican 13.6%, Black 9.1%, White 7.9%, and Latin@/Hispanic, 5.9. In *children* it is overall 8.4%, Puerto Rican 13.9%, Black 13.4%, Latin@/Hispanic 8.0, and White 7.4%. Puerto Rican and Black children have the two highest rates of asthma. The prescribed medications for asthma, inhaled steroids, may lead to yeast infections on the vocal folds and cause dryness and decreased voice quality.

Additional readings on voice and voice disorders in diverse populations can be found in Holland and DeJarnette, (2002) and Salas-Provance (1996). In these texts, historical information on vocal fold pathologies, oral and nasal pathologies, and health issues related to voice dysfunction in culturally diverse groups are presented. Additional summarized studies on perceptual features, fundamental frequency, and format frequencies for African American children and adults are found in these readings.

There are other ways that our voices are measured beyond the examination protocol reviewed earlier. An individual's voice carries a significant amount of sociocultural information. Voice can depict gender, age, weight, height, health status, sexual orientation, personality, physical attractiveness, emotional and mental status, social class, economic status, and even the ethnicity of the speaker (Baugh, 2003; Munson, 2007).

Another area to consider is how paralinguistic cues of volume or loudness are received across cultures. The use of volume, whether it is too loud or too soft for the setting, may be a product of biology (our body dictates our natural volume), pathology (change in anatomy or physiology from disease, illness, aging, etc.), personality (a loud or soft voice is the character of the person), or culture (strict rules dictate voice volume). There are sociocultural norms for speech volume, and simplistically speaking, we may be using an "outside" voice when we should be using an "inside" voice, or vice versa. Schoolchildren have been well trained to use these two voices appropriately for school culture. It may be considered a crime to talk above a certain decibel level in some cultures, and there may be a noise ordinance for "disturbing the peace" in other cultures. The way we control the volume of our voice is a product of our experience, the way we were brought up. But how it is perceived is based on another set of cultural rules set by the listener. For example, the "teacher voice" has one expectation, the "church voice" has another. In some religious gatherings it is appropriate to have a loud voice and is part of the spiritual experience where the use of voice is very culturally mandated, such as the "call-and-response" format in the African American community where a pastor may call out for a jubilant response from the congregation (Foster, 2001). While in another religious practice (e.g., in some Catholic religions), the sociocultural norm would be the use of a voice no louder than a murmur, soft whisper, if not complete silence in the church building or during the service. The silent Catholic Church is very possibly a rare event in Catholic communities today (Pope, 2013). However, our ability to use our voice according to the mores of the group is another way in which we are judged.

A speaker should be aware of the effect their voice is having on the listener, especially since it has been found that assumptions and judgments are made in less than a second after hearing a person's voice (McAleer, Tadorov, & Belin, 2014). Listeners, including SLPs, should also be aware of our own biases as we listen to the voices of the people that we serve. We review a few of the ways our voices are interpreted by others.

John Baugh (2003) coined the phrase *linguistic profiling*, referring to discriminatory practices against persons or in favor of persons on the basis of the sound of their voice. Linguistic profiling is based on auditory cues (Baugh, 2003, p. 158), and Baugh has found that persons of color, specifically African Americans and Latin@s/Hispanics, have been discriminated against based on the sound of their voice. Much of Baugh's work has focused on housing discrimination and discrimination experienced in the U.S. court systems. Some groups in the United States have received preferential treatment due to the sound of their voice. Such voices include French and British accents (Baugh, 2003).

Gender designation of male or female is clearly marked by our voice and is controlled by anatomical and physiological factors (Tietze, 1989). Vocal folds in males are usually longer and heavier, resulting in a lower pitch. Females have shorter and lighter vocal folds resulting in a higher-pitched voice, with children having the highest of pitch due to the child-size vocal folds. In addition, the shape of the vocal tract may influence how speech is perceived, with the variations in male and female vocal space projecting different acoustic information.

We are perceived to be a certain gender based on the interplay of these anatomical and physiological factors that shape our voice along with other aspects of articulation, language, and pragmatics (Hannah & Murachuer, 1999; Holmes & King, 2017; Newman, Groom, Handelman, & Pennebaker, 2008; Wood, 2009). In the LGBTQIA community, which is large and culturally diverse, there may be individuals who seek surgical and therapeutic intervention to change their voices to better match their sexual orientation and to transition well as a member of their new social group. There are broad characterizations of how an LGBTQIA individual should sound linguistically with accompanying behaviors. For example, the effeminate voice with a lisp has been part of a long-standing history of popular-culture stereotypes. It is important that research and clinical practice resist the temptation to reinforce the stereotypes, and provide evidence-based and culturally responsive care.

Individuals may transition from male to female (MtF) or female to male (FtM). For MtF individuals, medical interventions to raise pitch have included cricothyroid approx-

imation, anterior commissure advancement, and injection of triamcinolone into the vocal folds (Gross, 1999). Male to female transsexuals may also seek anterior glottal web feminization surgery. One Turkish study (Yilmaz, Kuscu, Sozen, & Suslu, in press) reported on 27 cases that underwent this surgery. They found a 74% patient satisfaction rate and 85% of the patient voices were rated as feminine post-surgery by medical students. Of the approximately 25% who were unsatisfied with the surgery, the voice was found to feel "tight" and too high in pitch, almost like a child.

The SLP may be in a position to assist in the care of the transgender voice patient by providing a comprehensive voice evaluation with follow-up voice therapy (Hancock & Garabedian, 2013; McCready, Campbell, Crutchley, & Edwards, 2011). That assessment should include a comprehensive systems approach keeping in mind the needs of the individual and whether he or she has transitioned from MtF or FtM. In the individual who transitions from MtF, the following assessment protocol can lead directly into intervention strategies. Examination of the respiratory system can show the patient the need for a breathier voice, which can increase feminization. Measurement of loudness levels can show how decreased voice volume may be preferred as a softer voice is often attributed to females. The phonatory system exam can reveal voice quality and the need to decrease glottal fry or other factors that may be lowering pitch. Examination of pitch can lead to pitch variability tests and the use of inflection in speech to produce a more feminine voice. Examination of the resonatory system should review tongue placement and lip posture. Carrying the tongue forward and spreading the lips can affect vocal resonance in a positive way for the MtF individual. Finally, the articulatory system exam should include coordinated movement and articulator precision for vowel and consonant production. Subtle changes in vowel or consonant production may provide more feminine cues for the listener. Other parts of the assessment should include a review of language, both pragmatics and syntax, to identify gender-specific options in this area. For the FtM individual, the hormone replacement therapy may lower the voice. The individual should also receive a thorough examination.

Listener perception studies of gay, lesbian, and transgender individuals reveal their speech can be distinguished on certain acoustical parameters (Munson, McDonald, DeBoe, & White, 2006). It was found that gay/bisexual men could be distinguished from heterosexual men by the unique pattern of negative /s/ skewness for this sibilant fricative. They were identified acoustically with a higher F_1 frequency of low front vowels /ɛ/ and /æ/. Lesbian/bisexual women had a lower F_1 frequency for low front vowel /ɛ/ and lower F_2 frequency for back vowel /oʊ/. Generally the gay or bisexual male is reported as having dynamic intonation, lisping, and high pitch, while the lesbian or bisexual female has a more exaggerated monotone voice. The assessment of voice for individuals from the LGBTQIA community should be individualized for the needs of each client.

In the instance of serving the LGBTQIA community, it is not only necessary to have the clinical tools to evaluate the voice and speech (Adler, 2012), it is also important to reflect upon our personal feelings about gender identity and gender expression (Kanamori & Cornelius-White, 2016; Kite & Wiley, 1996; Reading, 2014) to provide culturally responsive services. The clinician should refer the LGBTQIA patient (or any other patient) to another service provider if he or she is unable to provide treatment without bias (ASHA, 2016).

Voice parameters can be interpreted differently across cultures. It is well known that there is pragmatic intent in the use of pitch. The rising F_o contour can signal the request for a response for some cultural groups, while a fall intonation may signal a request for a response in others. The flat or falling F_o can depict a flat emotional state. The use of a loud or soft voice can also relay meaning such as generating anger or commanding attention. The voice is used in tonal languages to extract lexical meaning. Over half of the world's languages are tonal to some degree, and all spoken languages will manipulate fundamental frequency at some level for word stress, phrase stress, or pragmatic purposes (Hyman, 2001). Some languages use systems of complex tones such as those that can be found in some African countries (Bantu language), where "I" versus "You" has a different meaning depending on the tone. Strong tonal languages are seen in Asia (Mandarin Chinese, Vietnamese, Thai, and Hmong) where tones have a contour, with a rising tone of the same length meaning one thing and a falling tone another. Depending on the inflection, [ma] could mean scold, rough, horse, or mother. Many Indo-European languages are tonal, as well as First Nations languages such as Navajo (Campbell, 1991).

How voice intent is interpreted culturally is learned over time as we become more familiar with the people and their customs. A listing of each culture's intent in the use of vocal parameters would be susceptible to stereotyping of that culture. When entering a culture different from your own, it is more important to be a listener and an observer of behavior and learn from that experience. Having a preconceived notion of vocal intent can result in cross-cultural misunderstandings and confusion.

Finally, it is important to know how health care disparities affect our patients' ability to receive the care they need in the area of voice disorders. This information applies to all speech, language, hearing, and swallowing disorders. There is substantial evidence to support the notion that implicit ethnic and racial bias may present barriers to the access and delivery of health care (Blair, Steiner, & Havranek, 2011; CDC, 2011; Ellis, Mayo, Mayo, & Holt, 2016; Hayes, Riley, Radley, & McCarthy, 2015; Smedley, Stith & Nelson, 2003). The National Healthcare Quality and Disparities Report (AHRQ, 2015) revealed that Blacks, Latin@s/Hispanics, First Nations/American Indians, and Alaskan Natives received worse health care than Whites for 40% of five quality measures. The quality measures included person-centered care, patient safety, healthy living, effective treatment, and care coordination. An example of health care disparity with African Americans was provided at the beginning of this section regarding the use of laryngeal preservation management for laryngeal cancer. The African American patients were opting for the total laryngectomy more often than the laryngeal preservation. The laryngeal preservation surgery represents a significant quality of life improvement that is not being utilized.

Access to specialized medical care, as would be necessary for assessment of voice disorders, may be difficult for racially and ethnically diverse families given the information in the AHRQ 2015 report. Economic factors are a significant barrier to access health care. The number of uninsured in diverse populations in poverty decreased from 2010 to 2015. Yet, Latin@s/Hispanics and Blacks still remain more likely to be uninsured than Whites (AHRQ, 2015). Without insurance or sufficient insurance, the ability to pay for a large battery of tests, as would be required in a voice assessment, is unlikely. Professionals should be aware of these barriers to health care for diverse populations and seek alternatives for their patients and students with voice disorders and other communication disorders. Voice disorders have also been found in indi-

viduals with cleft palate, which is reviewed in the following section.

Cleft Lip and Palate

Campinha-Bacote (2002) describes a model of cultural competence in the delivery of health care that allows the health care provider to work within the cultural context of the culturally and linguistically diverse patient. This allows a doctor–therapist–patient relationship to develop that is mutually beneficial and where the best health care can be provided. Knowledge of the individual characteristics of each patient with cleft lip and palate will guide our practices to more responsibly meet the needs of culturally and linguistically diverse populations. Overall, cleft lip and palate are found in approximately 1:700 live births in the United States and 1:500 live births worldwide. However, if we look further, a strong cultural variation can be found in the prevalence rates of cleft lip with or without cleft palate and cleft palate alone (Croen, Shaw, Wasserman, & Tolarova, 1998; Tinanoff, 2007). In Table 10–10, you can see that African Americans (0.62 and 0.54) are lowest in both types of clefts, while persons from First Nations have the highest prevalence in both areas (1.99 and 1.11). Interestingly, the prevalence rate for Latin@s/Hispanics is higher for cleft lip with and without cleft palate (1.05) than for cleft palate alone (0.56). It is known that cleft alone is more common in females. With a lower prevalence of Latin@s/Hispanics with isolated clefts, Latin@s/Hispanic females and African American females will be represented in smaller numbers in this group.

We may want to look further into why the First Nations population has the highest prevalence of cleft palate with or without cleft lip and isolated cleft palate, and why the lowest prevalence is found in the African American population. The CDC reports that the

TABLE 10–10. Prevalence Rates of Cleft Lip and Palate or Cleft Palate Alone per 1,000 from Lowest to Highest

Cleft Lip With or Without Cleft Palate		Cleft Palate Alone	
African American	0.62	African American	0.54
Pacific Islander	0.83	Hispanic	0.56
Chinese	0.96	Chinese	0.56
Japanese	1.05	Pacific Islander	0.89
White	1.05	Japanese	0.77
Hispanic	1.05	White	0.72
East Indian	1.14	East Indian	1.06
First Nation	1.99	First Nation	1.11

exact cause of cleft lip and palate is unknown (CDC, 2016b), but it is known that both genetic and environmental factors may be involved. Therefore, when studying this high rate of incidence in the First Nations population, one can look at multifactorial causes that have been generally reported, including genetic predisposition and environmental risk factors such as poor prenatal care, dietary factors (e.g., folate deficiency in Wehby & Murray, 2010), the use of drugs, or high levels of alcohol consumption in a community (Dixon, Marazita, Beaty, & Murray, 2011). American Indian/First Nations report more binge drinking episodes per month and higher alcohol consumption per episode than other groups (CDC, 2011).

There has not been conclusive evidence to explain the low prevalence in African Americans. In ancient times, congenital deformities were a sign of the child being infused with an evil spirit. These children were removed from their cultural unit to die in the wilderness. This is thought to still occur in some African groups (Bhattacharya, Khanna, & Kohli, 2009). Few children and adults with cleft lip and palate may have been part of the slave trade due to the practices of infanticide in some countries (Abrahams et al., 2016; Mathews, Abrahams, Jewkes, Martin, & Lombard (2013). It is likely that individuals with a physical abnormality would not have been perceived as slaves for whom slave traders could have demanded a high price. In addition, during the forced displacement to America, 12% to 13% of the enslaved succumbed to rampant disease and epidemics. A smaller gene pool of cleft may be one of the explanations for the lower incidence of cleft lip and palate in African Americans (Mwiti, 2015). Further study is needed to investigate this phenomenon.

As part of the case interview, the family may discuss their understanding of the causes of cleft lip and palate from their cultural perspective, as discussed in Chapter 6. For example, in some South American countries, the families feel that the cause of the cleft was "el rayo" [εl raɪo] (lightening). In some cultures, a cleft lip is thought to be caused by the mother looking up at a lunar eclipse, which is called "a bite on the moon." To protect herself, the mother must wear something metallic, such as a safety pin, under clothing during pregnancy. This folk belief has been reported by many

South American parents who have children with cleft lip and palate, and can be traced back to the Aztecs (Nutlall, 1897; Torres, 2006). In the Mexican (Catholic) and Hindu cultures a red bracelet or string (pulsera kalava) is worn by the mother and later the baby to keep the evil spirits away. In some African cultures a talisman or charm is put on infants to ward off evil spirits. Loh and Ascoli (2011) found that Chinese, African, and Indian families included spirits (supernatural powers in the child), diets (eating poisoned rabbit food), and fate (act of God) as part of their belief systems regarding cleft lip and palate. It is important to respond appropriately to these narratives of cultural traditional beliefs and be supportive, while at the same time offering the correct information on the causes of cleft lip and palate. There are many traditional attitudes and perceptions about cleft lip and palate. It is critical for a family, no matter the cultural background, to know that a cleft lip and palate has a strong hereditary component. Families should receive genetic counseling as appropriate after the birth of their first child with cleft lip and palate.

In assessing the nasality in the speech of patients with cleft palate, it is important to use the available normative data for diverse populations. There are data available for Mexican males and females, Spanish-speaking females, and Greek monolinguals (Anderson, 1996; Nichols, 1999; Okalidous, Karathanasi, & Grigoraki, 2011). There are nasalance scores available across many languages, including English, Spanish, Swedish, Japanese, Maranthi, and Thai, among others (Mayo & Mayo, 2011).

Beyond the assessment of the speech resonance of patients with cleft palate, the assessment will include typical procedures and tools for speech and language evaluations. The suggestions provided throughout this chapter can be integrated in the assessment for culturally and linguistically diverse patients. Kuehn and Henne (2000) have provided a report in both English and Spanish of the assessment and treatment practices for patients with cleft palate as an extension of their work with children with cleft lip and palate in Villahermosa, Mexico. The report serves as a concise guide for use by SLPs and other professionals who may be providing speech pathology services both in the United States and in medical missions abroad. The final disorder discussed will be swallowing disorders. ASHA's 2015 Healthcare Survey reported that the SLPs in adult settings spend 41% of their time providing swallowing intervention, while SLPs in pediatric settings spend 13% of their time in swallowing intervention. This is an important practice area in the profession.

Swallowing Disorders

Assessment for a patient with swallowing disorders should follow appropriate protocols established for the severity of the disorder (Arvedson & Brodsky, 2002; Groher & Crary, 2015; Riquelme, 2015). There also may be some cultural factors to take into consideration when selecting the diet preferences of the individual (Riquelme, 2007, 2013). Use of a language that facilitates understanding is critical, and an interpreter may be needed. Of course, if there are language or speech concerns, whether related to use of English as a second language or use of language and speech production following a stroke, those issues must be addressed appropriately for the individual. Kohnert (2008) and Riquelme (1997) address assessment of neurological disorders in individuals who use English as a second language. It is important to know that some bilingual adults may have well-developed language proficiency in two languages, while others will have some variation on this continuum, whether we are speaking of normal bilinguals or those with a language disorder due to aphasia. In order to provide a culturally responsive assessment, the intricacies of bilingualism must be understood well for the adult population. It is known that some bilinguals may revert to their original language after a stroke. A review of the assessment of patients with neurological disorders is beyond the scope of this chapter. We refer you to ASHA's Practice Portals on neurological disorders, aphasia, and other adult neurogenic disorders. Here you will find current assessment practices and references for further study in this area (ASHA, 2017).

In closing the review of the assessment of communication disorders, we go back to the beginning of this chapter and the importance of knowing the cultural background of the patient with swallowing disorders. We present the 10 questions and provide a second opportunity for you to work through these questions in a case scenario (Table 10–11).

In this case, the patient is a 72-year-old Korean male, Mr. Hwan Kang, who goes by "Henry." He has been in the United States since he was 14 years of age. He completed 2 years of community college after high school and then worked as a computer analyst. He remained with the same company for over 30 years until his retirement at 65 years of age. He is married and has four daughters who are all college educated. He stays busy painting and with other quiet hobbies around the house. His English proficiency allows him to communicate well, but he prefers to speak Korean at home with his family and friends.

By using the set of questions provided above, we know that the patient has lived and worked in the United States for many years, which assumes a certain level of acculturation to the mainstream. He has raised four daughters in the United States; they are highly educated and bilingual speakers who still communicate with their father using the Korean language. It appears that the family is middle socioeconomic level as suggested by Mr. Kang's posi-

TABLE 10–11. Questions on Cultural and Linguistic Background for English as a Second Language Speaker

1. How long has the family been in the country?

2. How long has the patient been in the United States?

3. What is the language(s) spoken at home?

4. What is the patient's level of exposure to English?

5. What is the language skill of other family members?

6. What is the patient's language development history in each language?

7. What is the education level of the family?

8. What has been the acculturation pattern of the family?

9. What is the economic level of the family?

10. What is the family's cultural dynamic?

tion and work career. They have managed the health care system well, evident by the comments made by the daughters that his care has been handled professionally and efficiently. There does not seem to be any undue anxiety about his medical situation from the family or the patient. Another sign of acculturation is that Mr. Kang has taken on the Americanized name of Henry. But, he prefers to be with his Korean friends and to keep a low profile around the house during his retirement.

As you begin your consultation with Mr. Kang, it is important to get an idea of the correct communication style, whether it will be formal or relaxed. In this family dynamic, it is unclear which one will be the best. Thus, the clinician will need to take cues from the family so as not to have a cultural misstep from the start. Next you will want to ask other questions that will facilitate your examination:

Who in the family will be the person in charge of approving or carrying out the care plan? Can you take charge of the assessment as soon as you enter the room or should you wait? The taking of a meal is culturally mandated, influenced by traditions, religion, and family (Meigs, 1997), not only in terms of what we eat, but how the food is served and who is included in the meal. When a patient is being assessed for a swallowing disorder, this entire ritual is upset. The patient is many times being fed by someone he or she does not know and being fed foods that are not acceptable to him or her (puree and other textures). Generally, the clinician should make sure to get permission from the patient and family to begin the evaluation, as feeding of another person is quite invasive as you enter closely in the patient's personal space. The patient may want another family member to take on this role, but of course this could only occur if safety has been assured. There are many culturally determined practices of personal care. Feeding oneself is a basic need that an adult has been doing independently the majority of his or her life. Thus, it is important to enter this assessment arena with a significant amount of cultural humility knowing that, yes, you are the expert and know what needs to occur to complete an effective bedside swallow, but the cultural space you have entered must be respected, especially in this critically important clinical environment.

In some cultures, there are strict rules of family hierarchy for making decisions in these situations. Sometimes it is the father, but in this case he is not able to be the spokesperson for his family. It could be a first-born son, but again, there are four daughters. Is it the oldest or the most educated child? The daughter who is married? In most situations, the best policy is to ask the family of their preferences regarding to whom you should direct your communication. There is much information available in the literature on practices specific to a culture (Battle, 2012). This information

could be helpful in a general sense. It is important to remember that each group dynamic is unique, and the level of acculturation of the group, like in this instance, Korean, may have shifted to more mainstream practices. The use of an individual's cultural mores can range from strict adherence to traditional practices to complete acceptance of mainstream practices. For that reason, it is more important to have a global sense of cultural sensitivities that can be used in all of your interactions with individuals from different cultural groups than a list of cultural behaviors that may be incorrect for the patient. Should you need to provide counseling during your treatment of this patient, some techniques appropriate for a culturally diverse patient are provided in the final section of this chapter.

Activity 10–3

1. Using the 10 cultural background questions, identify the information presented in the scenario that could be used to answer those questions.
2. Are there other cultural questions that should be asked, specifically for a patient with a swallowing disorder?
3. How successful do you think you would be in managing this patient's swallowing disorder within the cultural framework of this family?

COUNSELING

If counseling is provided during the assessment, it is important to be aware of personal limitations in this area and to be cognizant of the issues that would best be treated by a trained counselor. Successful counseling requires not only the necessary counseling techniques, but it is based on being able to establish good relationships. In fact, its outcome may hinge on the relationship between therapist and client (Rivera, Phan, Maddeux, Wilbur, & Arredondo, 2006). There may be cultural issues that come into play in building the relationship (Salas-Provance, 2010). Many studies have found that the experiences of individuals vary as a result of their cultural, racial, and ethnic backgrounds and do, in fact, impact their response to the counseling process (Constantine, 2002; Twohey, 2004). It has been noted that ethnically diverse groups use counseling services less often than other groups (Gladding, 2009; Sue & Sue, 2002). One reason for this may be related to the issue of cultural mistrust (Benkert, Peters, Clark, & Keves-Foster, 2006; Terrell & Terrell, 1984). In addition, views on the use of help-seeking behaviors may differ across cultures (Kim, 2004; Lee, 2008). One Hispanic family was found to rely more on prayer and on their immediate family when dealing with issues related to disabilities (Salas-Provance, Erickson, & Reed, 2002). The expectation was that these concerns were not discussed outside of the family and that the best advice came from within the family. Marino (1996) conducted an informal survey and found that counselors were not considered to be "real" by diverse groups because they could not understand issues beyond those in their own White culture. Rivera, Phan, Maddeux, Wilbur, and Arredondo (2006) further studied the concept of being "real" and found that in multicultural counseling, honesty and being real were closely related. It was as important to teach the dynamics of honest relationships to counseling students in training as it was to teach the technical skill of counseling. They reported that "ethnic minority clients may often see through the politically correct evasions of multicultural counselors who are too skills-oriented" (p. 43).

The assessment period is stressful for families and more so for the individual being assessed. The testing environment places them in a vulnerable position, which can limit their ability to perform at their optimum. The use of culturally responsive practices makes it more likely that the clinician is able to report the impact of the disability beyond the effects of confounding cultural variables. It is important to identify unique ways to communicate with diverse individuals to achieve the best outcomes of our assessments. Westby (2009) describes the use of skilled dialogue to assist in understanding an individual's cultural background and perspective. A third space (Patterson, Grenny, McMillan, & Switzler, 2002) is created where clarity occurs, allowing the building of trusting relationships necessary for successful dialogue. Westby refers to having an "anchored understanding" of the individual's culture (p. 283), which brings to mind words such as firm, reinforced, and strong. One can envision a rope between therapist, family, and client that is woven and becomes thicker over time. The thick rope, or the anchor of understanding, grows stronger as the commitment to becoming culturally responsive increases and we move away from stereotypes and generalizations.

CHAPTER SUMMARY

This review of assessment protocols for populations from culturally and linguistically diverse populations reveals that there are many tools that can be used to conduct a culturally responsive assessment. It is possible, however, that even with the correct tools, the assessment can be unsuccessful. If the clinician enters the process without a caring and sensitive viewpoint, the outcome will be failure for the student, patient, family, therapist, and the entire educational and health care system. Biases, stereotypes, and generalizations must be discarded at the door. The ultimate goal is to conduct an assessment that will provide the clinician enough information to make appropriate recommendations and intervention decisions. Culturally responsive practices are evidence-based practices because they are responsive to the needs of the patient, student, or client. The clinician may need to make adaptations during the assessment to get the information necessary. It may take a greater effort and more time to get prepared, to assess, and then to write the report for a patient from a diverse culture or a patient who uses a language other than English. However, the time will be well spent and will be the basis of a solid assessment with important, relevant, and beneficial results.

FURTHER READING

Danahy Ebert, K., & Scott, C. M. (2014). Relationships between narrative language samples and norm-referenced test scores in language assessments of school-age children. *Language, Speech, and Hearing Services in Schools, 45,* 337–350.

Fabiano, L. C. (2007). Evidence-based phonological assessment of bilingual children. *Perspectives on Communication Disorders and Sciences in Culturally and Linguistically Diverse Populations, 14,* 21–23.

Gutierrez-Clellan, V. F., & Peña, E. (2001). Dynamic assessment of diverse children: A tutorial. *Language, Speech, and Hearing Services in Schools, 32*(4), 212–224.

Roseberry-McKibbin, C. (2014). *Multicultural students with special language needs: Practical strategies for assessment and intervention* (4th ed.). Oceanside, CA: Academic Communication Associates.

REFERENCES

Abrahams, N., Mathews, S., Martin, L. J., Lombard, C., Nannan, N., & Jewkes, R. (2016). Gender differences in homicide of neonates, infants, and children and 5 y in South Africa: Results from the cross-sectional 2009 National Child Homicide Study. *PLOS Medicine, 13*(4), 1–15.

Adler, N. E., Boyce T., Chesney, M. A., Cohen, S., Folkman, S., Kahn, R. L., & Syme, L. (1994). Socioeconomic status and health. The challenge of the gradient. *American Psychologist, 49,* 15–24.

Adler, R. K., Hirsch, S., & Mordaunt, M. (2012). *Voice and communication therapy for the transgender/transsexual client: A comprehensive clinical guide* (2nd ed.). San Diego, CA: Plural.

Agency for Healthcare Research and Quality (AHRQ). (2015). *2015 National healthcare quality and disparities report and 5th anniversary. Update on the national quality strategy.* Retrieved from https://www.ahrq.gov/research/findings/nhqrdr/nhqdr15/quality.html

Alim, H. S. (2005). Critical language awareness in the United States: Revisiting issues and revising pedagogies in a resegregated society *Educational Researcher, 34*(7), 24.

American Heart Association (AHA). (2017). AHA statistical update: Heart disease and stroke statistics—2017 update: A report from the American Heart Association. *Circulation, 135*(10), e146–e603. Retrieved from http://circ.ahajournals.org/content/135/10/e146

American Speech-Language-Hearing Association (ASHA). (1998). *Training guidelines for laryngeal videoendoscopy/stroboscopy.* Rockville, MD: Author.

American Speech-Language-Hearing Association (ASHA). (2003). *American English dialects* [Technical report]. Retrieved from http://www.asha.org/policy

American Speech-Language-Hearing Association (ASHA). (2005). *Evidence-based practice in communication disorders* [Position statement]. Retrieved from http://www.asha.org/policy

American Speech-Language-Hearing Association (ASHA). (2007). *Consensus auditory-perceptual evaluation of voice (CAPE-V).* Retrieved from http://www.asha.org/about/membership-certification/divs/div_3.htm

American Speech-Language-Hearing Association (ASHA). (2015). *ASHA SLP health care survey 2015: Caseload characteristics.* Retrieved from http://www.asha.org

American Speech-Language-Hearing Association (ASHA). (2016). *Code of ethics* [Ethics]. Retrieved from http://www.asha.org/policy/

American Speech-Language-Hearing Association (ASHA). (2017). *ASHA practice portals.* Retrieved from http://www.asha.org/practice-portal/

Anderson, R. (1996). Nasometric values for normal Spanish-speaking females: A preliminary report. *Cleft Palate and Craniofacial Journal, 36*(4), 333–336.

Andrianopoulous, M. V., Darrow, K. N., & Chen, J. (2001a). Multimodal standardization of voice among four multicultural populations: Formant structures. *Journal of Voice, 15*(1), 61–77.

Andrianopoulous, M. V., Darrow, K. N., & Chen, J. (2001b). Multimodal standardization of voice among four multicultural populations: Fundamental frequency and spectral characteristics. *Journal of Voice, 15*(2), 194–219.

Aronson, A. E., & Bless, D. M. (2009). *Clinical voice disorders.* New York, NY: Thieme Medical.

Arvedson, J. C., & Brodsky, L. (Eds.). (2002). *Pediatric swallowing and feeding: Assessment and management* (2nd ed.). San Diego, CA: Singular.

Barkan, E. (1992). *The retreat of scientific racism: Changing concepts of race in Britain and the United States between the World Wars.* Cambridge, UK: Cambridge University Press.

Battle, D.E. (2002). *Communication disorders in multicultural populations* (3rd ed.). Oxford, UK: Butterworth-Heinemann.

Battle, D. E. (2012). *Communication disorders in multicultural and international populations* (4th ed.). New York, NY: Elsevier Health Services.

Baugh, J. (2000). *Beyond Ebonics: Linguistic pride and racial prejudice.* New York, NY: Oxford University Press.

Baugh, J. (2003). Linguistic profiling. In S. Makoni, G. Smitherman, A. F. Ball, & A. K. Spears (Eds.), *Black linguistics: Language, society and politics in Africa and the Americas* (pp. 155–168). New York, NY: Routledge.

Bedore, L. M., Fiestas, C. E., Peña, E. D., & Nagy, V. J. (2006). Cross-language comparisons of maze use in Spanish and English in functionally monolingual and bilingual children. *Bilingualism: Language and Cognition, 9,* 233–247.

Bedore, L. M., Peña, E. D., Gillam, R. B., & Ho, T. (2010). Language sample measures and language ability in Spanish English bilingual kindergarteners. *Journal of Communication Disorders, 43*(6), 498–510.

Behlau, M., & Murray, T. M. (2012). International and intercultural aspects of voice and voice disorders. In D. E. Battle (Ed.), *Communication disorders in multicultural and international popu-* *lations* (4th ed., pp. 174–202). New York, NY: Elsevier Health Services.

Benkert, R., Peters, R., Clark, R., & Keves-Foster, K. (2006). Effects of perceived racism, cultural mistrust and trust in providers on satisfaction of care. *Journal of the National Medical Association, 98*(9), 1532–1540.

Benninger, M. S., Holy, C. E., Bryson, P. C., & Milstein, C. F. (2017). *Prevalence and occupation of patients.* Retrieved from https://www.ncbi.nlm.nih.gov/pubmed/28416083

Bernstein Ratner, N. (2011). Fluency. In B. Goldstein (Ed.), *Language development: A focus on the Spanish-English speaker* (2nd ed.). Baltimore, MD: Brookes.

Bhattacharya, S., Khanna, V., & Kohli, R. (2009). Cleft lip: The historical perspective. *Indian Journal of Plastic Surgery, 42,* S4–S8.

Bilodeau, B. L., & Ren, K. A. (2005). Analysis of LGBT identity development models and implication for practice. *New Directions for Student Services, 111,* 25–39.

Blair, I. V., Steiner, J. F., & Havranek, E. P. (2011). Unconscious (Implicit) Bias and healthcare disparities: Where do we go from here? *Permanente Journal, 15*(2), 71–78.

Bland-Stewart, L. M. (2005). Difference or deficit in speakers of African American English?: What every clinician should know . . . and do. *ASHA Leader, 10,* 6–31.

Bliss, L., & McCabe, A. (2012). Personal narratives: Assessment and intervention. *Perspectives on Language Learning and Education, 19,* 130–138.

Blood, G. W., & Blood, I. M. (2016). Long-term consequences of childhood bullying in adults who stutter: Social anxiety, fear of negative evaluation, self-esteem, and satisfaction with life. *Journal of Fluency Disorders, 50,* 72–84.

Boone, D. R., McFarlane, S. C., Von Berg, S. L., & Zraick, R. I. (2010). *The voice and voice therapy.* Boston, MA: Allyn & Bacon.

Borsel, J. V., Maes, F., & Foulon, S. (2001). Stuttering and bilingualism: A review. *Journal of Fluency Disorders, 26*(3), 179–220.

Boshoff, P. H. (1945). The anatomy of the South African Negro larynges. *South African Journal of Medical Sciences, 10,* 35–50.

Boyle, M. P., Daniels, D., Hughes, C., & Buhr, A. (2016). Considering disability culture for culturally competent interactions with individuals who stutter. *Contemporary Issues in Communication Sciences and Disorders, 43*, 11–22.

Brackenbury, T., & Pye, C. (2005). Semantic deficits in children with language impairments: Issues for clinical assessment. *Language, Speech and Hearing Services in Schools, 36*, 5–16.

Bullock, L. (2006, August 16). *Testers posing as Katrina survivors encounter "linguistic profiling."* San Francisco, CA: New America Media.

Burns, F., de Villiers, P., Pearson, B. Z., & Champion, T. B. (2012). Dialect neutral indices of narrative cohesion and evaluation. *Language, Speech and Hearing Services in Schools, 43*, 132–152. (clauses)

Byrd, C. T., Bedore, L. M., & Ramos, D. (2015). The disfluent speech of bilingual Spanish–English children: Consideration for differential diagnosis of stuttering. *Language, Speech, and Hearing Services in the Schools, 45*(1), 30–43.

Campbell, G. L. (1991). *Compendium of the world's languages, Vol. 1–2.* London, UK and New York. NY: Routledge.

Campbell, T., Dollaghan, C., Needleman, H., & Janosky, J. (1997). Reducing bias in language assessment: Processing-dependent measures. *Journal of Speech, Language, and Hearing Research, 40*, 519–525.

Cavalli-Sforza, L. L., & Cavalli-Sforza, F. (1995). *The great human diasporas: The history of diversity and evolution.* Boston, MA: Addison-Wesley.

Campinha-Bacote, J. (2002). The process of cultural competence in the delivery of healthcare services: A model of care. *Journal of Transcultural Nursing, 13*, 181.

Centers for Disease Control and Prevention (CDC). (2011). CDC health disparities and inequalities report—United States, 2011 [monograph on the Internet]. Atlanta, GA: Author; *MMWR Surveillance Summary 2011 Supplement.* Retrieved from https://www.cdc.gov/mmwr/pdf/other/su6001.pdf

Centers for Disease Control and Prevention (CDC). (2016a). *Reported tuberculosis in the United States, 2015.* Atlanta, GA: U.S. Department of Health and Human Services. Retrieved from http://www.cdc.gov/tb/statistics/reports/2015

Centers for Disease Control and Prevention (CDC). (2016b). *Facts about cleft lip and palate.* Retrieved from https://www.cdc.gov/ncbddd/birthdefects/cleftlip.html

Champion, T. B. (1998). 'Tell me something good': A description of narrative structures among African American children. *Linguistics and Education, 9*, 251–286.

Charity, A. H. (2008). African-American English: An overview. *Perspectives on Communication Sciences and Disorders in Culturally and Linguistically Diverse Populations, 15*(2), 33–42.

Chow, J. C-C., Jaffe, K., & Snowden, L. (2003). Racial/ethnic disparities in the use of mental health services in poverty areas. *American Journal of Public Health, 93*, 792–797.

Chun, E. W. (2001). The construction of White, Black, and Korean American identities through African American vernacular English. *Journal of Linguistic Anthropology, 11*(1), 52–64.

Colton, R. H., Casper, J. K., & Leonard, R. (2011). *Understanding voice problems: A physiological perspective for diagnosis and treatment* (4th ed.). Baltimore, MD: Lippincott Williams and Wilkins.

Constantine, M. G. (2002). Predictors of satisfaction with counseling: Racial and ethnic minority clients' attitudes towards counseling and ratings of their counselors' general and multicultural counseling competence. *Journal of Counseling Psychology, 49*, 255–263.

Coussens, A. K., Wikinson, R. J., Nikolajevskyy, V., Elkington, P. T., Hanifa, Y., Islam, K., . . . Martineau, A. R. (2013). Ethnic variation in inflammatory profile tuberculosis. *PLOS Pathogens, 9*(7), 1–15.

Craig, H. K., & Grogger, J. T. (2012). Influences of social and style variables on adult usage of African American English features. *Journal of Speech and Hearing Research, 55*(5), 1274–1288.

Croen, L. A., Shaw, G. M., Wasserman, C. R., & Tolarova, M. M. (1998). Racial and ethnic variations in the prevalence of orofacial clefts in California, 1983–1992. *American Journal of Medical Genetics, 79*(1), 42–47.

Crystal, D. (1997). *English as a global language.* Cambridge, UK: Cambridge University Press.

Cummins, J. (2008). BICS and CALP: Empirical and theoretical status of the distinction. In B. Street & N. H. Hornberger (Eds.), *Encyclopedia of Language and Education* (2nd ed., Vol. 2, pp. 71–83). New York, NY: Springer Science + Business Media.

Current Population Survey (CPS). (2016). Labor force statistics from the current population survey. *Bureau of Labor Statistics*. Retrieved from https://www.bls.gov/cps/demographics .htm#race

Danahy Ebert, K., & Scott, C. M. (2014). Relationships between narrative language samples and norm-referenced test scores in language assessments of school-age children. *Language, Speech, and Hearing Services in Schools, 45,* 337–350.

Dawson, J. L., Stout, C. E., & Eyer, J. A. (2003). *Structured Photographic Expressive Language Test.* 3rd ed. DeKalb, IL: Janelle.

Debose, C., & Faraclas, N. (1993). An Africanist approach to the linguistic study of Black English: Getting to the African roots of the tense/ aspect/modality and copula systems in Afro-American. In S. Mufwene (Ed.), *Africanisms in Afro-American language varieties* (pp. 364–387). Athens, GA: University of Georgia Press.

DeJarnette, G., Rivers, K. O., & Hyter, Y. D. (2015). Pragmatic language of African American children and adolescents: A systematic synthesis of the literature. *Topics in Language Disorders, 35*(1), 8–45.

Dixon, M. J., Marazita, M. L., Beaty, T. H., & Murray, J. C. (2011). Cleft lip and palate: Synthesizing genetic and environmental influences. *Nature Reviews Genetics, 12,* 168–178.

Duff, M. C., Proctor, A., & Yairi, E. (2004). Prevalence of voice disorders in African American and European American preschoolers. *Journal of Voice, 18,* 348–353.

Eddey, G. E., & Robey, K. L. (2005). Considering the culture of disability in cultural competence education. *Academic Medicine, 80*(7), 706–712.

Edwards, W., & Winford, D. (Eds.). (1991). *Verb phrase patterns in Black English and Creole.* Detroit, MI: Wayne State University Press.

Ellis, C., Mayo, R., Mayo, C. M., & Holt, Y. F. (2016). The multidimensional nature of disparities in health-related outcomes: Contributions of patients, providers and health systems. *ECHO: Journal of the National Black Association for Speech-Language and Hearing, 2*(11), 8–21.

Erickson, J., & Iglesias, A. (1986). Assessment of communication disorders in non-English proficient children. In O. Taylor (Ed.), Nature of communication disorders in culturally and linguistically diverse populations [pp. 181–217). San Diego, CA: College-Hill Press

Fabiano, L. C. (2007). Evidence-based phonological assessment of bilingual children. *Perspectives on Communication Disorders and Sciences in Culturally and Linguistically Diverse Populations, 14,* 21–23.

Feldman, H. M., Campbell, T. F., Kurs-Lasky, M., & Rockette, H. E. (2005). Concurrent and predictive validity of parent reports of child language. *Child Development, 76*(4), 856–868.

Fuerstein, R., Fuerstein, R. S., Falik, L., & Rand, Y. (2006). *Creating and enhancing cognitive modifiability: The Feuerstein instrumental enrichment program by Reuven Feuerstein.* Retrieved from https://www.thinkingconnections.org/theory/ MLE.shtml

Fiscella, K., Franks, P., Gold, M. R., & Clancy, C. M. (2000). Inequality in quality: Addressing socioeconomic, racial, and ethnic disparities in healthcare. *Journal of the American Medical Association, 17*(19), 2579–2584.

Foster, M. (2001), Pay Leon, Pay Leon, Pay Leon, Paleontologist: Using call-and-response to facilitate language mastery and literacy acquisition among African American Students. In S. Lanehart (Ed.), *Sociocultural and historical contexts of African American English, varieties of English around the world.* Amsterdam: John Benjamin.

Gaither, S. E., Cohen-Goldberg, A. M., Gidney, C. M., & Maddox, K. B. (2016). Sounding Black or White: Priming identity and biracial speech. *Frontiers in Psychology, 6,* 1–11.

Gladding, S. T. (2009). *Counseling: A comprehensive profession* (6th ed.). Boston, MA: Pearson.

Glanz, K., Rimer, B. K., & Lewis, F. M. (2002). *Health behavior and health education: Theory, research, and practice.* San Francisco, CA: Jossey-Bass.

Goldman, R., & Fristoe, M. (2015). *Goldman Fristoe Test of Articulation 3.* San Antonio, TX: Pearson.

Goldstein, B. (2000). *Cultural and linguistic diversity resource guide for speech-language pathologists.* San Diego, CA: Singular.

Goldstein, B. (2012). *Bilingual language development and disorders in Spanish-English speakers* (2nd ed.). Baltimore, MD: Brookes.

Goldstein, B., & Gildersleeve-Neumann, C. (2012). Phonological development and disorders. In B. Goldstein (Ed.), *Bilingual language development and disorders in Spanish-English speakers* (2nd ed., pp. 285–311). Baltimore, MD: Brookes.

Green, L. (1990). *African American English: A linguistic introduction.* Cambridge, UK: Cambridge University Press.

Green, L. (2002). African American English speech and intonation. In C. Ferguson & E. Finegan (Eds.), *Language in the USA: Themes for the twenty-first century* (pp. 76–91). Cambridge, UK: Cambridge University Press.

Groher, M., & Crary, M. (2015). *Dysphagia: Clinical management of adults and children* (2nd ed.). St. Louis, MO: Elsevier.

Gross, M. (1999). Pitch raising surgery in male to female transsexuals. *Journal of Voice, 13*(2), 246–250.

Gutierrez-Clellan, V. F. & Quinn, R. (1993). Assessing narratives in diverse cultural/linguistic populations: Clinical implications. *Language, Speech, and Hearing Services in Schools, 24,* 2–9.

Gutierrez-Clellan, V. F., & Peña, E. (2001). Dynamic assessment of diverse children: A tutorial. *Language, Speech, and Hearing Services in Schools, 32*(4), 212–224.

Hall, E. T. (1976). *Beyond culture.* New York, NY: Random House.

Haller, R. M., & Thompson, E. A. (1975). Prevalence of speech, language, and hearing disorders among Harlem children. *Journal of the National Medical Association, 67*(4), 298–301.

Hancock, A. B., & Garabedian, L. (2013). Transgender voice and communication treatment: A retrospective chart review of 25 cases. *International Journal of Language and Communication Disorders, 48*(1), 54–65.

Hancock, A. B., Stutts, H. W., & Bess, A. (2015). Perceptions of gender and femininity based on language: Implications for transgender communication therapy. *Language and Speech, 58*(3), 315–333.

Hannah, A., & Murachver, T. (1999). Gender and conversational style as predictors of conversational behavior. *Journal of Language and Social Psychology, 19*(2), 153–174.

Harris, K. L., & Morgan, M. J. (2006). Phonological features exhibited by children speaking African American English at three grade levels. *Communication Disorders Quarterly, 27*(4), 195–205. Retrieved from http://jslhr.asha.org/

Hayes, S., Riley, P., Radley, D. C., & McCarthy, D. (2015). Closing the gap: Past performance of health insurance in reducing racial and ethnic disparities in access to care could be an indication of future results. *The Commonwealth Fund, 5,* 1–12.

Hedberg, N., & Westby, C. (1993). *Analyzing story telling skills: Theory to practice.* Tucson, AZ: Communication Skill Builders.

Hegde, M. N., & Freed, D. (2016). *Assessment of communication disorders in adults: Resources and protocols* (2nd ed.). San Diego, CA: Plural.

Hegde, M. N., & Pomaville, F. (2016). *Assessment of communication disorders in children: Resources and protocols* (3rd ed.). San Diego, CA: Plural.

Hernstein, R. J., & Murray, C. (1994). *The bell curve: Intelligence and class structure in American life.* New York, NY: Free Press Paperback.

Herrera, S. G., Murry, K. G., & Cabral, R. M. (2012). *Assessment accommodations for classroom teachers of culturally and linguistically diverse students* (2nd ed.). New York, NY: Pearson.

Heyer, E., Balaresque, P., Jobling, M. A., Quintana-Murci, L., Chaix, R., Segurel, L., . . . Hegay, T. (2009). Genetic diversity and the emergence of ethnic groups in Central Asia. *BMC Genetics, 10*(1), 10–49.

Holland, R. W., & DeJarnette, G. (2002). Voice and voice disorders. In D. E. Battle (Ed.), *Communication disorders in multicultural populations* (3rd ed., pp. 299–333). Woburn, MA: Butterworth-Heinemann.

Holmes, J., & King, B. W. (2017). Gender and sociopragmatics. In A. Barron, G. Yueguo, & G. Steen (Eds.), *Routledge handbook of pragmatics* (pp. 121–138). London, UK: Routledge.

Horton-Ikard, R., & Miller, J. F. (2004). It is not just the poor kids: The use of AAE forms by African American school-aged children from middle SES communities. *Journal of Communication Disorders, 37*(6), 467–487.

Hou, W. H., Daly, M. E., Lee, N. Y., Farwell, D. G., Luu, Q., & Chen, A. M. (2012). Racial disparities in use of voice preservation therapy for locally advanced laryngeal cancer. *Archives of Otolaryngology Head and Neck Surgery, 138*(7), 644–649.

Hudson, A., & Holbrook, A. (1981). A study of the reading fundamental frequency of young Black adults. *Journal of Speech and Hearing Research, 24*, 197–201.

Hudson, A., & Holbrook, A. (1982). Fundamental frequency characteristics of young adults: Spontaneous speaking and oral reading. *Journal of Speech and Hearing Research, 25*, 25–28.

Hughes, D. L., McGillivray, L., & Schmidek, M. (1997). *Guide to narrative language: Procedures for assessment.* Eau Claire, WI: Thinking Publications.

Hyman, L. (2001). Tone systems. In M. Haspelmath, E. König, W. Oesterreicher, & W. Raible (Eds.), *Language typology and language universals: An international handbook* (Vol. 2, pp. 1367–1380). New York, NY: Walter de Gruyter.

Hyter, Y. D. (1994). *A cross-channel description of reference in the narratives of African, American vernacular English speakers* (Unpublished doctoral dissertation). Temple University, Philadelphia, PA.

Hyter, Y. D. (2014). A conceptual framework for responsive global engagement in communication sciences and disorders. *Topics in Language Disorders, 34*(2), 103–120.

Jenson, J. M. & Fraser, M. W. (2015). *Social policy for children and families: A risk and resilience perspective.* Thousand Oaks, CA: Sage.

Jones, R., & Mayo, R. (2001). Voices of African Americans: Do we need clinical norms? *Perspectives on Communication Disorders and Sciences in Culturally and Linguistically Diverse Populations, 7*(2), 7–11.

Kanamori, Y., & Cornelius-White, J. H. D. (2016). Big changes, but are they big enough? Healthcare attitudes toward transgender persons. *International Journal of Transgenderism, 3*(3–4), 165–175.

Karnell, M. P. (1994). *Videoendoscopy: From velopharynx to larynx.* San Diego, CA: Singular.

Kempster, G. B., Gerratt, B. R., Abbott, K. V., Barkmeier-Kraemer, J., & Hillman, R. E. (2009). Consensus auditory-perceptual evaluation of voice: Development of a standardized clinical protocol. *American Journal of Speech-Language Pathology, 18*, 124–132.

Kim, J. M. (2004). Ethnic minority counselors as cultural brokers: Using the self as an instrument to bridge the gap. *VISTAS Online, 16*, 77–79.

Kite, M. E., & Whitley, B. E., Jr. (1996). Sex differences in attitudes toward homosexual persons, behavior, and civil rights. *Personality and Social Psychology Bulletin, 22*, 336–353.

Kleinman, A., & Benson, P. (2006). Anthropology in the clinic: The program of cultural competency and how to fix it. *PLOS Medicine, 3*(10), e294.

Kling, J. R., Sanbonmatsu, L., Sanchez-Ordoñez, A. E., Sciandra, M., Thomas, E., & Ludwig, J. (2015). Neighborhood effects on use of African-American vernacular English. *Proceedings of the National Academy of Sciences of the United States of America, 112*(38), 11817–11822.

Kohnert, K. (2008). *Language disorders in bilingual children and adults.* San Diego, CA: Plural Publishing.

Kohnert, K. (2013). *Language disorders in bilingual children and adults* (2nd ed.). San Diego, CA: Plural.

Kratcoski, A. M. (1998). Guidelines for using portfolios in assessment and evaluation. *Language, Speech, and Hearing Services in Schools, 29*, 3–10.

Kuehn, D. P., & Henne, L. J. (2002). Speech evaluation and treatment for patients with cleft palate. *American Journal of Speech-Language Pathology, 12*, 103–109.

Labov, W. (1968). The reflections of social processes in linguistic structures. In J. A. Fishman (Ed.), *Language in sociocultural change* (pp. 240–251). Redwood City, CA: Stanford University Press.

Labov, W., Cohen, P., Robins, C., & Lewis, J. (1968). *A study of the non-standard English of Negro and Puerto Rican speakers in New York City.* U.S. Office of Education Final Report, Research Project 3288. Columbia University, New York, NY.

Laing, S. P., & Kamhi, A. (2003). Alternative assessment of language and literacy in culturally and linguistically diverse populations. *Language, Speech, and Hearing Services in Schools, 34,* 44–55.

Lanehart, S. (2015). *The Oxford handbook of African American languages.* Oxford, UK: University Press.

Langdon, H. (2008). *Assessment and intervention for communication disorders in culturally and linguistically diverse populations.* Clifton Park, NY: Thomson Delmar Learning.

Lass, N. J., Almerino, C. A., Jordan, J. F., & Walsh, J. M. (1980). The effect of filtered speech on speaker race and sex identifications. *Journal of Phonetics, 8,* 101–112.

Lass, N. J., Tecca, J., Mancuso, R., & Black, W. (1979). The effect of phonetic complexity on speaker race and sex identifications. *Journal of Phonetics, 7,* 105–118.

Lee, A. S., Robb, M. P., Ormond, T., & Blomgren, M. (2014). The role of language familiarity in bilingual stuttering assessment. *Clinical Linguistics and Phonetics, 28*(10), 723–740.

Lee, C. C. (2008). *Elements of culturally competent counseling* (ACAPCD-24). Alexandria, VA: American Counseling Association.

Lee, L., Stemple, J. C., Glaze, L., & Kelchner, L. N. (2004). Quick screen for voice and supplementary documents for identifying pediatric voice disorders. *Language, Speech, and Hearing Services in Schools, 35*(4), 308–319.

Lemert, E. M. (1962). Stuttering and social structure in two Pacific societies. *Journal of Speech and Hearing Disorders, 27,* 3–10.

Lieberman, L., Kirk, R. C., & Littlefield, A. (2003). Perishing paradigm: Race—1931–1999. *American Anthropology, 105,* 110–113.

Lieberman, L., & Reynolds, L. T. (1978). The debate over race revisited: An empirical investigation. *Phylon, 39,* 333–343.

Lippi-Green, R. (2012). *English with an accent: Language ideology and discrimination in the United States* (2nd ed.). New York, NY: Routledge.

Loh, J., & Ascoli, M. (2011). Cross-cultural attitudes and perceptions towards cleft lip and palate deformities. *World Cultural Psychiatry Research Review, 6*(2), 127–134.

Long, S. H., Fey, M. E., & Channell, R. W. (2004). *Computerized profiling (version 9.6.0).* Cleveland, OH: Case Western Reserve University.

Loury, G. C. (2005). Racial stigma and its consequences. *FOCUS, 24*(1), 1–6.

Loustaunau, M. O., & Soho, E. J. (1997). *The cultural context of health, illness and medicine.* Carvey, CT: Berin and Westport.

Makoni, S., Smitherman, G., Ball, A. F., & Spears, A. K. (2003). Introduction. In S. Makoni, G. Smitherman, A. F. Ball, & A. K. Spears (Eds.), *Black linguistics: Language, society and politics in Africa and the Americas* (pp. 1–18). New York, NY: Routledge.

Manning, H. W., & DiLollo, A. (2017). *Clinical decision making in fluency disorders* (4th ed.). San Diego, CA: Plural.

Marino, T. W. (1996). The challenging task of making counseling services relevant to more populations: Reaching out to communities and increasing the cultural sensitivity of counselors-in-training seen as crucial. *Counseling Today,* 1–6.

Masterson, J., & Berndardt, B. (2006). *Computerized Articulation and Phonology and Evaluation System (CAPES).* San Antonio, TX: Harcourt Assessment.

Masuda, T. (2016). The relation between language, culture, and thought. *Current Opinion in Psychology, 8,* 70–77.

Mathews, S., Abrahams, N., Jewkes, R., Martin, J. L., & Lombard, C. (2013). The epidemiology of child homicides in South Africa. *Bulletin of the World Health Organization. 91,* 562–568.

Matthews, K. A., & Gallow, L. C. (2011). Psychological perspectives on pathways linking socioeconomic status and physical health. *Annual Review of Psychology, 62,* 501–530.

Mattes, L. J. & Omark, D. R. (1991). *Speech and language assessment for the bilingual handicapped.* Oceanside, CA: Academic Communication Associates.

Mayo, C. M., & Mayo, R. (2011). Normative nasalance values across languages. *ECHO, 6*(1), 22–32.

Mayo, R. (1990). *Fundamental frequency and vowel formant frequency characteristics of normal African-American and European American adults*

(Unpublished doctoral dissertation). Memphis State University, Memphis, TN.

Mayo, R., & Grant, W. C. (1995). Fundamental frequency, perturbation, and vocal tract resonance characteristics of African-American and white American male speakers. *Journal of National Black Association Speech-Language Hearing, 17,* 32–33.

Mayo, R., & Manning, W. H. (1994). Vocal tract characteristics of African American and European-American adult male speakers. *Texas Journal of Audiology and Speech Pathology, 20,* 33–36.

Mayo, R., Manning, W. H., & Hudson, A. I. (1989). *Formant frequency characteristics of adult African-American male and female speakers.* Paper presented at the annual convention of the American Speech-Language-Hearing Association, St. Louis, MO.

McAleer, P., Todorov, A., & Belin, P. (2014). How do you say "Hello"?: Personality impressions from brief novel voices. *PLoS ONE, 9*(3), e90779.

McCauley, R. J. (1996). Familiar strangers: Criterion-referenced measures in communication disorders. *Language, Speech, and Hearing Services in Schools, 27,* 122–131.

McCready, V., Campbell, M., Crutchley, S., & Edwards, C. (2011). Doris: Becoming who you are: A voice and communication group program for a male-to-female transgender client. In S. Chabon & E. Cohn (Eds.), *The communication disorders casebook: Learning by example* (pp. 518–532). Upper Saddle River, NJ: Pearson Education.

McLeod, S. (2012). *Multilingual speech assessments.* Bathurst, NSW, Australia: Charles Sturt University. Retrieved from http://www.csu.edu.au/research/multilingual-speech/speech-assessments

McLeod, D. S., Caturegli, P., Cooper, D. S., Matos, P. G., & Hutfless, S. (2014). Variation in rates of autoimmune thyroid disease by race/ethnicity in US military personnel. *Journal of the American Medical Association, 311*(15), 1563–1565.

McLeod, S., & Verdon, S. (2014). A review of 30 speech assessments in 19 languages other than English. *American Journal of Speech-Language Pathology, 23*(4), 708–723.

Mehta, D., & Hillman, R. E. (2007). Use of aerodynamic measures in clinical voice assessment. *Perspectives on Voice and Voice Disorders, 17,* 14–18.

Meigs, A. (1997). Food as a cultural construction. In C. Counihan & P. Van Esterik (Eds.), *Food and culture: A reader* (pp. 95–106). New York, NY: Routledge.

Mohammadzadeh, A., Heydari, E., & Aziz, F. (2011). Speech impairment in primary hypothyroidism. *Journal of Endocrinology Investigation, 34*(6), 31–33.

Munson, B. (2007). The acoustic correlates of perceived sexual orientation, perceived masculinity, and perceived femininity. *Language and Speech, 50,* 125–142.

Munson, B., McDonald, E. C., DeBoe, N. L., & White, A. R. (2006). The acoustic and perceptual bases of judgments of women and men's sexual orientation from read speech. *Journal of Phonetics, 34*(2), 202–240.

Musu-Gillette, L., Robinson, J., McFarland, J., Kewal-Ramani, A., Zhang, A., & Wilkinson-Flicker, S. (2016). Status and trends in the education of ethnic and racial groups 2016. *National Center for Educational Statistics. U.S. Department of Education.* Retrieved from https://nces.ed.gov/pubs2016/2016007.pdf

Mutsmi, I., Kanero, J., & Masuda, T. (2016). The relation between language, culture, and thought. *Current Opinion in Psychology, 8,* 70–77.

Mwiti, L. (2015). *13 facts about slavery in Africa.* Retrieved from http://mgafrica.com/article/2015-03-10-13-fascinating-facts-about-slavery-in-africa-for-one-european-slaves-were-cheaper-but-africans-sold-their-own-more-readily

Nelson, N. W. (1989). Curriculum-based language assessment and intervention. *Language, Speech and Hearing Services in Schools, 20,* 170–184.

Nelson, N. W., & Van Meter, A. M. (2002). Assessing curriculum-based reading and writing samples. *Topics in Language Disorders, 22,* 35–59.

Newman, M. L., Groom, C. J., Handelman, L. D., & Penebaker, J. W. (2008). Gender differences in language use: An analysis of 14,000 text samples. *Discourse Processes, 45,* 211–236.

Nichols, A. C. (1999). Nasalance statistics for two Mexican populations. *Cleft Palate and Craniofacial Journal, 36*(1), 57–63.

Nutlall, Z. (1897). Mexican superstitions. *Journal of American Folklore, 39*(10), 265–281.

Ogundare, A. A. (2012). *Multicultural stuttering and treatment: A cross-cultural analysis.* Research Paper 301. Southern Illinois University, Carbondale, IL.

Okalidous, A., Karathanasi, A., & Grigoraki, E. (2011). Nasalance norms in Greek adults. *Clinical Linguistics and Phonetics. 25*(8), 671–688.

Oller, D., & Delgado, R. (2000). *Logical international phonetics program (LIPP).* Miami, FL: Intelligent Hearing Systems.

Ortega, P. (2016). *Spanish and the medical interview: A textbook for clinically relevant medical Spanish* (2nd ed.). Philadelphia, PA: Elsevier.

Oetting, J. B., & Newkirk, B. L. (2011). Children's relative clause markers in two non-mainstream dialects of English. *Clinical Linguistics & Phonetics, 25*, 725–740.

Patterson, K., Grenny, J., McMillan, R., & Switzler, A. (2002). *Crucial conversations: Tools for talking when stakes are high.* New York, NY: McGraw-Hill.

Pearson, B. Z., Velleman, S. L., Bryant, T. J., & Charko, T. (2009). Phonological milestones for African American English-speaking children learning mainstream American English as a second dialect. *Language, Speech, and Hearing Services in Schools, 40*, 229–244.

Pearson, R. (2002). The debate on race: A problem of semantics rather than of biology. *Mankind Quarterly, 42*, 419–440.

Peña, E. D. (2000). Measurement of modifiability in children from culturally and linguistically diverse backgrounds. *Communication Disorders Quarterly, 21*(2), 87–97.

Peña, E. D., & Iglesias, A. (1992). The application of dynamic methods to language assessment: A nonbiased procedure. *Journal of Special Education, 26*, 269–280.

Peña, E. D., Gillam, R. B., & Bedore, L. M. (2014). Dynamic assessment of narrative ability in English accurately identifies language impairment in English language learners. *Journal of Speech, Language, and Hearing Research, 57*(6), 2208–2220.

Petersen, D. B., Chanthongthip, H., Ukrainetz, T. A., Spencer, T. D., & Steeve, R. W. (2017). Dynamic assessment of narratives: Efficient accurate identification of language impairment in bilingual students. *Journal of Speech, Language, and Hearing Research, 60*(4), 983–998.

Pollock, K., Bailey, G., Berni, M., Fletcher, D., Hinton, L. N., Johnson, I., . . . Weaver, R. (1998). *Phonological features of African American Vernacular English (AAVE).* Child Phonology Laboratory, University of Alberta. Retrieved from http://www.rehabmed.ualberta.ca/spa/phonology/features.htm

Pope, C. (2013, September 22). Pastoral perspectives on silence in church [Blog post]. Retrieved from http://blog.adw.org/2013/09/pastoral-perspectives-on-silence-in-church/

Reading, W. (2014). Separating out gender identity from gender expression. *Everyday Feminism.* Retrieved from http://everydayfeminism.com/2014/05/separating-identity-expression/

Rickford, J. R. (1999). *African American vernacular English: Features, evolution, and educational implications.* Oxford, UK: Blackwell

Rickford, J. R., Duncan. G. J., Gennetian, L. A., Gou, R. Y., Greene, R., Katz, L. F., . . . Ludwig, J. (2015). Neighborhood effects on use of African-American vernacular English. *Proceedings of the National Academy of Sciences of the USA (PNSD), 112*(38), 11817–11822.

Rickford, J. R., & Rickford, R. J. (2000). *Spoken soul: The story of Black English.* New York, NY: Wiley.

Riquelme, L. F. (1997). Practical applications and case presentations: Clinical management of a bilingual Hispanic American adult with dysphagia and dysarthria. In G. Wallace (Ed.), *Multicultural neurogenics: A clinical resource for speech-language pathologists providing services to neurologically impaired adults from culturally and linguistically diverse backgrounds* (pp. 397–402). Tucson, AZ: Communication Skills Builders.

Riquelme, L. F. (2007). The role of cultural competence in providing services to persons with dysphagia. Invited manuscript to *Topics in Geriatric Rehabilitation, 25*(3), 228–239.

Riquelme, L. F. (2013). Cultural competence for everyone: A shift in perspectives. *Perspectives on Gerontology, 18*(2), 42–49.

Riquelme, L. F. (2015). Clinical swallow examination (CSE): Can we talk? *Perspectives on Swallowing and Swallowing Disorders, 24*(1), 34–39.

Rivera, E. T., Phan, L. T., Maddeux, C. D., Wilbur, J. R., & Arredondo, P. (2006). Honesty in multicultural counseling: A pilot study of the counseling relationship. *Inter-American Journal of Psychology, 40*(1), 37–45.

Roseberry-McKibbin, C. (2014). *Multicultural students with special language needs: Practical strategies for assessment and intervention* (4th ed.). Oceanside, CA: Academic Communication Associates.

Roy, N., Barkmeier-Kraemer, J., Eadie, T., Sivasankar, M. P., Mehta, D., Paul, D., & Hillman, R. (2013). Evidence-based clinical voice assessment: A systematic review. *American Journal of Speech-Language Pathology, 22*, 212–226.

Roy, N., Merrill, R. M., Gray, S. D., & Smith, E. M. (2005). Voice disorders in the general population: Prevalence, risk factors, and occupational impact. *Laryngoscope, 115*(11), 1988–1995.

Salas-Provance, M. B. (1996). Orofacial, physiological, and acoustic characteristics: Implications for the speech of African American children. In A. G. Kamhi, K. E. Pollock, & J. L. Harris (Eds.), *Communication development and disorders in African American children: Research, assessment, and intervention* (pp. 155–187). Baltimore, MD: Brookes.

Salas-Provance, M. B. (2010). Counseling in a multicultural society: Implications for the field of communication sciences and disorders. In L. Flasher & P. Fogel (Eds.), *Counseling skills for speech-language pathologists and audiologists* (pp. 159–189). Clifton Park, NY: Delmar.

Salas-Provance, M. B., Erickson J. G., & Reed, J. (2002). Disabilities as viewed by four generations of one Hispanic family. *American Journal of Speech Language Pathology, 11*(2), 151–162.

Sanchez, K., & Wood, C. (2016). Perceptions of disability: Families from culturally and linguistically diverse backgrounds. *Perspectives of the ASHA Special Interest Groups, 1*, 38–46.

Seymour, H. N., Bland-Stewart, L., & Green, L. (1998). Difference versus deficit in child African American English. *Language, Speech, and Hearing Services in Schools, 29*, 96 – 108.

Seymour, H. N., & Seymour, C. M. (1977). A therapeutic model for communicative disorders among children who speak Black English vernacular. *Journal of Speech and Hearing Disorders, 42*, 247–256.

Seymour, H. N., Roeper, T. W., & de Villiers, J. (2003). *Diagnostic Evaluation of Language Variation Criterion Referenced.* San Antonio, TX: The Psychological Corporation.

Seymour, H. N., Roeper, T. W., & de Villiers, J. (2005). *Diagnostic Evaluation of Language Variation Norm Referenced.* San Antonio, TX: The Psychological Corporation.

Shenker, R. C. (2011). Multilingual children who stutter: Clinical issues. *Journal of Fluency Disorders, 36*(3), 186–193.

Smalls, D. L. (2004). Linguistic profiling and the law. *Stanford Law Review, 15*, 579.

Smedley, B. D., Stith, A. Y., & Nelson, A. R. (2003). *Unequal treatment: Confronting racial and ethnic disparities in healthcare.* Washington, DC: National Academy Press.

Steinsapir, C., Former, L., & Stemple, J. (1986). *Voice characteristics among black and white children: Do differences exist?* Paper presented at the annual convention of the American Speech-Language-Hearing Association, Detroit, MI.

Stemple, L. L., Glaze, J. C., & Kelchner, L. N. (2004). Quick screen for voice and supplementary documents for identifying pediatric voice disorders. *Language, Speech, and Hearing Services in Schools, 35*, 308–319.

Steuer, C. E., Deiry, M. E., Parks, J. R., Higgins, K. A., & Saba, N. F. (2017). An update on laryngeal cancer. *California Cancer Journal, 67*, 31–50.

Stewart, B. W., & Semmler, P. C. (2002). Establishing causation of laryngeal cancer by environmental tobacco smoke. *Medical Journal of Australia, 176*, 113–116.

Stewart, J. L. (1960). The problem of stuttering in certain North American Indian societies. *Journal of Speech and Hearing Disorders, Monograph Supplement 6.*

Stockman, I. J. (1996). Phonological development and disorders in African American children. In A. G. Kamhi, K. E. Pollock, & J. L. Harris (Eds.), *Communication development and disorders in African American children: Research, assessment, and intervention* (pp. 117–153). Baltimore, MD: Brookes.

Stockman, I. J. (1996). The promises and pitfalls of language sample analysis as an assessment tool for linguistic minority children. *Language, Speech and Hearing Services in Schools, 27,* 355–366.

Stockman, I. J. (2008). Toward validation of a minimal competence phonetic core for African American Children. *Journal of Speech, Language, and Hearing Research, 51,* 1244–1262.

Stockman, I. J. (2010). A review of developmental and applied language research on African American children: From a deficit to difference perspective on dialect differences. *Language, Speech and Hearing Services in Schools, 41*(1), 23–38.

Stockman, I. J., Guillory, B., Seibert, M., & Boult, J. (2013). Toward validation of a minimal competence core of morphosyntax for African American children. *American Journal of Speech-Language Pathology, 22*(1), 40–56.

Stockman, I. J., Newkirk-Turner, B. L., Swartzlander, E., & Morris, L. R. (2016). Comparison of African American children's performances on a minimal competence core for morphosyntax and the index of productive syntax. *American Journal of Speech-Language Pathology, 25,* 80–96.

Sue, D. W., & Sue, D. (2002). *Counseling the culturally diverse: Theory and practice.* New York, NY: Wiley.

Sulpizio, S., Fasoli, F., Maass, A., Paladino, M. P., Vespignani, F., Eyssel, F., & Bentler, D. (2015). The sound of voice: Voice-based categorization of speakers' sexual orientation within and across languages. *PLoS ONE 10*(7), e0128882.

Tarone, E. (1972). A suggested unit for interlingual identification in pronunciation. *TESOL Quarterly, 6,* 325–331.

Tarone, E. (1973). Aspects of intonation in Black English. *American Speech, 1/2,* 29–36.

Terrell, F., & Terrell, S. (1984). Race of counselor, client sex, cultural mistrust level, and premature termination from counseling among Black clients. *Journal of Counseling Psychology, 31,* 371–375.

Terrell, J. E., Fisher, S. G., & Wolf, G. (1998). Long term quality of life after treatment of laryngeal cancer. *Archives of Otolaryngology–Head and Neck Surgery, 124*(9), 964–971.

Theis, S. M. (2010). Pediatric voice disorders: Evaluation and management. *ASHA Leader, 15*(14), 12–15.

Thomas, E. R. (2015). Prosodic features of African American English. In J. Bllomquist, L. J. Green, & S. L. Lanehart (Eds.), *The Oxford handbook of African American languages* (pp. 421–435). Oxford, UK: University Press.

Thomas, E. R., & Carter, P. M. (2006). Prosodic rhythm and AAE. *English World-Wide, 27*(3), 331–355.

Tinanoff, N. (2007). Cleft lip and palate. In R. M. Kliegman et al. (Eds.), *Nelson textbook of pediatrics* (18th ed., pp. 1532–1533). Philadelphia, PA: Saunders Elsevier.

Titze, I. R. (1989). Physiologic and acoustic differences between male and female voices. *Journal of the Acoustical Society of America, 85,* 1699–1707.

Toliver-Weddington, G., & Meyerson, M. D. (1983). Training paraprofessionals for identification and intervention with communicatively disordered bilingual. In Omark, D. R. and Erickson, J. G. (Eds.). The bilingual exceptional child. (pp. 379–395). Austin, TX: PRO-ED.

Torres, E. (2006). *Healing with herbs and rituals: A Mexican tradition.* Albuquerque, NM: UNM Press.

Trosborg, A. (Ed.). (2010). *Pragmatics across languages and culture.* New York, NY: De Gruyter Mouton.

Twohey, D. (2004). American Indian perspectives of Euro-American counseling behavior. *Journal of Multicultural Counseling and Development, 32,* 320–331.

U.S. Department of Health and Human Services (USDHHS). (2014). *The health consequences of smoking—50 years of progress: A report of the Surgeon General.* Department of Health and Human Services, Centers for Disease Control and Prevention, National Center for Chronic Disease Prevention and Health Promotion, Office on Smoking and Health. Retrieved from https://www.cdc.gov/tobacco/disparities/low-ses/index.htm

Van Hofwegen, J., & Wolfram, W. (2010). Coming of age in African American English: A longitudinal study. *Journal of Sociolinguistics, 14*(4), 427–455.

Van Keulen, J. E., Weddington, G. T., & DeBose, C. E. (1998). *Speech, language, learning, and the African American child.* Boston, MA: Allyn & Bacon.

Van Riper, C. (1982). *The nature of stuttering* (2nd ed.). Englewood Cliffs, NJ: Prentice-Hall.

Vargo, R. A. (2012). *Acoustic and perceptual analyses of the fundamental frequencies of African American and Caucasian males and females* (Unpublished thesis). Cleveland State University, OH.

Verdolini, K., & Ramig, L. O. (2001). Review: Occupational risks for voice problems. *Logopedics, Phoniatrics, Vocology, 26,* 37–46.

Vygotsky, L. (1978). *Mind in society: The development of higher psychological processes.* Cambridge, MA: Harvard University Press.

Walton, J. H., & Orlikoff, R. F. (1994). Speaker race identification from acoustic cues in the vocal signal. *Journal of Speech, Language, and Hearing Research, 37,* 738–745.

Washington, J. A., & Craig, H. K. (1998). Socioeconomic status and gender influences on children's dialectal variations. *Journal of Speech, Language, and Hearing Research, 41,* 618–626.

Wehby, G. L., & Murray, J. C. (2010). Folic acid and orofacial clefts: A review of the evidence. *Oral Disease, 16*(1), 11–19.

Westby, C. (1990). Ethnographic interviewing. *Journal of Childhood Communication Disorders, 13,* 110–118.

Westby, C. (2009). Considerations in working successfully with culturally/linguistically diverse families in assessment and intervention of communication disorders. *Seminars in Speech and Language, 30*(4), 279–289.

Widome, R., Brock, B., Noble, P., & Forster, L. (2013). The relationship of neighbor demographic characteristics to point-of-sale tobacco advertising and marketing. *Ethnicity and Health, 18*(2), 136–151.

Williams, R. (1975). *Ebonics: The true language of Black folks.* St. Louis, MO: The Institute of Black Studies.

Williams, R. (1997). The Ebonics controversy. *Journal of Black Psychology, 23*(3), 208–214.

Wolfram, W. (2011). The African American English canon in sociolinguistics. In A. Curzan (Ed.), *Contours of English and English language studies* (34–52). Ann Arbor, MI: University of Michigan Press.

Wolfram, W., & Fasold, R., (1974). *The study of social dialects in American English.* Englewood Cliffs, NJ: Prentice-Hall.

Wood, J. T. (2009). *Gendered lives* (8th ed.). Boston, MA: Wadsworth Cengage Learning.

Wyatt, T. A. (2017). Assessing the language skills of African American English child speakers: Current approaches and perspectives. In S Lanehart (Ed.), *The Oxford handbook of African American Language* (pp. 526–543). Oxford, UK: Oxford University Press.

Xue, S. A., Hao, G. J. P., & Mayo, R. (2006). Volumetric measurements of vocal tracts for male speakers from different races. *Clinical Linguistics and Phonetics, 20*(9), 691–702.

Yilmaz, T., Kuscu, O., Sozen, T., & Suslu, A. E. (in press). Anterior glottic web formation for voice feminization: Experience of 27 patients. *Journal of Voice.* Retrieved from http://www.sciencedirect.com/science/article/pii/S0892199717300619

Zimmerman, I. L., Steiner, V. G., & Pond, R. A. (2011). *The Preschool Language Scale-5.* San Antonio, TX: Pearson.

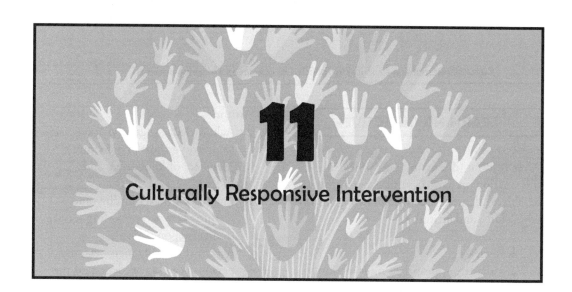

11

Culturally Responsive Intervention

In this chapter we review strategies for the provision of intervention services in a culturally responsive manner. The most critical factor in intervention and a strong predictor of its effectiveness will be that the speech-language pathologist (SLP) and audiologist have used reflective practice to clearly understand and accept the cultural background of the individual well beyond the superficial physical layer of culture. Remember the iceberg analogy from Chapter 2. There is so much more to the individual than what you see before you. This is a good time to review both the Salas-Provance *Hierarchy of Cultural Knowledge* and the Hyter *Model of Cultural and Global Responsiveness* to conduct the difficult task of facing outright, and attempting to understand any implicit biases that you may hold toward the race, culture, or language of individuals under your care. This is a practice that we can all use as we prepare to provide the most culturally responsive intervention. Another important factor that is critical to the success of intervention is the inclusion and empowerment of the family caregivers in the intervention process. Consider whether the caregivers are supportive of the intervention strategy recommended and whether they have time and resources to support this intervention by meeting with the professional and carrying out the hard work of supporting the therapy process at school, hospital, clinic, or home. They may have cultural beliefs that differ strongly from the professional's, in terms of traditions regarding family relationships and hierarchy, child-rearing practices, time dedicated to and available for supporting the person and his or her disabling condition, their understanding and personal beliefs on disability, or their beliefs on the importance or lack of importance of speech-language therapy. Making the effort to communicate with the caregiver prior to the beginning of intervention will help assure that there is a successful outcome in therapy. Including the caregivers in planning the goals and objectives of the intervention allows them to be true partners in this endeavor. It motivates and empowers them by allowing them to clearly understand their family member's or child's needs and their role in the partnership. There are a multitude of cultural aspects that come into play in the intervention process. These aspects are discussed here.

LEARNING OBJECTIVES

After reading, discussing and processing the information presented in this chapter, you will be able to demonstrate the following knowledge, skills, and attitudes:

1. Knowledge
   a. Identify appropriate intervention practices for bilingual children with language disorders.
   b. Identify appropriate intervention practices for bilingual adults with aphasia.
   c. Be aware of five important cultural aspects to consider in all intervention practices.
2. Skills
   a. Recognize that culturally and linguistically diverse (CLD) children can be overrepresented or underrepresented in caseloads and address the issue appropriately.
   b. Use culturally responsive practices to inform CLD families of the value of speech, language, and hearing services.
   c. Use current evidence-based practices with diverse clients.
   d. Learn to use an interpreter to facilitate your success in intervention with linguistically diverse individuals.

3. Attitudes
   a. Acknowledge that service provision to diverse groups may require a "new" set of knowledge and skills.
   b. Practice cultural humility and reciprocity when providing services to diverse populations.
   c. Accept the family members, the person receiving services, and the interpreter as key members of your educational and health care team to provide services to linguistically diverse individuals.
   d. Allow a culture- and family-centered process to guide your service provision.

KEY CONCEPTS

Key concepts addressed in this chapter are presented in Table 11–1.

CULTURALLY RESPONSIVE INTERVENTION

Intervention is a microcosm and extension of the family dynamic and cannot function well

TABLE 11–1. Key Concepts

Under- and overidentification	Cross-linguistic transfer
	Bilingual aphasia
Cultural mismatch	Theories of bilingualism
Second language learning	Bidialectal African American English (AAE) and standard American English (SAE)
Bilingual approach	
Cross-linguistic approach	Cultural-linguistic broker

as a separate entity. The therapist, family, student, patient, or client must function as one unit to meet the goals of therapy, so that learning will occur and treatment outcomes will be achieved. Without this interdependence, the hopes for successful intervention with culturally and linguistically diverse individuals are diminished.

We begin by considering children and their inclusion in caseloads at all levels. It has long been reported that there may be overrepresentation of racially, culturally, and linguistically diverse individuals in our caseloads, but recent research speaks to a concern of underrepresentation of these populations in special education (Artiles & Trent, 1994; Artiles, Harry, Reschy, & Chinn, 2001; Hibel, Farkas, & Morgan, 2010; Morgan et al., 2015). Morgan et al. (2016) examined the characteristics of children who received speech and language services in the first 5 years of life. They reviewed secondary data from the Early Childhood Longitudinal Study-Birth Cohort of the U.S. Department of Education, for infants born in the United States in 2001 at 9, 24, 48, and 60 months of age. The data included parent interviews where they were asked if their child received services for special needs, including speech and language services. The findings showed that children with the following characteristics were at risk for needing SLP services (e.g., underrepresented in service delivery), including: (a) racial identification as Black; (b) early low vocabulary use reported at 24 months of age; (c) low birth weight; (d) history of learning disability in the family; (e) history of maternal depression; and (f) a language other than English spoken at home, especially for Latin@/Hispanic children. They note that one limitation of the study was that parents may be underreporting the use of services, which could explain the disparities found for the Black and Latin@/Hispanic children receiving services.

Underrepresentation of CLD students in speech, language, and hearing services may be due to the hesitation of diverse parents to start the process that begins with a referral of their children for an evaluation. As with medical advice, these parents may take educational/therapeutic advice from their extended family members rather than professionals. These medical practices could influence participation in speech, language, and hearing services. A PEW study (Livingston, Minnushkin, & Cohn, 2008) found that for 32% of Latin@s, *most* of their health care information came from professionals. The remaining 68% of information came from nonprofessional sources such as television (23%), family, and friends (20%) with the remaining 25% spread among the Internet, print, radio, churches, or community group sources. Specifically, Latin@s/Hispanics, First Nations, and Native Alaskans may use medical professionals for advice less often because they represent the three largest groups of uninsured in the United States (27% uninsured) (Barnett, & Vornovitsky, 2016). They may not have access to a professional resource to consult for medical issues. Economic factors, language barriers, or reluctance in exposing an undocumented immigrant status that could affect the use of medical services all may impact the use of other health care services like speech, language, and hearing services resulting in underutilization of services by CLD persons.

There are also many cultural factors that affect access and use of health care and other services, even among the educated and middle class in these diverse groups. There are anecdotal reports that indicate that for some ethnically diverse individuals, if they do seek services, they may have limited adherence to the treatment regimen, including discontinuing services as soon as their symptoms are resolved (Al-Krenawi & Graham, 2000; Antshel, 2002). There appears to be an emphasis on short-term treatment for some. This could explain why some students, patients, or clients may not complete the number of recommended treatment sessions. It has been found that those with stronger social and family support tend to be more compliant with treatment recommendations (DiMatteo, 2004). What may seem like a noncompliance issue may be a practice determined by social, economic, or even cultural reasons. Other cultural factors that may affect the use of medical or other services are fear and distrust in medical or other professionals (which was discussed in Chapter 6), reliance on home remedies or practices, and the use of an alternative network of health professionals (Machado, 2014; Salas-Provance, Erickson, & Reed, 2002). Dr. Salas-Provance had a personal experience where an elderly patriarch of the family passed away within days after a surgery that he had strongly resisted. He had avoided hospitals and distrusted doctors all his life as he truly believed (as did his friends) that "doctors will kill you." This is a tragic end to a cultural story that plays out in real lives and reinforces set cultural beliefs. Many of these aspects of low use or avoidance of medical services due to cultural aspects may transfer over to the use of speech, language, and hearing services. To be true to culturally responsive practice, we must remember that although certain cultural behaviors have been reported in an ethnic group, they may not be found in students, patients, or clients of the same ethnic group. There is great diversity within the same ethnic groups, and among ethnic groups. Whenever you have a question about a behavior, the best practice is to determine whether a behavior is related to a cultural practice common in their family. This determination can be made by engaging in an ethnographic interview, for example (see Chapter 7). This is where you will always find the best answer.

Underidentification of linguistically diverse individuals for services may also be based on the issue that SLPs may easily dismiss a child with accented speech or language variation, such as African American English (AAE), believing their speech is typical for their group. However, without an extensive examination of the difference versus disorder aspect of second language speakers and AAE speakers, the SLP may miss a significant disorder (Stockman, 2010). Without a complete understanding of the rules of AAE, the African American child with a language disorder could be inaccurately diagnosed as having typical AAE speech patterns. Another reason reported by Hibel et al. (2010) for underidentification of CLD students was that some SLPs may decrease number of referrals, so as not to appear racist and to avoid the error of overidentification. It is important to consider that there may be an implicit bias in the way that referrals are made for services for diverse children.

As noted earlier in this chapter, overidentification of children for special education services has been a common practice for diverse children including those who use AAE. Stockman (2010) stated the following, "the more work that listeners must do to understand a speaker, the more likely is that speaker to be judged as unclear, if not communicatively impaired by professionals who are unaccustomed to hearing AAE" (p. 25). There are some SLPs who provide services to modify an accent. However, this intervention is considered an option that would not be eligible for insurance coverage in most instances (American Speech-Language-Hearing Association [ASHA], 2017a), especially in the public school system where most children are served. Accent modification (i.e., helping someone learn a different accent) and dialect modification (e.g., helping an AAE speaker learn an additional dialect and/or language variation) are optional services, and fall under the prevention and wellness activities in which SLPs can be involved (ASHA, 2016). The ability to accurately distinguish a dialectal difference from a language disorder is a critical skill that a SLP should possess (Levey & Sola, 2013) in order to appropriately enroll or exclude children for intervention services.

Inaccurate assessment practices can also create underrepresentation, such as CLD children not receiving the services they need (Morgan et al., 2016) if they are *not* referred for services when they should be. Chapter 10 describes culturally responsive assessment practices that can be used as a basis for making appropriate referrals. Researchers also have found that CLD preschoolers with communication problems (Black and Latin@/Hispanic) are identified less often for early childhood special education services (Morgan et al., 2012). For many years, studies have consistently identified the influence of socioeconomic factors on test outcomes, such as the impact of maternal education on a child's language development (Dollaghan et al., 1999; Hoffe, 2003). The children of mothers with high levels of education appear to have better speech and language skills as compared to children of mothers with limited educational experiences and opportunities. However, there are many examples of less-educated mothers who have raised children with age-appropriate speech and language skills and who have gone on to become highly educated individuals. There are many facets to this issue that must be considered. Many research studies on speech and language do control for the mother's level of education as it remains an important consideration.

Understanding that individuals from culturally and linguistically diverse groups may be over- or underrepresented in our caseloads demands that we are vigilant in carefully and appropriately examining those diverse individuals who are referred to us for services. We should be aware that there may be a child or adult from a CLD population that needs our services who has not been referred. Parents of culturally and linguistically diverse children

should have knowledge of "how" and "when" to access services for their children. Professionals can offer CLD families information about the availability, importance, and benefit of speech, language, and hearing services by reaching out to them using traditional and untraditional methods such as through schools, community social events, faith-based organizations, and health fairs, to name a few. One practice that has worked well for the medical professions is the training of community health workers (health promoters/promatoras) to talk to families in their homes about their medical needs. These programs initially targeted areas such as obesity and diabetes in Latin@/Hispanic populations as well as promotion of lifestyle changes (Koskan et al., 2013). These health promoters could also provide information about services for children with speech, language, and hearing issues while they are in the home for other health issues (Youdelman & Perkins, 2005). Community health workers addressing communication impairments is a growing area of focus in the international realm of speech-language and hearing sciences (Wickenden, 2013).

Both underrepresentation and overrepresentation of diverse children in our caseloads have been attributed to errors in assessment. In overrepresentation, excessive referrals are based on the use of assessment practices that are not appropriate for their cultural or linguistic group (Dollaghan et al., 1999; Peña & Fiestas, 2009). High numbers of diverse children may also be found on our caseloads due to their low socioeconomic levels. It has been found that a greater number of severe speech and language impairments are found among those children who live in impoverished situations. As a result, they may be referred for speech and language services at a higher rate. Children who are impoverished are more often from groups of color (Proctor, Semega, & Kollar, 2016), with the poverty rate for Blacks at 24.1%, Latin@s/Hispanics at

21.4%, Asian at 13.1%, and Whites at 11.6% (Institute for Research on Poverty, 2015). In these instances, communication disorders may result from less cognitive stimulation at home, stressful and unsafe living conditions (e.g., exposure to toxins from a bus terminal being located in the neighborhood, or exposure to lead from paint found in older housing) that may attribute to slower development overall, an unstable family dynamic, and parenting styles that are culturally different from White middle-class parenting interaction styles, which are consistent with expectations in academic settings, for example (Damron, 2015). However, a thorough and accurate evaluation is imperative before placing children in special education services, as not all children who are impoverished will meet this profile or exhibit a speech, language, or hearing disorder.

Apart from these earlier aspects of service provision patterns and cultural aspects, there are other important areas to consider in the intervention process. There are five areas that will generalize across disorders. As you consider students, patients, and clients and their various disorders, reflect on these five areas to provide culturally responsive intervention services. First, and most important, is working with an interpreter in the intervention session. The level of interpreter assistance should have been identified during the assessment. Review Chapter 9 on Interpreters for more extensive information on how to work with an interpreter. Second, materials in the appropriate language of the individual should be used. The materials you are accustomed to using with English-speaking patients can be translated, or you can purchase materials in the language needed. If you cannot complete the translation yourself, the interpreter or a translation company can do this for you. In fact, we have observed that sometimes family members are anxious to help during the intervention session. With regard to therapy

materials, family members can help identify those materials that will be in sync with their cultural backgrounds/beliefs. Pictures should include individuals who "look" like your student, patient, or client and who are engaged in activities that would be typical for the background of the CLD individual. In order to avoid stereotyping in material selection, get to know the student, patient, or client as quickly as possible by asking him or her and the family questions about their background and preferences. Third, some individuals may feel reluctant to engage in personal conversations when they first meet you, so neutral materials should be used until you are sure that the CLD individual will associate with the culturally specific materials you present. It may not be possible to have only culturally specific materials, but an attempt should be made to include them to the greatest extent possible. For the initial intervention session, the use of materials readily available in the immediate environment is the most plausible choice. As intervention progresses, materials are added as needed, always keeping in mind the cultural appropriateness of the materials. Fourth, there may be culturally specific communication and pragmatic issues that must be addressed. For example, the male adult patient from a certain culture with a swallowing disorder may not be comfortable being fed by a female SLP, and there may be some negotiations that must be made. A male family member may be the only one allowed to feed the patient, or the female therapist may be allowed to do the feeding only with a male family member present. These types of unique arrangements cannot be predicted ahead of time for a specific cultural group. It is always best to be flexible and attentive to the communication that is occurring among the patient and the family to glean knowledge. If this is not possible, then you must describe what you are planning to do in detail and get agreement from the family, student, patient, or client to continue. This is the time to consider cultural factors in terms of nonverbal and verbal communication. Identify where you should sit, how you should maintain eye contact, or whether you should praise often or touch the person in encouragement. You may need to learn these factors through trial and error, but using ethnographic methods to determine family practices would be appropriate and help you avoid cultural missteps. If you are a female and the patient is a male, there may be some gender practices to which you must abide in terms of levels of respect (addressing by Mr., Mrs., or a professional title), where you sit, or who speaks first or last. Erring on the side of formality with regard to forms of address is always a good course of action regardless to whom you are talking. Of course, it is always necessary to be respectful and allow as much dignity as possible to all individuals (children and adults), including those with a communication disorder. Family involvement in the intervention session may be determined by cultural traditions. You should have a discussion with the student or patient and his or her family to decide the best family model for intervention. Evaluate both the cultural preference of the individual and their family and your knowledge on the best intervention environment for success. Sometimes it may be necessary to have only the professional and the student, patient, or client in the intervention session, and other times inclusion of a combination of family members is necessary. Never exclude the family members if they feel that they must be present in the therapy session. Exclusion would be a disrespectful choice and could undermine the success of all future intervention. If the CLD individual speaks English as a second language, there is a legal mandate by Culturally and Linguistically Appropriate Services (CLAS) Standards and a strong recommendation from JACO that

family-centered and culturally and linguistically appropriate services be provided.

A fifth aspect to consider is the differences in acceptance of intervention by individuals from different cultural groups. The ideas of cultural mistrust and stigma were discussed earlier in Chapter 6. These are very real phenomena that can derail the best of intentions by the professional in intervention. This is a particular consideration for intervention with adults, but may also affect the intervention with children through their parents, especially if treatment is conducted in the home. You will not know immediately if what you are doing during your intervention is acceptable to the individual. This is something that will take time to present itself, but initially, you should ask the CLD person or the family outright about their beliefs regarding intervention. Using some of the questions from Kleinman's explanatory model may be useful in this case (see Chapter 6, Table 6–3, for examples). Their information can help you avoid initial pitfalls and set you on the path to success. In addition to Kleinman's questions, other questions to ask initially include the following: (a) Tell me about how you would like to be addressed. (b) Tell me about your communication style and preferences (listen for information regarding whether or not it is acceptable to stand close or to touch the CLD person). (c) Would you like for your [e.g., friend, family member] to be with you in the room, or to leave the room? (d) Can I address the male patient if I am a female? (e) Tell me about your role in your family (listen for the hierarchy of the CLD person in his or her family). These questions are appropriate across all racial and ethnic groups. It may be that you are starting services in a hospital and then following the patient to his or her home for continued services. What the CLD person allowed to occur in a hospital may not be the same at home. Once home, he or she may feel that the family is capable of providing services needed. This is not unusual, and this decision should be respected. Review and reflect on the story below.

Box 11–1

In one story, an elderly Hispanic woman who was being seen in the hospital for therapy was now to continue therapy at home. The woman was very happy to be receiving the services; in fact, she was dressed up and waiting for the therapist with her daughters in the front room of the house, which was only open to special visitors. The first misstep was that the therapist was late. The second misstep was that she wore scrubs and tennis shoes for the therapy session in the home (which the patient interpreted as "wearing pajamas"). She became too casual too quickly (calling the patient by her first name and bypassing the greeting phase "la platica" in Spanish) to get right to work. She used a very directive approach and tone, rather than being family-centered. The patient followed the exercise instructions very diligently and was friendly to the therapist. Needless to say, however, the therapist did not return to the home. This patient was Dr. Salas-Provance's mother. The family members were relegated to conduct all therapy sessions in the future.

If you are engaged in home-health services for children or adults, the best practice is to use cultural humility (recognizing that there are cultural variabilities and that all of these variabilities are legitimate and valuable) and cultural reciprocity (learning and being able to: [a] communicate the cultural values and beliefs of our professional practice so that we can explain them to others, [b] name the cultural values and beliefs of those being served, and then being able to [c] partner with the client in developing intervention processes that synthesize these possibly divergent values and beliefs). Both cultural humility and cultural reciprocity are defined and discussed in Chapter 2. All individuals, not just those from CLD groups, are protective of their home environment with its many culturally specific and socially determined rules. The best practice is to ask to enter, even if they are expecting you, be slow to enter, and ask where they want you to sit. Never make assumptions. You should state what you need, as well as have them identify if they would like specific numbers of family members in the room. This is a very unusual and uncomfortable situation for most families and one that must be traversed lightly with great respect. More than one therapist has been asked to leave or not return because of a cultural mismatch that offended the family, as noted in the earlier story. Many times, unfortunately, the therapist may not know what he or she did. The goal is to provide successful intervention. The home should be the ideal environment for the CLD person, but it is one in which the professional must be invited to participate, no matter whether they "should" be there according to a doctor, school, or agency referral.

A final point to make is that the use of the current evidence-based intervention practices in our field applies to all of our students, patients, and clients. Thus, it goes without saying, that when we are providing services to CLD populations we are using evidence-based practices (Frattali et al., 2002; Gillam & Gillam, 2006; Yorkston et al., 2001), and the most current and effective intervention models mandated by health or educational institutions (e.g., Response to Intervention [RtI], transdisciplinary models, or curriculum-based assessment and interventions). Yet, there may be cultural variables, as described earlier, that will impact intervention and require cultural adaptations (ASHA, 2014a, 2017b). Intervention services for bilingual individuals may require new knowledge and skills (ASHA, n.d.c; Kohnert & Derr, 2012; Yu, 2013). We are guided by our professional association (ASHA, 2017b) with the following words, "if a professional feels unprepared to serve an individual on the basis of cultural and linguistic differences, then the option of an appropriate referral should be utilized." The information that follows in this chapter provides guiding principles for the use of culturally responsive practices in intervention. It is ultimately the decision of the clinician, educator, supervisor, student, or researcher as to whether he or she can provide these services in an ethical manner or whether a referral to a bilingual or culturally knowledgeable clinician is in order.

Services to Bilingual Clients

The SLP or audiologist must have the knowledge and skills necessary to provide intervention services to bilingual clients. Following a culturally responsive assessment, the mode of communication best suited for the person should be identified. If the decision is made that treatment must be provided in a language other than English, those professionals without native or near-native proficiency in the target language should work with an interpreter or make an appropriate referral for a bilingual professional. Service to bilingual individuals can include services related to the acquisition of the second language, the loss of language in a bilingual person, and speech disorders (ASHA, n.d.c).

Identify Intervention Services for CLD Children With Language Disorders

A typically developing child learning a second language (L2) plateaus and regresses in his or her first language (L1) as he or she learns the second language. However, the child eventually has an explosion in development of L2 while maintaining L1. For the child with primary or specific language impairment (PLI), he or she is reported to have slower growth in L2 and appears to decline in home language use (L1) (Anderson, 2004; Restrepo, 1998). Bilingual children with PLI may have language difficulty in both languages with delayed vocabulary acquisition; language problems in lexical, semantic, and morphosyntax; as well as code switching problems during conversation. In addition, language processing skills that may present difficulty are nonword repetitions, rapid naming, and novel morpheme learning (Restrepo & Gutiérrez-Clellen, 2012). Two main intervention approaches for bilingual children with language disorders have been reported (Durán et al. 2016; Kohnert & Derr, 2012; Kohnert et al., 2005). They include the bilingual approach (where attention is given to common skills across the two languages) and the cross-linguistic approach (where only a specific aspect/error of either one language or the other [e.g., English or Spanish] is targeted). For example, using the bilingual approach with a young bilingual Spanish-speaking child, intervention could focus on those phonemes such as /p/, /b/, /k/, /g/ that are shared across the Spanish and English languages. As cluster reductions occur often in both languages, this also may be a first intervention target. The cross-linguistic approach would focus on errors that occur only in Spanish, such as the trill sound. This could be a later intervention target. It is important to note that dialectal differences would not be treated. In using the cross-linguistic intervention approach, the SLP is utilizing the bidirectional capability of the bilingual brain, where L1 skills support L2 skills, and vice versa with L2 supporting L1. Cross-linguistic transfer of skills has been shown in the transfer of early literacy skills of letters and sounds (Cárdenas-

Hagan, Carlson, & Pollard-Durodola, 2007), phonological awareness (Dickinson, McCabe, Clark-Chairelli, & Wolf, 2004), and syntactic structures (Paradis and Navarro, 2003).

One study describes the use of three treatment approaches with a group of 59 school-age children with primary language disorder (Ebert et al., 2014) who learned Spanish at home in the United States as their first language and English as their second language. They used three treatment approaches, including: (a) language focus using English, (b) language focus using English–Spanish combined, and (c) a nonlinguistic cognitive processing approach. A fourth group did not receive treatment as part of the study but continued to receive their usual SLP treatment services in the schools. Refer to Ebert et al. (2014) for the details of the intervention within each group. Generally, the language intervention was computer based and traditional therapy based targeting common problems found in PLI children as noted earlier. The nonlinguistic cognitive intervention was focused on tasks for sustained selective attention, speech processing, and working memory. Several important findings were revealed. Those trained in English had a significant change on half of the English measures. The bilingual group gained in both English and Spanish measures, but statistical significance was reached in English only in the training mode. There was generalization from treated to untreated areas as found in the speech therapy being received outside of the experimental treatment. When the children received only English treatment, there were small gains in Spanish. Although not statistically significant, this shows that L2 training has a minimal effect on L1. There appeared to be cross-linguistic transfer to both L1 to L2. An important finding is that the influence of the cognitive linguistic training alone showed some small gains in language skills transferred to both L1 and L2. Although the results are mixed, the finding of even small gains through this intervention approach is

hopeful for the English-only clinician providing treatment to bilingual children using this treatment domain (Ebert, Rentmeester-Disher, & Kohnert, 2012). Overall, there were smaller gains in Spanish versus English. This can be attributed to the reported plateau in L1 and to the use of greater amounts of English for instruction in schools. This shows that intervention in L1 should not be abandoned. Further, when bilingual services are provided, there is an improvement in both L1 and L2. The authors speak to the issue of the preponderance of English-only (EO) treatment for bilingual children with PLI that may be due in part to the small numbers of available bilingual SLPs. At the current time, only 7% of ASHA members identify themselves as bilingual service providers. Of this group, approximately 7,000 SLPs provide services in Spanish (ASHA, 2017c). Although the English language is the focus of education in the United States, and mastery of English will improve academic and social outcomes, there still remains insufficient evidence to support the exclusive use of English-only treatment with bilingual children. It is important to build on their strength in L1.

A clinical survey (Jordaan, 2008) conducted of the 10 member countries of the International Association of Logopedics and Phoniatrics, reported that 80% of services for bilingual children are offered in the language of the majority community in which they live, in spite of recommendations that bilingual children should receive services in both languages or their stronger language (Fredman, 2006; Gutierrez-Clellen, 1999). Guiberson (2013) provides an extensive review of the literature that dismisses the "myth" that learning two languages can be confusing to the child. Additionally, anecdotally, we know that the majority of people in the world grow up learning and becoming proficient in more than one language, without any difficulties at all. Cummins (2005) showed that when a child develops two languages, they are not in competition with each other. Learning a second language does not take away skills from the first language. The evidence continues to build that intervention for bilingual children should utilize both languages in order to provide the child with the best opportunity for success (Paradis et al., 2011). The following summary is provided by Kohnert (2008) regarding bilingual children with language disorder (LD) (pp. 105–106):

- "Bilingualism does not cause LD
- Reverting to monolingualism will not cure LD
- Bilingual children with LD can and do learn two languages
- Level of proficiency in each of the languages . . . will vary with the opportunities and experiences
- Monolingual children need **one** language to be successful in their . . . communicative environments . . .
- Bilingual children with LD need **two** languages to be successful in their . . . communicative environments . . . "

IDENTIFY INTERVENTION STRATEGIES FOR CLD ADULTS WITH LANGUAGE DISORDERS

Bilingual adults with language disorders usually represent those individuals who have lost their language as a result of a neurological impairment, such as a cerebrovascular accident (CVA) or traumatic head injury. A place to start with a CLD patient or client is to review the five areas of preparation in Table 11–2, including: (a) use of an interpreter, (b) use of translated written materials, (c) use of culturally appropriate pictures and objects, (d) addressing of cultural communication and pragmatic issues, and (e) identification of cultural views on intervention. Once these aspects are in place, it is time to consider the use of evidence-based practices for the patient's disorder, in this case, bilingual aphasia (Centeno, 2005, 2009). There are many general resources that can provide the background information on intervention practices for adults with neurological impairment across the board (Darley, Aronson & Brown, 1969; Davis, 2007; Hallowell & Chapey, 2008) and the ASHA Portals (ASHA, n.d.b) and evidence maps are excellent resources for evidence-based practices in this area. It is as important to understand the patient's cultural background as it is to know the specifics of the impairment to assure a successful intervention. Just as we want what is familiar around us when we are in a "new" situation, including the patient's or client's traditional cultural practices may be the perfect way to ease into "new" intervention services with CLD students, patients, and clients. The cultural information becomes an overarching framework for the

TABLE 11–2. Five Areas of Preparation for Culturally Responsive Intervention

1. Most importantly, use an interpreter as needed
2. Use materials in the appropriate language
3. Use culturally responsive pictures and objects
4. Understand relevant communication and pragmatic practices for culture
5. Consider and respect CLD person's level of acceptance of intervention processes

therapeutic work on the disorder. You may have learned in conversation with the family that the patient's family dynamic preference is to have the oldest daughter as the decision maker. Knowing this, you would make sure that the daughter is present in your first therapy session. The daughter may offer the encouragement and support needed should the patient be resistant or confused about the therapeutic requests. The patient may not understand why, for example, she is being asked to name simple words repeatedly in two languages. The daughter could explain the purpose in a more family-centered manner, knowing the personality of her parent. In one study (Nordehn, Meredith, & Bye, 2006), patients, their families, as well as focus groups, were asked what was needed to achieve patient-centered communication (PCC) (as required by the Joint Commmission patient-centered and cultural competence standards). The two most important findings for PCC were the desire to be treated with respect and the need for sufficient time for the patient to communicate. Interestingly, little was noted about the impairment and the therapeutic strategies. Most importantly the daughter would not be used as the interpreter, if there is a second language issue to address. We continue to belabor the point about the use of an interpreter as anecdotal information and published studies continue to tell us that very small numbers of professionals use an interpreter, although this is a critical piece if the linguistically diverse patient is to receive culturally responsive treatment. There must be an interpreter available, if necessary. The intervention may be in English, in the second language, or in a combination of the two. Whichever the case, it is important to be prepared for the patient's language needs throughout the session. Materials also may need to be presented in both languages as needed.

As we may see with any other individual learning a second language, a client with a neurological problem may produce speech that includes dialectal variations. These varia-tions should be considered a difference and not a disorder, but a thorough assessment should still be completed. It is likely there are going to be many other speech, language, or cognitive needs that will be of greater importance to address beyond a dialectal variation for the neurologically impaired patient.

Aphasia has an extensive body of literature that spans several decades (Darley, 1982; Freed, 2000; Hegde, 1998; Holland & Halper, 1996; LaPointe, 1997; Papathanasiou & Coppens, 2017; Yorkston, Beukelman, Strand, & Bell, 1999). The majority of individuals in the United States with bilingual aphasia are Spanish speakers. They represent the largest group of second language speakers in the United States at approximately 38 million individuals (U.S. Census, 2015). Today there is more clinical demand for treating patients with bilingual aphasia than ever before (Centeno, Ghazi-Saidi, & Ansaldo, 2017; Fabbro, 2001). Refer to Lorenzen and Murray (2008) for a comprehensive theoretical and clinical review of bilingual aphasia. Faroqi-Shah et al. (2010) provided a systematic review of 14 studies (45 patients) on best practices for rehabilitation of individuals with bilingual aphasia. They reported on the following areas: (a) the results of language therapy when provided in the secondary (less-dominant) language (L2), (b) the extent of cross-language transfer (CLT) and variables that influence CLT, and (c) outcomes when language therapy is mediated by a language broker. They found that there are positive outcomes when therapy is provided in the second language and that there was crossover to the other language for over half of the patients. The same results were found by Kiran et al. (2013) for 17 Spanish–English bilinguals, in Miertsch et al. (2009) for one German–English–French trilingual, and in Goral et al. (2010, 2012) for a Spanish–German–French–English speaker.

Because the majority of rehabilitation for bilingual aphasics is provided by monolingual speech-language pathologists in English, the studies reporting transfer of learned information for L2 to L1 are valuable and encouraging. There have been other studies that showed only language-specific improvements with no crossover (Amberder, 2012). There is expectation that trained items in L1 or L2 will show improvement in the targeted language. There is now evidence that untrained items in those same languages will also show improvement. The most important findings are that there will be translation from L2 to L1 or L1 to L2 in both trained and untrained items. There does appear to be variation in generalization by type of treatment provided.

The treatment protocol that focuses on naming deficits is most responsive to the transfer phenomena. L1 and L2 semantic systems connections are possible according to the revised hierarchical model (Kroll et al., 2010). The strength of the connection varies by dominance of language with larger *semantic* links found in the L1 with its larger pool of vocabulary. *Lexical* links are the opposite with stronger links found from L2 to L1. We present an example of the use of two languages (bilingualism) to explain this phenomenon.

Dr. Salas-Provance was a simultaneous bilingual in English and Spanish, hearing and speaking both languages from birth. However, being the youngest of seven children, English was brought into the home from her siblings since birth, with the oldest sibling being in middle school at that time. As a result, she became a dominant English speaker very early and a "hesitant" Spanish speaker, although able to comprehend the Spanish language with full proficiency. As a result of numerous professional affiliations in Spanish-speaking countries and clinical work in these countries, she now uses her Spanish more often. However, she is not a balanced bilingual at the highest level of the language proficiency scale. There is still effort needed in some situations to recall the Spanish lexicon and to use it seamlessly. Her lexicon for L1 English is much larger than the L2 Spanish lexicon. Therefore, the stronger lexical associations from L2 to L1 are evident when speaking Spanish on a daily basis. To hear the following words in Spanish quickly brings associations with the English word, rosa:rose; increíble:incredible; asociación:association; *final* ("i" is "ee" in Spanish) and *final* ("i" is /aɪ/ in English) and asistente:assistant. There is little association with the words comer:eat; hablar;speak: camino:road; azul:blue. These words simply need to be memorized as there is no lexical association. However, there are some Spanish words that have been used so regularly in English it seems as if they are English words, such as camino (road) "Camino Real"; colorado (red) Colorado; santa fe (Holy Faith); Santa Fe. One theory of bilingualism purports that it takes much effort to translate from the stronger language to the weaker language because the stronger language must be inhibited to access the target language (Costa, Santesteban, & Ivanova 2006). For Dr. Salas-Provance the weaker language is Spanish; thus, it is not difficult to inhibit the Spanish language when speaking in English, but it is difficult to inhibit English when speaking in Spanish. The bilingual speaker is not aware of this inhibition process, which is an automatic cognitive process, but there are taxing moments when a word or words are not readily available in Spanish; thus, English seems to be the only language accessible. During these times, there is an asymmetry to the switching of language use from L1 to L2 and the use of two languages becomes conscious. This reveals, also, how semantic system links are stronger to L1 than to L2 (Costa, La Heij, & Navarrete, 2006). In attempting to produce a word such as "computer" in Spanish, the process is that both L1 and L2 semantic and phonological systems are activated simultaneously without preference to either system to produce the word in Spanish such as "computadora." This is similar in principle to the inhibition theory, whereby the L1 is inhibited to use the L2 (Green, 1998).

It is important to review the semantic-based naming treatment and findings by Kiran et al. (2013) more closely. Seventeen Spanish–English bilinguals with aphasia were each given three sets of stimuli for the English language and for the Spanish language to complete a naming task. The English items were translated into Spanish. The English and Spanish items in Set 2 were semantically related to those in Set 1. Set 3 contained control items that were unrelated to Set 1 or Set 2. Treatment was conducted in only one language. There was within-language improvement for 14 of 17 participants, with 10 of the 14 showing within-language generalization to untrained similar semantic items. There were five participants who showed improvement across languages in the trained items, and six participants showed improvement in the untrained items. According to the authors, this shows evidence of the theoretical processes noted earlier in bilingualism of an "interplay between facilitation (generalization) and inhibition" (p. 300). Training in Spanish (the native language of all participants) showed the best outcomes compared to training in English, although there was improvement in both languages. The generalization effects of the therapy were influenced by language use, language dominance, and language impairment. It appeared that patients with better semantic processing abilities showed the best improvement. Interestingly, seven of the 17 patients were trained in their weaker language, and four of them showed within- and between-language generalization. Research continues in this promising area of translation of learned information from one language to another in bilingual aphasics to identify reliable and consistent treatment protocols.

Another promising treatment protocol was used by Kohnert (2004) with one English–Spanish bilingual with nonfluent aphasia include training in linguistic and nonlinguistic tasks. This cognitive-based treatment utilized visual scanning tasks, categorizing tasks, and simple arithmetic problem solving. The linguistic tasks included cross-linguistic training of cognates similar in meaning and form like *rose* and *rosa* and noncognates with similar meaning but different form like *mesa* and *table*. Results showed small gains in both English and Spanish for the cognitive-based treatment. The linguistic task showed transference of language skills for the cognate-based task. Both of these findings are promising for monolingual clinicians working with bilingual patients.

To provide treatment to a bilingual person with aphasia requires knowledge of the most current evidence in treatment protocols for this group. ASHA provides needed information in this area (ASHA, n.d.a). One of the main questions to address is whether to offer the treatment in one language or two languages (Centeno, 2005; Kohnert, 2004). There are proponents for both. As mentioned earlier in the section on bilingual treatment for children, currently there is not sufficient evidence to show that treatment in one language is sufficient for bilingual children. Bilingual therapy is recommended. The one or two language treatment debate brings to the forefront an oft used, but misguided and *incorrect* recommendation for bilingual parents that they should refrain from using both languages in the home with their language impaired child—that the use of one language is best. There is now significant evidence that supports that a child raised in a bilingual home is not at a disadvantage in terms of language development when both languages are used simultaneously in the home. In fact, if the child has a language delay, this is the most suitable environment for language development. It seems then, that treatment in two languages for the bilingual person with aphasia may warrant many benefits beyond the improvement of the communication disorder. A few reports show that there is generalization and cross-linguistic transfer, from the language of treatment to the nontreated language for some study participants, which may be a function of shared neural networks (Edmonds & Kiran, 2006; Kohnert, 2009). The study by Kiran et al. (2013) shows that it is possible for bilingual training to result in improvement in only one language. The systematic review by Faroqi-Shah et al. (2010) provides state-of-the-art information in this area from 1980 to August 2009. This review is comprehensive and provides clinical guidelines for treatment from the 14 studies. There is continued support for the use of two languages in treatment. The review did not identify any studies reporting the feasibility of using language brokers during bilingual treatment. This is an area ripe for research. The clinician should review these studies carefully for information that may be pertinent to their unique case. At this time there does not appear to be a standard treatment protocol that can be recommended for patients with bilingual aphasia. Farocqui-Shah and colleagues (2010) point to the following as areas to control in future treatment research: (a) spontaneous recovery in the treatment process; (b) modality of treatment such as expression, comprehension, and reading; (c) language domain; (d) influence of L2 acquisition age; (e) premorbid proficiency; and (f) daily usage patterns, among others. As you conduct your treatment in a culturally responsive manner, these are some issues to consider that can provide direction to your treatment. It appears that the evidence to support the use of specific treatment protocols in the area of bilingual aphasia remains preliminary.

IDENTIFY INTERVENTION STRATEGIES FOR CLD CHILDREN WITH SPEECH SOUND DISORDERS

Children who speak English as a second language may have disorders of speech in either their first or second language or both languages. Before we speak to the specific issues related to speech sound disorders, be sure to review the five points of preparation for intervention with CLD persons found in Table 11–2 as a way to set the foundation for culturally responsive treatment of CLD clients. The points include: (a) use of an interpreter, (b) use of translated written materials, (c) use of culturally appropriate pictures and objects, (d) addressing cultural communication and pragmatic issues, and (e) identifying cultural views on intervention. Once these aspects are in place, it is time to consider the use of evidence-based practices for the client's or student's disorder—in this case, speech sound disorders. The first step is to identify the typical sound system for the child's first language. McLeod (2007) provides extensive information on the speech acquisition development profiles of children from many languages around the world. ASHA provides resources of phonemic inventories across languages (ASHA, n.d.f). Some sound system information was provided for Spanish in the earlier assessment in Chapter 10 (Fabiano-Smith & Goldstein, 2010). If an articulation disorder has been identified during the assessment, then an intervention program should be put into place. Treatment practices for articulation therapy should be similar across all children no matter their racial or ethnic background. An articulation disorder is a type of motor learning where the articulators move into various positions to produce the speech sound during the production of language. Proper articulation for speech utilizes the systems of articulation, resonation, phonation, and respiration. Articulation requires speed, mobility, and precision over a designated time period. There are universal principles for use of speech sounds in terms of the manner of production, place of articulation, and voicing. We should expect the linguistically diverse children to perform in a similar fashion to the English speakers. There should not be an alternate expectation in articulation because students are bilingual or monolingual. Articulation disorder can be remediated using established speech therapy principles (Van Riper, 1963). The training usually begins with a listening task or speech sound discrimination task followed by sound production in isolation, syllables, multisyllables, words, phrases, sentences, ending with the use of the correct speech sounds in connected speech. A multisensory approach is used and can include sound amplification, tactile cues, visual cues, gestures and more recently palatography, ultrasound imaging, and tactile biofeedback (Byen & Hitchock, 2012; Dagenais, 1995; Hodson, 2010; Preston, Brick, & Landi, 2013; Shriberg, 1980). This traditional approach to remediation of articulation errors has been used for almost 50 years. Treatment approaches can include such variations as the context utilization approach (Bernthal et al., 2013), contrast therapy (Gierut, 1982), core vocabulary approach (Dodd et al., 2006), and distinctive feature therapy (Blache & Parsons, 1980), among others. There are many resources that can provide the background information on articulation therapy including the ASHA Portals and evidence maps (ASHA, n.d.g). For bilingual or multilingual children, the clinician will need to know the consonants and vowels in each of the child's languages. There may be sounds that are similar among the languages and some sounds that are unique to each language. Sounds in L1 may influence how sounds in L2 are produced (Dickinson et al., 2004). It is important to differentiate an accent associated with the first language from a true articulation disorder (ASHA, 2017a; Bernthal & Bankson, 1994). In Spanish, a child may use a rolled /r/ rather than the consonant /r/. As a carryover from the sound system of their first language, this would not be considered an error, and remediation would not be necessary. If the clinician is unable to serve as a good speech model for the child, other measures must be considered such as the use of an interpreter or a bilingual clinician in the child's language (Goldstein &

Gildersleeve-Newman, 2012; Goldstein & Fabiano, 2007). It is important to go one step further and evaluate the phonological system and how these speech sounds interact during language (Hua & Dodd, 2006; Lowe, 1994). There may be contextual variation for the bilingual or multilingual children that must be considered. There may be rule-governed patterns of speech sounds in one language that transfer to English. For example, the /t/ and /d/ are dentalized in Spanish and are not released (Melgar de González, 2007; Merino, 1982, 1983). The child may replace the English lingua alveolar placement for /t/ with the Spanish dentalized version. Sounds change when they are in different phonetic contexts, and this must be considered, especially when there is cross-language variation. For example, the production of the /s/ phoneme changes in the words "sing" and "shows." The Spanish-speaking child does not produce a /z/, thus, in the prior example, the final /s/ in the word "shows" will be produced as an /s/ and not a /z/. The production will be /ʃows/ and not /ʃowz/. A thorough examination of the phonemic system within various contexts is needed. Phonological disorders are systemic, so it is important to look system-wide for patterns of errors. An entire body of knowledge is dedicated to phonological disorders including fronting errors, voicing errors, final consonant deletions, among others (Bernthal, Bankson, & Flipsen, 2013). One of the most common therapy procedures for phonological disorders is the cycle approach (Hodson, 2010, Prezas & Hodson, 2010). Most words in Spanish end in vowels. The only final consonants used in Spanish are /n, l, d, r, s/ (Jimenez, 1987). A phonological processing disorder of final consonant deletion could incorrectly be diagnosed in a Spanish-speaking child because of this phenomenon. Because the majority of SLPs are solely English speakers, the intervention will most likely focus on improving the speech sound disorder in the English language of those sounds not attributed to a dialectal variation. If there is an articulation or phonological disorder in the first language, a bilingual SLP could address those issues.

The SLP must also be knowledgeable of the variations in speech for children who use African American English (AAE). Refer to Chapters 5 and 10 for background information on the use of AAE. To provide appropriate intervention, it is important to first identify typical patterns of AAE development and use (Bland-Stewart, 2003; Cole, 1980; Craig, 2016; Harris & Moran, 2006). Stockman (2010) provides a review of studies on AAE phonological development. To provide culturally responsive practice, the clinician must learn the unique features of AAE. Similar to the use of an interpreter for second language speakers, the SLP may need an AAE cultural-linguistic broker who understands well the AAE patterns of speech and can assist the SLP in this process. When addressing speech sound differences, the therapy principles, strategies, and treatments will be similar to what was mentioned earlier in this section. Because AAE is also a language system that incorporates morphology, semantics, syntax, and pragmatics, standard language therapy evidence-based principles should be used (ASHA, n.d.e; Cirrin & Gillam, 2008; Steele, 2014; Taylor-Goh, 2005).

The SLP should have established the child's skill level for the use of AAE and GAE during the assessment phase. The use of AAE should be considered additive to the child's GAE linguistic repertoire, not subtractive. AAE plus GAE is evidence of dual dialectal proficiency, a skill that should be valued. It is *not* a matter of comparing the child's skills in GAE to their skills in AAE, with GAE used as the standard. A child's AAE skills should be compared to the skills of a typically developing AAE speaking child and GAE skills to GAE speakers, just as we would not compare a child's first language, of Korean for example, to English. These are two different and separate linguistic systems. There may be some similarities and many differences. But one is not set as the standard for the other; however, the language structures of one may influence the language structures of the other. When this occurs, intervention is *not warranted*. This is evidence of the "difference" between the two dialects or the two languages. However, when a disorder is identified (which can be in one dialect/language alone, or in both dialects/languages), intervention *would be warranted*.

We mentioned earlier in this chapter that a child who speaks the Spanish language (which has few final consonants) and proceeds to use this same phonological rule of omission of final consonants in English does not have a phonological disorder. There is a "difference" in the two languages, and the child may simply need more experience adding final consonants to words. A similar situation occurs in AAE with, for example, the use of the plural inflection of a noun (Stockman, 2010). Its absence in AAE speakers should not always be noted as an error. The use of *two shoe* instead of *two shoes* would not be counted as an error, because it is an accurate use of this AAE feature. Yet, an AAE child who says "I have shoe" (failure to use an article or failure to add plural inflection) would be considered to have made an error in both AAE and GAE. Intervention for the bidialectal GAE and AAE child is not simply a matter of making sure they adhere to GAE standards with the same intervention goals and objectives used with GAE-speaking students. These children use both language variations within the rule-governed systems of each dialect as part of their everyday lives. It is highly unlikely that the child who uses AAE is aware that there is a second set of sound system and language rules in GAE to which they should abide in some circumstances. Children should be provided with structured guidance to differentiate between the "home" or "heritage" language and the "school" language

(Craig, 2016). It requires a culturally responsive mindset to complete the rigorous work of addressing each of the dialects, including their unique and overlapping contributions. Review Bland-Stewart (2005) for other examples of AAE and GAE that should be taken into consideration when establishing therapy goals. One intervention strategy that has been recommended is the use of noncontrastive targets (those shared by both dialects, e.g., GAE and AAE) *before* intervention with contrastive targets (those unique to each dialect) (Bland-Stewart, 2005; Stockman, 2010). It appears that "AA children with and those without impairment will both use the AAE and SAE[1] contrastive patterns that are typical of the dialect" (p. 31). Knowing that the child is having difficulty with the AAE features shared with GAE (noncontrastive targets) will allow you to better distinguish the child with a difference versus the child with a disorder (Seymour, Bland-Stewart, & Green, 1998).

There are several advantages to the use of AAE. Children who use extensive amounts of AAE have been reported to have complex syntax (Craig & Washington, 1994). If this level of dense use of AAE is not understood by the clinician, the child may be diagnosed with a disorder and placed in special education services inappropriately. We discussed this issue of overidentification or underidentification for special education services earlier in the chapter. There also could be underidentification of AAE speakers for services when a thorough evaluation is not completed and the children are passed on as "just" having AAE speech. It is important to reiterate Stockman's (2010) statement that when the listener cannot understand the speaker, he or she will conclude that he or she is a poor speaker, or will go as far as thinking the person has disordered speech. Yet, studies have found that when African American children use AAE in narrative storytelling, their stories are richer (Godley et al., 2006; Schachter & Craig, 2013). Students who used more AAE in oral language tasks had better literacy skills (Connor & Craig, 2006). Including and encouraging the use of AAE in therapy appears to be a positive intervention strategy. Similar to how bilingual students can have a disorder in their first language, African American students who are using AAE could have a disorder in AAE as well as in GAE. Viewing the use of AAE as an advantage rather than a disadvantage will allow clinicians to rethink the use of AAE and possibly reset a long-held bias of AAE as something to eradicate. As with all children, it is important to make a connection between the "home" language (AAE) and the "school" language (GAE) in order to provide services that are responsive to the needs of the students.

Identify Intervention Strategies for CLD Persons Who Stutter

As noted in Chapter 10, it is important to know if there is a true stuttering disorder (Manning, 2017) or if the dysfluency of a linguistically diverse student, patient, or client is due to the transition when learning two languages. Once this is resolved, the treatment will focus on the individual with a true stuttering problem in his or her first or second language or both. In terms of cultural and linguistic background, the typical intervention strategies used to correct dysfluent speech should be the same for CLD individuals. However, a large portion of the intervention for dysfluency is working with the "person" and his or her social adjustment. It is this area that we discuss as it relates

---

[1]SAE refers to standard American English. It is used here because it was used in a direct quote. In this text, we are using GAE, general American English, to avoid the implication that SAE is some *standard* to which other language variations should be measured.

to culturally responsive practice. The first area to address is the attitudes toward stuttering by different cultural groups. To avoid stereotyping that a person within a cultural group will behave in a certain way, we say that there may be differences among diverse groups; however, there are many within-group and across-group differences. Thus, it is hard to pinpoint the "beliefs" of one group. Depending on the cultural attitudes toward stuttering for the CLD client, it may be a personal issue that you will need to address in therapy (Daniels, 2008; Ogundare, Ambrose, & Franca, 2011; Tellis & Tellis, 2003). Generally speaking, some of the cultural beliefs that have been reported about stuttering include that it is God's will, caused by something you ate, caused by "el ojo" the evil eye, caused from the baby being dropped at birth, or is the fault of the parent who is being punished for a transgression (Ogundare, 2012). Beliefs will also vary depending on whether the person with stuttering (PWS) is a long-term resident of the United States or a recent immigrant. It is good to look back at the process of cultural humility and cultural reciprocity as a best practice when learning cultural information of this type. If the attitudes about stuttering are upsetting to the PWS, then it is something that should be discussed in therapy as part of your counseling; otherwise, it will not be of consequence in the specific intervention protocol. However, if there are deep-rooted problems for your client with the attitudes of others toward (cultural or social) or the act of stuttering itself, a referral to a trained mental health professional may be appropriate.

Generally, individuals who stutter are stigmatized for the behavior and suffer significant personal consequences (Langevin, 1997). In today's era of "political correctness," it is hoped that individuals with disabilities are not outwardly shamed and that there is more than a modicum of acceptance of diversity. Refer to Chapter 2 where we alluded to the comments of the candidate for president in 2016 who mocked both a disabled individual and the entire Latin@/Hispanic population. It appears that there is still a long way to go in both of these areas. This is especially important for diverse individuals who stutter, as they carry a dual burden. Several years ago, the Public Opinion Survey of Human Attributes (POSHA-E) was developed and distributed worldwide (St. Louis, 2005). The overall finding regarding stuttering was that individuals would not want to have this condition, but almost all felt that persons who stutter could lead normal lives.

Because stuttering therapy involves quite a large degree of counseling, general counseling techniques used in speech, language, and hearing sciences would also be helpful for the diverse patients (Flasher & Fogel, 2011; Salas-Provance, 2011). Some of this counseling will be directed to the ethnically and linguistically diverse parents of young children who stutter. Early intervention is readily used to achieve the best outcomes in these children (Kellman & Nicholas, 2008; Yairi & Ambrose, 2005). Family-centered intervention is culturally appropriate intervention. An issue that is critical to address for early treatment of diverse children who stutter is the family's access to services. This is especially important for the large number of racially and ethnically diverse children who live in poverty or at low-socioeconomic levels. This one factor places them at a great disadvantage for their ability to receive the appropriate treatments that can make an effect on the long-term outcome of their lives. Because group therapy is used often with children (Stewart & Turnball, 2007), the involvement of parents from racial and ethnic backgrounds is appropriate. However, this could present a challenge due to the reported desire, by some ethnic groups, to keep family matters in the family, not to be shared with others outside the home (Boyle & Andrews, 1989; Campinha-Bacote, 1998). The psychoanalysis aspect of stuttering therapy may deter some parents whose cultural beliefs may include to reject the idea of mental illness in their family (Snowden, 2007), or at least the refusal to talk about it to others. Hunt and colleagues (2014) in an extensive study on beliefs of mental health by various racial groups showed little differences by race and ethnicity in terms of their health care beliefs. These findings contradict other research (see Chapter 6 for references by Glanz et al., 2006; Harris et al., 2012; Kleinman, 1978; Kleinman & Benson, 2006; Kleinman, Eisenberg, & Good, 2006). Yet, there are many anecdotal stories that support the existence of differences in beliefs across CLD persons.

Of course, CLD families will want what is best for their children and family members. However, opening up about their feelings regarding their child's stuttering to strangers in a group may be difficult. This can also occur in adults from CLD groups. However, the collaborative and consultative model of therapy (Zebrowski & Cilek, 1997) is similar to how many ethnic families live their lives within their extended families. Communication in groups is not unfamiliar to them. They want to talk with teachers and clinicians about how to best support their children. Many hold educational and medical professionals in high regard, especially when it comes to their children, and will follow their advice. However, for school-aged children, it may be difficult to have parents who work long schedules with few days off to meet with the clinician and participate in therapy. This is a challenge for all parents in this situation, not only those from CLD backgrounds. It will take creative arrangements to include parents in school therapy sessions. Before-school or after school sessions could be options for all working parents. There are many opportunities through electronic mediums, such as Face Time or Skype, which could be used with families whose transportation, work, or family commitments and restrictions make it a challenge to meet with the clinician and participate in therapy.

Adults may also be involved in group therapy, but in addition, they will be focused on modifying the stuttering itself. A culturally responsive practice would attempt to alleviate the power differential in these sessions where the responsibility of the session is transferred to the client as to not impose the clinician's beliefs on the diverse client. A relationship or reciprocity model (Buriski & Haglund, 2001) may be more typical of the familial structure of the diverse client. It is important to consider that the CLD person may be more inclined to silence as a cultural norm and feel more comfortable speaking little and being more reflective, working through the dysfluencies at a different pace. It has been reported that SLPs, because their job is to talk, tend to overexplain and fill in the silence. There may be a "letting go" of the client that may be needed as a cultural alternative (Ezrati-Vinacour & Weinstein, 2011). Clinicians are taught to anticipate how a student or client might feel, or to "know what is going on in our clients' minds" (p. 181). It is important to be sensitive and attentive to our clients, but when it comes to a client or student who has a cultural or linguistic background different from our own, we may not "know" what they are thinking. We may need to try a new path with them in therapy with them as the cultural guide. Consider the iceberg analogy from Chapter 2. The stuttering we hear is only the tip of the iceberg. It is well known that stuttering is a multidimensional problem (Guitar, 2014), but with the addition of cultural and language variations, stuttering takes on yet another dimension, which requires the SLP to learn about the person who stutters.

Another area of intervention for adults who stutter is cognitive therapy (Yairi & Seery, 2011). Here the patient is involved in self-analysis in order to change and improve their lives and thus decrease their dysfluent behavior. Rather than think about stuttering negatively, they become in control of their behaviors, especially when they are anxious and experience the stuttering events. It is essentially a cognitive reframing (Fry & Cook, 2004). This type of treatment requires a great deal of trust between the clinician and the client. The area of client-caregiver trust has been difficult for many diverse clients based on past experiences where they have been marginalized or exploited as a group (Clark, 1998; Martin, 2012). If you are engaging in this type of intervention with the diverse client, it is important to consider that there may be some resistance or at least trepidation by the client initially, until the trusting relationship is established.

Stuttering is a debilitating disorder for both young children and adults, but effective treatment allows them to manage the disorder and live good lives. There may be cultural aspects that affect the treatment. Take the time to learn the cultural background for the student or client and identify any adjustments you may need to make in the therapy process. Be open to the opportunity to unlock a hidden cultural gem that may make the difference between success and failure of the intervention.

VOICE DISORDERS

Most intervention strategies used in voice disorders (Boone et al., 2013) are applicable to all students, patients, and clients no matter their cultural background. The manner in which these strategies are used, however, may have a cultural component. Many voice disorders are the result of vocal abuse and require voice therapy to improve vocal parameters such as pitch, quality, and loudness. Similar to what was discussed in the stuttering section, many of the strategies to improve the perceptual

symptoms of the voice disorder are universal. The clinician should use the best evidence-based practices available, and the ASHA portal (ASHA, n.d.h) is a good place to begin. For individuals with voice disorders, as with fluency disorders, there are many layers to the person that are represented below the tip of the iceberg that must be addressed to achieve the best outcomes.

Access to care remains a significant problem for individuals from diverse backgrounds who may be from low socioeconomic backgrounds. Therefore, there may be a limited number of patients in your voice caseloads from racial and ethnic groups in lower socioeconomic status (SES) levels. Children will receive services in schools, but more and more, children with voice disorders represent a small percentage of the school-based caseload (ASHA, 2014b). From 2004 to 2014 the percentage of SLPs treating students with voice or resonance disorders decreased from 32% to 22%. Many of the children with voice disorders who receive voice therapy will be attending private therapy. This type of therapy is out of reach for the majority of diverse students from low SES backgrounds. It is important to be cognizant of this health care disparity should there be an opportunity to assist either children or adults from low SES backgrounds with voice disorders.

As with all types of speech therapy, there may be gender roles to consider in terms of the client and patient relationship. This is more applicable to adults than to children, generally. If there is to be a therapeutic intervention where the individual is touched for demonstration purposes, such as laryngeal massage or breathing exercises, the gender and cultural roles should be respected. The best practice, again, is to ask. Dr. Salas-Provance observed a physician who was going to listen to a woman's heartbeat, ask her if he could move her "holy thing" aside so he could touch her skin with a stethoscope. He was very caring and gentle when he moved aside her scapular. A scapular is a necklace made of cloth with pictures of saints on the squares on the front and back end of the necklace. The importance of the scapular is that some believe that if you pass away with the scapular on your person, you will immediately rise to heaven. This is a strong belief held among some, and if the doctor would have touched or removed it without asking, it would have been a serious cultural misstep. In fact, it has been reported that Pope John Paul II requested that his scapular stay on his body during a surgical procedure (Edmisten, 2017).

Psychogenic voice disorders may require the clinician to address them from a cultural basis. A patient of Dr. Salas-Provance had a conversion dysphonia and was without voice except for an occasional whisper. This male adult was from a culture that valued machismo (e.g., cultural value on male virility and superiority) and all men in the family had been members of the police force. During the course of treatment, he revealed that he did not want to become a policeman but had gone through the police academy to please his father. He developed conversion dysphonia at the end of his schooling, thus placing him at a desk job, rather than the street, after graduation. It was a cultural journey with many complicated layers to manage. Although it is not possible to know every aspect of a culture, once you begin the therapy process, be attentive to the morsels of information that you receive about cultural values and traditions. Most individuals are proud of their racial and ethnic backgrounds and will talk about them. As we advised earlier, simply use ethnographic methods to seek information from clients or patients regarding any cultural aspects that you should consider in the therapy process. It is likely that this one piece of information will result in helpful information. Although the information may not come in the first session, it will come naturally and

willingly as you build the relationship and trust. Then, it is important to listen without judgment.

An important part of voice intervention is the opportunity to provide preventive care. Smoking is known to cause laryngeal cancer, yet cigarettes are advertised more often in stores in low SES areas and smoking is more prevalent, as well. See more information on this subject in Chapter 10 under voice assessment. An effort to educate families who may be vulnerable to voice disorders because of their lifestyle should be included as part of an outreach intervention protocol. Environmental pollutants, air quality, water quality, healthy sleeping patterns, and good nourishment, among others, are all important to vocal health. Some diverse groups may be challenged because of SES to achieve these good voice hygiene standards. Yet, there are individuals from all ethnic backgrounds who make poor choices in terms of aspects that may affect their vocal health. One of the most serious issues to address in terms of health care disparity is the reported high incidence of smoking in low SES groups (DeSantis, Naishadham, & Jemal, 2013). It is commonly known that the combination of smoking and alcohol leads to laryngeal cancer. The highest incidence of laryngeal cancer is found in African American males and White males. There may be cultural aspects to address when providing services to patients.

CLEFT LIP AND PALATE

We addressed many cultural aspects of cleft lip and palate in Chapter 10 on assessment. The majority of children with cleft lip and palate will have normal language development (Peterson-Falzone et al., 2010). However, should there be a CLD child with cleft palate with a language disorder, the disorder should be addressed as discussed earlier in this chapter. Therapy for the compensatory articulation errors associated with cleft lip and palate should be addressed using standard articulation protocols and additional strategies specific to cleft palate (Golding-Kushner, 2001; Peterson-Falzone et al., 2005). A child with English as a second language may have articulation errors specific to their language along with errors specific to the cleft palate. The cleft-related speech errors, such as compensatory articulations (e.g., glottal stops), depressurized consonants, and backing of sounds should be corrected following standard speech articulation protocols, which were discussed earlier in this chapter. The resonance issues related to cleft palate are universal in terms of air flows and air pressures. The appropriate surgical interventions and therapeutic protocols should be followed to remediate the resonance disorder in a CLD child with cleft palate (Kummer, 2014).

The incidence of cleft lip and palate has a strong cultural component. As discussed in Chapter 10, First Nation and Alaskan Natives having the highest incidence of cleft lip and palate. Should you have children from these ethnic groups in your caseload, appropriate counseling should be provided for the family about the genetic component of cleft lip and palate. A referral should be made to a geneticist, if needed.

The amount of speech therapy a CLD child is able to receive may be related to his or her SES. Many CLD children come from low SES backgrounds. This can limit their access to care as a result of cost for therapy and transportation, among other factors. It is important, however, for families to receive information about the value of team care and encouraged to seek services from a cleft palate team. They may need more support and guidance to access care from a cleft palate team. Team care is critical to ensure the best clinical outcomes for the child with cleft lip and palate. Team care is long-term comprehensive

care, which includes at the minimum, a SLP, surgeon, and orthodontist. All children should have the advantage of team treatment. Many times, families who do not access team care are just not aware of its availability.

Another aspect that is of concern for some diverse and/or low SES families is the lack of access to early intervention services. A child with cleft lip and palate will have lip surgery any time between 3 and 6 months of age in the United States, followed by palate surgery around 1 year of age. There is much work to do in that first year of life that is related to the speech, language, and hearing development of children with cleft lip and palate, but many parents do not access services in this first year for many reasons. For many families, the most important event in the first year of life is repair of the cleft lip if their child has a cleft lip and a cleft palate. Also, many families are not aware of the importance of this first year to the development of speech and language skills. They may find it confusing that a child who cannot talk would need speech and language intervention. Culturally determined child-rearing practices may dictate the amount of therapy a family feels is appropriate for their child. A concerted effort must be made to help all families understand the importance of early speech and language intervention during the first 12 months. Because these services with young children are conducted in the home, it is important to consider culturally responsive practices as described throughout this text. A conversation with parents from CLD backgrounds on their child-rearing practices and beliefs may be beneficial and help support your intervention goals.

In the first year of life, intervention services for the child with cleft lip and palate should focus on strategies for language stimulation, which predominantly involves the parent and child. In addition, the SLP should counsel the parents to focus on oral productions versus glottal productions due to the overuse of glottal stops in children with cleft palate. The remediation of any ear problems for children with cleft palate is critical to support speech. Children with cleft palate have been found to have a universal tendency toward middle ear disease, which may be accompanied with a conductive hearing loss in the first year of life (Jordan & Sidman, 2014; Stool & Randall, 1967). There are excellent resources on cleft lip and palate on ASHA's portal (ASHA, n.d.d) and ASHA's Special Interest Group 6 on Craniofacial and Velopharyngeal Disorders. The American Cleft Palate and Craniofacial Association (http://www.acpa-cpf.org/) and the Cleft Palate Foundation are excellent resources for both professionals and families.

CHAPTER SUMMARY

This chapter has described the culturally responsive intervention practices for children and adults. We took a broad view of culture and did not attempt to identify what each cultural group would do differently in each situation. Rather, we addressed practices that would cut across all cultures, keeping in mind that individuals from CLD backgrounds are highly represented in low SES levels. This economic disadvantage makes access to intervention difficult for many of these families and places them at a disadvantage in terms of their therapeutic outcomes. We considered specific and important factors for children who are developing speech in a bilingual environment. A dual language focus is paramount. To stop the use of the first language as the second language is developing is not advised, nor is it an appropriate culturally responsive practice. A child is capable of developing multiple languages well, even a child with a speech and language disorder. We reviewed important aspects for intervention with bilingual children and

bilingual adults with language disorders and the unique characteristics of these therapeutic procedures. We showed how speech sound disorders of bilingual children are treated with traditional articulation and phonological therapy protocols, keeping in mind that there may be influences of one sound system on the other for bilingual persons. The language variations of African American children who use African American English (AAE) are considered from an additive perspective in reference to Standard American English rather than a subtractive reference, as has often been done in the past. The rule-governed features of AAE are seen in many children, not only African American children. The SLP must be prepared to address these differences versus disorders issues. Finally, stuttering, voice disorders, and cleft palate have many therapeutic aspects that will remain constant regardless of the linguistic or cultural aspect of the student or client. However, there are many psychosocial aspects and access issues that must be addressed in all three of these speech disorders from a cultural perspective.

FURTHER READING

American Speech-Language-Hearing Association (ASHA). (2016). *Scope of practice in speech-language pathology.* Retrieved from http://www.asha.org/policy/SP2016-00343/

American Speech-Language-Hearing Association (ASHA). (2017a). *Accent modification.* Retrieved from http://www.asha.org/public/speech/development/accent-modification/

American Speech-Language-Hearing Association (ASHA). (2017b). *Cultural and linguistic competence.* Retrieved from http://www.asha.org/Practice/ethics/Cultural-and-Linguistic-Competence/

American Speech-Language-Hearing Association (ASHA). (2017d). *Evidence maps.* Retrieved from http://www.asha.org/Evidence-Maps/

REFERENCES

Al-Krenawi, A., & Graham, J. P. (2000). *Culturally sensitive social work practices with Arab clients in mental health settings.* National Association of Social Workers. Retrieved from http://www.socialworkers.org/pressroom/events/911/alkrenawi.asp

American Speech-Language-Hearing Association (ASHA). (n.d.a). *Aphasia.* Retrieved from http://www.asha.org/EvidenceMapLanding.aspx

American Speech-Language-Hearing Association (ASHA). (n.d.b). *Aphasia* [Practice portal]. Retrieved from http://www.asha.org/Practice-Portal/Clinical-Topics/Aphasia/

American Speech-Language-Hearing Association (ASHA). (n.d.c). *Bilingual service delivery* [Practice portal]. Retrieved from http://www.asha.org/Practice-Portal/Professional-Issues/Bilingual-Service-Delivery

American Speech-Language-Hearing Association (ASHA). (n.d.d). *Cleft lip and palate* [Practice portal]. Retrieved from http://www.asha.org/PRPSpecificTopic.aspx?folderid=8589942918&section=Treatment

American Speech-Language-Hearing Association (ASHA). (n.d.e). *Compendium of EBP guidelines and systematic reviews.* Retrieved from http://www.asha.org/Evidence-Maps/

American Speech-Language-Hearing Association (ASHA). (n.d.f). *Phonemic inventories across languages.* Retrieved from http://www.asha.org/practice/multicultural/Phono/

American Speech-Language-Hearing Association (ASHA). (n.d.g). *Speech sound disorders: Articulation and phonology* [Practice portal]. Retrieved from http://www.asha.org/PRPSpecificTopic.aspx?folderid=8589935321&section=Treatment

American Speech-Language-Hearing Association (ASHA). (n.d.h). *Voice disorders* [Practice portal]. Retrieved from http://www.asha.org/Practice-Portal/Clinical-Topics/Voice-Disorders/

American Speech-Language-Hearing Association (ASHA). (2014a). *Cultural competence* [Practice portal]. Retrieved from http://www.asha.org/Practice-Portal/Professional-Issues/Cultural-Competence/

American Speech-Language-Hearing Association (ASHA). (2014b). *Schools survey report: Caseload characteristics trends, 1995–2014.* Retrieved from http://www.asha.org

American Speech-Language-Hearing Association (ASHA). (2016). *Scope of practice in speech-language pathology.* Retrieved from http://www.asha.org/policy/SP2016-00343/

American Speech-Language-Hearing Association (ASHA). (2017a). *Accent modification.* Retrieved from http://www.asha.org/public/speech/development/accent-modification/

American Speech-Language-Hearing Association (ASHA). (2017b). *Cultural and linguistic competence.* Retrieved from http://www.asha.org/Practice/ethics/Cultural-and-Linguistic-Competence/

American Speech-Language-Hearing Association (ASHA). (2017c). *Demographic profile of ASHA members providing bilingual services: March 2017.* Retrieved from http://www.asha.org/uploadedFiles/Demographic-Profile-Bilingual-Spanish-Service-Members.pdf

Anderson, R. (2004). First language loss in Spanish-speaking children: Patterns of loss and implications for clinical practice. In B. Goldstein (Ed.), *Bilingual language development and disorders in Spanish-English speakers.* Baltimore, MD: Brookes.

Antshel, K. M. (2002). Integrating culture as a means of improving treatment adherence in the Latino population. *Psychology, Health, and Medicine, 7*(4), 435–449.

Artiles, A. J., Harry, B., Reschly, D. J., & Chinn, P. C. (2001). *Overidentification of students of color in special education* (pp. 1–11). Monarch Center, University of Illinois at Chicago.

Artiles, A. J., & Trent, S. C. (1994). Overrepresentation of minority students in special education: A continuing debate. *Journal of Special Education, 4*(27), 410–437.

Barnett, J. C., & Vornovitsky, M. S. (2016). *Current Population Reports, P60-257(RV), Health Insurance Coverage in the United States: 2015.* Washington, DC: U.S. Government Printing Office.

Bernthal, J., & Bankson, N. (Eds.). (1994). *Child phonology: Characteristics, assessment, and inter-*

vention with special populations. New York, NY: Thieme Medical.

Bernthal, J., Bankson, N. W., & Flipsen, P., Jr. (2013). *Articulation and phonological disorders.* New York, NY: Pearson Higher Education.

Blache, S. E., & Parsons, C. L. (1980). A linguistic approach to distinctive feature training. *Language, Speech, and Hearing Services in the Schools, 11,* 203–207.

Bland-Stewart, L. M. (2003). Phonetic inventories and phonological patterns of African-American two-year-olds. A preliminary investigation. *Communication Disorders Quarterly, 24*(3), 109–120.

Bland-Stewart, L. M. (2005). Difference or deficit in speakers of African American English? What everyone should know and do. *ASHA Leader, 10,* 6–31.

Bloom, D. R., McFarlane, S. C., vonBerg, S. L., & Zraick, R. I. (2014). *The voice and voice therapy.* Boston, MA: Pearson.

Boyle, J., & Andrews, M. (1989). *Transcultural concepts in nursing care.* Boston, MA: Scott Foresman.

Buirski, P., & Haglund, P. (2001). *Making sense together: The intersubjective approach to psychotherapy.* Northvale, NJ: Jason Aronson.

Byun, T. M., & Hitchcock, E. R. (2012). Investigating the use of traditional and spectral biofeedback approaches to intervention for /r/ misarticulation. *American Journal of Speech-Language Pathology, 21*(3), 207–221.

Campinha-Bacote, J. (1998). *The process of cultural competence in the delivery of healthcare services: A culturally competent model of care* (3rd ed.). Cincinnati, OH: Transcultural C.A.R.E. Associates.

Cárdenas-Hagan, E., Carlson, C. D., & Pollard-Durodola, S. D. (2007). The cross-linguistic transfer of early literacy skills: The role of initial L1 and L2 skills and language of instruction. *Language, Speech, and Hearing Services in Schools, 38*(3), 249.

Centeno, J. (2009). Issues and principles in service delivery to communicatively impaired minority bilingual adults in neurorehabilitation. *Seminars in Speech and Language, 30,* 139–152.

Centeno, J. G. (2005, March). Working with bilingual individuals with aphasia: The case of a Spanish–English bilingual client. American

Speech-Language-Hearing Association Division 14. *Perspectives on Communication Disorders and Sciences in Culturally and Linguistically Diverse Populations, 12,* 2–7.

Centeno, J. G., Ghazi-Saidi, L., & Ansaldo, A. I. (2017). Aphasia in multilingual populations. In I. Papathanasiou & P. Coppens (Eds.), *Aphasia and related neurogenic communication disorders* (2nd ed., pp. 331–350). Boston, MA: Jones and Bartlett.

Cirrin, F. M., & Gillam, R. B. (2008). Language intervention practices for school-age children with spoken language disorders: A systematic review. *Language, Speech, and Hearing Services in Schools, 39*(1), S110–S137.

Clark, P. A. (1998). A legacy of mistrust: African-Americans, the medical profession, and AIDS. *The Linacre Quarterly, 65*(1), Article 8. Retrieved from http://epublications.marquette.edu/lnq/vol65/iss1/8

Cole, L. (1980). *A developmental analysis of social dialect features in the spontaneous language of preschool black children* (Unpublished doctoral dissertation). Northwestern University, Evanston, IL.

Connor, C. M., & Craig, H. K. (2006). African American preschoolers' language, emergent literacy skills, and use of African American English: A complex relation. *Journal of Speech, Language, and Hearing Research, 49,* 771–792.

Costa, A., La Heij, W., & Navarrete, E. (2006). The dynamics of bilingual lexical access. *Bilingualism: Language and Cognition, 9*(2), 137–151.

Costa, A., Santesteban, M., & Ivanova, I. (2006). How do highly proficient bilinguals control their lexicalization process? Inhibitory and language-specific selection mechanisms are both functional. *Journal of Experimental Psychology: Learning, Memory, and Cognition, 32*(5), 1057–1074.

Craig, H. K. (2016). *African-American English and the achievement gap: The role of dialectal code switching.* New York, NY: Routledge.

Craig, H. K., & Washington, J. A. (1994). The complex syntax skills of poor, urban, African-American preschoolers at school entry. *Language, Speech, and Hearing Services in Schools, 25,* 181–190.

Cummins, J. (2005). *Teaching for cross-language transfer in dual language education: Possibilities and pitfalls.* Paper presented at the TESOL Symposium on Dual Language Education: Teaching and Learning Two Languages in the EFL Setting, Boğaziçi University, Istanbul, Turkey. Alexandria, VA: TESOL.

Dagenais, P. A. (1995). Electropalatography in the treatment of articulation/phonological disorders. *Journal of Communication Disorders, 28*(4), 303–329.

Damron, M. (2015). *Brain drain: A child's brain on poverty.* Poverty Fact Sheet #8. Institute for Research on Poverty, University of Wisconsin–Madison. Retrieved from http://www.irp.wisc.edu/faqs/faq3.htm

Daniels, D. (2008). Working with people who stutter of diverse cultural backgrounds: Some ideas to consider. *SIG 4 Perspectives on Fluency and Fluency Disorders, 18,* 95–100.

Darley, F. (1982). *Aphasia.* Philadelphia, PA: W.B. Saunders.

Darley, F. L., Aronson, A. E., & Brown, J. R. (1969). Differential diagnostic patterns of dysarthria. *Journal of Speech and Hearing Research, 12,* 246–269.

Davis, G. A. (2007). *Aphasiology: Disorders and clinical practice* (2nd ed.). Needham Heights, MA: Allyn & Bacon.

DeSantis, C., Naishadham, D., & Jemal, A. (2013). Cancer statistics for African-Americans. *Cancer Journal Clinics, 63*(3), 151–166.

Dickinson, D. K., McCabe, A., Clark-Chiarelli, N., & Wolf, A. (2004). Cross-language transfer of phonological awareness in low-income Spanish and English bilingual preschool children. *Applied Psycholinguistics, 25*(3), 323–347.

DiMatteo, M. R. (2004). Social support and patient adherence to medical treatment: A meta analysis. *Health Psychology, 23*(2), 207–218.

Dodd, B., Holm, A., Crosbie, S., & McCormack, P. (2005). Differential diagnosis of phonological disorders. In B. Dodd (Ed.), *Differential diagnosis and treatment of children with speech disorder* (pp. 44–70). London, UK: Whurr.

Dollaghan, C. S., Campbell, T. F., Paradise, J. L., Feldman, F. M., Janosky, J. E., Pitcarin, D. N., & Kurs-Lasky, M. (1999). Maternal edu-cation and measures of early speech and language, *Journal of Speech, Language, and Hearing Research, 42,* 1432–1443.

Durán, L. K., Hartzheim, D., Lund, E. M., Simonsmeier, V., & Kohlmeier, T. L. (2016). Bilingual interventions with young dual language learners: A research synthesis. *Language, Speech, and Hearing Services in Schools, 47*(4), 347–371.

Ebert, K. D., Kohnert, K., Pham, G., Rentmeester Disher, J., & Payesteh, B. (2014). Three treatments for bilingual children with primary language impairment: Examining cross-linguistic and cross-domain effects. *Journal of Speech, and Hearing Research, 57,* 172–186.

Ebert, K. D., Rentmeester-Disher, J., & Kohnert, K. (2012). Nonlinguistic cognitive treatment for bilingual children with primary language impairment. *Clinical Linguistics and Phonetics, 26,* 485–501.

Edmiston, K. (2017). Discover the secrets of the scapular. *Catholic Digest.* Retrieved from http://www.catholicdigest.com/articles/faith/heritage/2009/01-01/discover-the-secrets-of-the-scapular

Edmonds, L., & Kiran, S. (2006). Effect of semantic naming treatment on cross-linguistic generalization in bilingual aphasia. *Journal of Speech, Language, and Hearing Research, 49,* 729–748.

Ezrati-Vinacour, R., & Weinstein, N. (2009). A dialogue among various cultures and its manifestation in stuttering therapy. *Journal of Fluency Disorders, 36,* 174–185.

Fabbro, F. (2001). The bilingual brain: Bilingual aphasia. *Brain and Language, 79*(2), 2001–2010.

Fabiano-Smith, L., & Goldstein, B. A. (2010). Phonological acquisition in bilingual Spanish-English–speaking children. *Journal of Speech, Language, and Hearing Research, 53*(1), 160–178.

Faroqi-Shah, Y., Frymark, T., Mullen, R., & Wang, B. (2010). Effect of treatment for bilingual individuals with aphasia: A systematic review of the evidence. *Journal of Neurolinguistics, 23*(4), 319–341.

Flasher, L. V., & Fogle, P. T. (2011). *Counseling skills for speech-language pathologists and audiologists* (pp. 159–190). New York, NY: Delmar Cengage Learning.

Frattali, C., Bayles, K., Beeson, P., Kennedy, M. R. T., Wambaugh, J., & Yorkston, K. M. (2002). Development of evidence-based practice guidelines: Committee update. *Journal of Medical Speech-Language Pathology, 11*(3), ix–xviii.

Fredman, M. (2006). Recommendations for working with bilingual children—Prepared by the Multilingual Affairs Committee of IALP. *Folia Phoniatrica et Logopaedica, 58*, 458–464.

Freed, D. (2000). *Motor speech impairments: Diagnosis and treatment.* San Diego, CA: Singular.

Fry, J., & Cook, F. (2004). Using cognitive therapy in group-work with young adults. In A. Packmanm, A. Meltzer, & H. F. M. Peters (Eds). *Proceedings of the Fourth World Congress on Fluency Disorders, 2003: Theory, research and therapy in fluency disorders* (pp. 63–68). Njimegen, The Netherlands: University of Njimegen Press.

Gierut, J. A. (1989). Maximal opposition approach to phonological treatment. *Journal of Speech and Hearing Research, 54*, 9–19.

Gillam, S. L., & Gillam, R. B. (2006). Making evidence-based decisions about child language intervention in schools. *Language, Speech, and Hearing Services in Schools, 37*(4), 304–315.

Godley, A. J., Sweetland, J., Wheeler, R. S., Minnici, A., & Carpenter, B. D. (2006). Preparing teachers for dialectally diverse classrooms. *Educational Researcher, 35*(8), 30–37

Golding-Kushner, K. (2001). *Therapy techniques for cleft palate speech and related disorders.* San Diego, CA: Singular.

Goldstein, B., & Fabiano, L. (2007). Assessment and intervention for bilingual children with phonological disorders. *ASHA Leader, 12*, 6–31.

Goldstein, B., & Gildersleeve-Neumann, C. (2012). Phonological development and disorders. In B. Goldstein (Ed.), *Bilingual language development and disorders in Spanish-English speakers* (2nd ed., pp. 285–309). Baltimore, MD: Brookes.

Goral, M., Levy, E., & Kastl, R. (2010). Cross-language treatment generalization: A case of trilingual aphasia *Aphasiology, 24*(2), 170–187.

Goral, M., Rosas, J., Conner, P. S., Maul, K. K., & Obler, L. K. (2012). Effects of language proficiency and language of the environment on aphasia therapy in a multilingual. *Journal of Neurolinguistics, 25*(6), 538–551.

Green, D. W. (1998). Mental control of the bilingual lexico-semantic system. *Bilingualism: Language and Cognition, 1*, 67–81.

Guiberson, M. (2013). Bilingual myth-busters series language confusion in bilingual children. *SIG 14 Perspectives on Communication Disorders and Sciences in Culturally and Linguistically Diverse (CLD) Populations, 20*, 5–14

Guitar, B. (2014). *Stuttering: An integrated approach to its nature and its treatment* (4th ed.). Baltimore, MD: Lippincott Williams & Wilkins.

Gutierrez-Clellen, V. (1999). Language choice in intervention with bilingual children. *American Journal of Speech-Language Pathology, 8*, 291–301.

Hallowell, B., & Chapey, R. (2008). Introduction to language intervention strategies in adult aphasia. In R. Chapey (Ed.), *Language intervention strategies in aphasia and related neurogenic communication disorders* (5th ed., pp. 1–19). Philadelphia, PA: Lippincott Williams & Wilkins.

Harris, K. L., & Moran, M. J. (2006). Phonological features exhibited by children speaking African American English at three grade levels. *Communication Disorders Quarterly, 4*(27), 195–205.

Hegde, M. (1998). *A coursebook on aphasia and other neurogenic disorder* (2nd ed.). San Diego, CA: Singular.

Hibel, J., Farkas, G., & Morgan, P. (2010). Who is placed into special education? *Sociology of Education, 83*, 312–332.

Hodson, B. (2010). *Evaluating and enhancing children's phonological systems: Research and theory to practice.* Wichita, KS: PhonoComp.

Hoffe, O. (2003). The specificity of environmental influence: Socioeconomic status affects early vocabulary development via maternal speech. *Child Development, 74*, 1368–1378.

Holland, A., & Halper, A. (1996). Talking to individuals with aphasia: A challenge for the rehabilitation team. *Top Stroke Rehabilitation, 2*(4), 27–37.

Hua, Z., & Dodd, B. (2006). *Phonological development and disorders in children: A multilingual perspective.* Clevedon, UK: Multilingual Matters.

Hunt, J., Sullivan, G., Chavira, D. A., Stein, M. B., Craske, M. G., Golinelli, D., . . . Sherbourne, C. D. (2013). Race and beliefs about mental health treatment among anxious primary care patients. *Journal of Nervous Mental Disorders. 201*(3), 188–195.

Institute for Research on Poverty. (2015). *Who is poor?* Retrieved from http://www.irp.wisc.edu/faqs/faq3.htm

Jimenez, B. (1987). Acquisition of Spanish consonants in children aged 3 to 5 years, 7 months. *Language, Speech, and Hearing Services in Schools, 18*, 344–356.

Jordaan, H. (2008). Clinical intervention for bilingual children: An international survey. *Folia Phoniatrica et Logopaedica, 60*, 97–105.

Jordan, V. A., & Sidman, J. D. (2014). Hearing outcomes in children with cleft palate and referred newborn hearing screen. *Laryngoscope. 124*(9), E384–E388.

Kellman, E., & Nicholas, A. (2008). *Practical intervention for early childhood stammering.* Milton Keynes, UK: Speechmark.

Kiran, S., Sanberg, C., Gray, T., Ascensp, E., & Kester, E. (2003). Rehabilitation in bilingual aphasia: Evidence for within and between-language generalization. *American Journal of Speech, Language Pathology, 22*, S298–S309.

Kohnert, K. (2004). Cognitive and cognate-based treatments for bilingual aphasia: A case study. *Brain and Language, 91*, 294–302.

Kohnert, K. (2008). *Language disorders in bilingual children and adults.* San Diego, CA: Plural.

Kohnert, K. (2009). Cross-language generalization following treatment in bilingual speakers with aphasia: A review. *Seminars in Speech and Language, 30*, 174–186.

Kohnert, K., & Derr, A. (2012). Language intervention with bilingual children. In B. Goldstein (Ed.), *Bilingual language development and disorders in Spanish-English speakers.* Baltimore, MD: Brookes.

Kohnert, K., Yim, D., Nett, K., Fong Kan, P., & Duran, L. (2005) Intervention with linguistically diverse preschool children. *Language, Speech, and Hearing Services in Schools, 36*, 251–263.

Koskan, A., Friedman, D. B., Hifinger Messias, D. K., Brandt, H. M., & Waisemann, K. (2013). Sustainability of promotora initiatives: Program planners' perspectives. *Journal of Public Health Management Practices, 19*(5), E1–E9.

Kroll, J. F., van Hell, J. G., Tokowicz, N., & Green, D. W. (2010). The revised hierarchical model: A critical review and assessment. *Bilingualism, Language and Cognition, 13*(3), 373–381.

Kummer, A. W. (2014). *Cleft palate and craniofacial anomalies* (3rd ed.). Clifton Park, NY: Delmar.

Langevin, M. (1997). Peer teasing project. *Journal of Fluency Disorders, 22*, 96.

LaPointe, L. (Ed.). (1997). *Aphasia and related neurogenic language impairments* (2nd ed.). New York, NY: Thieme.

Levey, S., & Sola, J. (2013). Speech language pathology students' awareness of language differences versus language disorders. *Contemporary Issues in Communication Sciences and Disorders, 40*, 8–14.

Livingston, G., Minnushkin, S., & Cohn, D'Vera. (2008). *PEW Research Center. Hispanic trends: Hispanics and healthcare in the United States.* Retrieved from http://www.pewhispanic.org/2008/08/13/iv-sources-of-information-on-health-and-health-care/

Lorenzen, B., & Murray, L. L. (2008). Bilingual aphasia: A theoretical and clinical review. *American Journal of Speech-Language Pathology, 17*(3), 299–317.

Lowe, R. J. (1994). *Phonology, assessment and intervention applications in speech pathology.* Baltimore, MD: Williams and Wilkins.

Machado, A. (2014). *Why many Latinos dread going to the doctor: How cultural barriers can be more important than income.* Retrieved from https://www.theatlantic.com/health/archive/2014/05/why-many-latinos-dread-going-to-the-doctor/361547/

Manning, W. H. (2017). *Clinical decision-making in fluency disorders* (3rd ed.). Clifton Park, NY: Delmar.

Martin, S. (2012). Exploring discrimination in American health care system: Perceptions/experiences of older Iranian immigrants. *Journal of Cross-Cultural Gerontology, 27*(3), 291–304.

McLeod, S. (2007). *The international guide to speech acquisition.* San Diego, CA: Delmar Learning.

Melgar de González, M. (2007). *Cómo detectar al niño con problemas del habla* [How to detect child with speech problems]. Mexico City, Mexico: Trillas.

Merino, B. J. (1983). Language development in normal and handicapped Spanish speaking children. *Hispanic Journal of Behavioral Sciences, 5,* 379–400.

Merino, B. J. (1992). Acquisition of syntactic and phonological features in Spanish. In H. W. Langdon & L. R. Cheng (Eds.), *Hispanic children and adults with communication disorders: Assessment and intervention* (pp. 57–98). Gaithersburg, MD: Aspen.

Miertsch, B., Meisel, J. M., & Isel, F. (2009). Nontreated languages in aphasia therapy of polyglots benefit from improvement in the treated language. *Journal of Neurolinguistics, 22*(2), 135–150.

Miller, A. A. (2012). Language intervention in French–English bilingual aphasia: Evidence of limited therapy transfer. *Journal of Neurolinguistics, 25*(6), 588–614.

Morgan, P. L., Farkas, G., Hillemeier, M. M., & Maczuga, S. (2012). Are minority children disproportionately represented in early intervention and early childhood special education? *Education Research, 41*(9), 339–351.

Morgan, P. L., Farkas, G., Hillemeier, M. M., Mattison, R., Maczuga, S., Li, H., & Cook, M. (2015, June 1). Minorities are disproportionately underrepresented in special education: Longitudinal evidence across five disability conditions. *Educational Researcher.*

Morgan, P. L., Hammer Scheffner, C., Farkas, G., Hillemeier, M. M., Maczuga, S., Cook, M., & Morano, S. (2016). Who receives speech/language services in the U.S. by 5 years of age? *American Journal of Speech-Language Pathology, 25,* 183–199.

Nordehn, G., Meredith, A., & Bye, L. (2006). A preliminary investigation of barriers to achieving patient-centered communication with patients who have stroke-related communication disorders. *Top Stroke Rehabilitation, 12*(1), 69–77.

Ogundare, A. A. (2012). *Multicultural stuttering and treatment: A cross-cultural analysis.* Research Papers. Paper 301. Southern Illinois University, Carbondale, IL. Retrieved from http://opensiuc.lib.siu.edu/gs_rp/301

Ogundare, A., Ambrose, N., & Franca, M. C. (2011, November). *Multicultural influences and perceptions of stuttering and their appreciation in therapy.* Poster session presented at the annual meeting of the American Speech Hearing Association (ASHA), San Diego, CA.

Papathanasiou, I., & Coppens, P. (Eds.). (2017). *Aphasia and related neurogenic communication disorders* (2nd ed., pp. 331–350). Boston, MA: Jones and Bartlett.

Paradis, J., Genesee, F., & Crago, M. B. (2011). *Dual language development and disorders: A handbook on bilingualism and second language learning* (2nd ed.). Baltimore, MD: Brookes.

Paradis, J., & Navarro, S. (2003). Subject realization and crosslinguistic interference in the bilingual acquisition of Spanish and English: What is the role of the input? *Journal of Child Language, 30*(2), 371–393.

Peña, E., & Fiestas, C. (2009). Talking across cultures in early intervention: Finding common ground to meet children's communication needs. *Perspectives on Language, Learning, and Education, 16,* 79–85.

Peterson-Falzone, S., Hardin-Jones, M., & Karnell, M. (2010). *Cleft palate speech* (4th ed.). St. Louis, MO: Mosby.

Peterson-Falzone, S., Trost-Cardamone, J., Karnell, M., & Hardin-Jones, M. (2005). *The clinician's guide to treating cleft palate speech.* St. Louis, MO: Mosby.

Preston, J. L., Brick, N., & Landi, N. (2013). Ultrasound biofeedback treatment for persisting childhood apraxia of speech. *American Journal of Speech-Language Pathology, 22*(4), 627–643.

Prezas, R. F., & Hodson, B. W. (2010). The cycles phonological remediation approach. In A. L. Williams, S. McLeod, & R. J. McCauley (Eds.), *Interventions for speech sound disorders in children* (pp. 137–158). Baltimore, MD: Brookes.

Proctor, B. D., Semega, J. L., & Kollar, M. A. (2016). *U.S. Census Bureau, Current population reports, P60-256(RV), income and poverty in the United States: 2015.* Washington, DC: U.S. Government Printing Office.

Restrepo, M. A. (1998). Identifiers of predominantly Spanish-speaking children with language impairment. *Journal of Speech, Language, and Hearing Research, 41,* 1398–1411.

Restrepo, M. A., & Gutiérrez-Clellen, V. F. (2012). Grammatical impairments in Spanish-English bilingual children. In B. Goldstein (Ed.), *Bilingual language development and disorders in Spanish-English speakers* (2nd ed., pp. 213–232). Baltimore, MD: Brookes.

Salas-Provance, M. B. (2011). Counseling in a multicultural society: Implications for the field of speech-language pathology. In L. V. Flasher & P. T. Fogle (Ed.), *Counseling skills for speech-language pathologists and audiologists* (pp. 159–190). New York, NY: Delmar Cengage Learning.

Salas-Provance, M. B., Erickson, J., & Reed, J. (2002). Disabilities as viewed by four generations of one Hispanic family. *Journal of Speech, Language, and Hearing Disorders, 11,* 151–162.

Schachter, R. E., & Craig, H. K. (2013). Students' production of narrative and AAE features during an emergent literacy task. *Language, Speech, and Hearing Services in Schools, 44,* 227–238.

Seymour, H., Bland-Stewart, L., & Green, L. J. (1998). Difference versus deficit in child African English. *Language, Speech, and Hearing Services in Schools, 29,* 96–108.

Shriberg, L. D. (1980). An intervention procedure for children with persistent /r/ errors. *Language, Speech, and Hearing Services in Schools, 11*(2), 102–110.

Steele, S. C. (2014). Effects of morphological-based intervention on vocabulary learning in school-age children with language learning difficulties. *EBP Briefs, 9*(2), 1–7.

Stewart, T., & Turnball, J. (2007). *Working with dysfluent children.* Brackley, UK: Speechmark.

St. Louis, K. O. (2005). A global project to measure public attitudes about stuttering. *ASHA Leader, 10,* 12–23.

Stockman, I. J. (2010). A review of developmental and applied language research on African American children: From a deficit to difference perspective on dialect differences. *Language, Speech, and Hearing Services in Schools, 41,* 23–28.

Taylor-Goh, S. (Ed.). (2005). *Royal College of Speech and Language Therapists clinical guidelines: 5.3 School-aged children with speech, language and communication difficulties.* Bicester, UK: Speechmark.

Tellis, G., & Tellis, C. (2003). Multicultural issues in school settings. *Seminars in Speech and Language, 24,* 21–26.

U.S. Census Bureau. (2015). *Detailed languages spoken at home and ability so speak English for the populations 5 years and over: 2009–2013.* Retrieved from https://www.census.gov/data/tables/2013/demo/2009-2013-lang-tables.html

Van Riper, C. (1963). *Speech correction: Principles and methods* (4th ed.). Englewood Cliffs, NJ: Prentice-Hall.

Wickenden, M. (2013). Widening the SLP Lens: How can we improve the well-being of people with communication disabilities globally. *International Journal of Speech-Language Pathology, 15*(1), 14–20.

Yairi, E., & Amrose, N. G. (2005). *Early childhood stuttering—For clinicians by clinicians.* Austin, TX: Pro-Ed.

Yairi, E., & Seery, C. H. (2011). *Stuttering—Foundations and clinical applications.* Upper Saddle River, NJ: Pearson.

Yorkston, K., Beukelman, D. R., Strand, E., & Bell, K. (1999). *Management of motor speech disorders in children and adults.* Austin, TX: Pro-Ed.

Yorkston, K. M., Spencer, K., Duffy, J., Beukelman, D., Golper, L. A., & Miller, R. (2001). Evidence-based medicine and practice guidelines: Application to the field of speech-language pathology. *Journal of Medical Speech-Language Pathology, 9*(4), 243–256.

Youdelman, M., & Perkins, J. (2005). *Providing language services in small healthcare provider settings: Examples from the field. Field Report.* New York, NY: The Commonwealth Fund.

Yu, B. (2013). Issues in bilingualism and heritage language maintenance: Perspectives of minority-language mothers of children with autism spectrum disorders. *American Journal of Speech-Language Pathology, 22,* 10–24.

Zebrowski, P. M., & Cilek, T. (1997). Stuttering therapy in the elementary school setting: Guidelines for clinician-teacher collaborations. *Seminar in Speech and Language, 18,* 329–340.

12

Global Engagement, Sustainability, and Culturally Responsive Practices

This chapter focuses on the next logical step in culturally responsive practices, which is the ability to provide effective services locally to immigrants and refugees migrating from their home countries to the United States, and globally, if opportunities arise for speech-language pathologists (SLPs) and/or audiologists to travel and/or live and work abroad. When working outside of one's own country, it is imperative to engage in sustainable practices, in culturally and linguistically responsive ways. This is an important consideration in this increasingly interconnected world. It has been shown that connectivity provides a psycho-logical boost to individuals and groups of people, expanding learning across borders brings intellectual growth, and sharing of health education improves and extends lives. There are more people than ever looking for ways to connect globally, and they are receiving the benefits of these experiences (Wearing & McGee, 2013).

LEARNING OBJECTIVES

After reading, discussing and processing the information presented in this chapter, you will be able to demonstrate the following knowledge, skills, and attitudes:

1. Knowledge
   a. Be able to explain the varied reasons people move from their home country to other countries.
   b. Describe some of the U.S. immigration legislation.
   c. Explain the international conventions and goals.
2. Skills
   a. Identify the relationship between the international conventions, goals, and SLP and AUD services to individuals and groups with disabilities.
   b. Employ critical thinking.
   c. Employ dialectical thinking.
   d. Begin to implement your conceptual framework for culturally responsive practices.
3. Attitudes
   a. Demonstrate awareness of the importance of the international conventions and documents discussed in this chapter.
   b. Demonstrate awareness of the importance of cultural and global humility, self-reflection, cultural responsiveness, and sustainable practices.

KEY CONCEPTS

Key concepts addressed in this chapter are presented in Table 12–1.

MOVEMENT OF PEOPLE AROUND THE WORLD

You learned about globalization in Chapter 2, and that it has both positive and negative effects on countries and the people who reside in them. One of those consequences is the movement of people from one location or country to another. Two terms that are frequently used to refer to people moving from one place to another are *immigrants* and *refugees*. Immigrants are persons who choose to move from their home country to another, usually in search of additional opportunities for advancement (Martinez & Marquez, 2014; Sorrellis, 2016). The important part of this definition is that groups of people make a choice to move. Immigrants are voluntary migrants (Martinez & Marquez, 2014). Refugees are forcibly displaced in that they are fleeing

TABLE 12–1. Key Concepts

Globalization	Sustainable practice
Ethics	Reciprocity
Human rights	Immigrants
Refugees	Extreme poverty
Poverty rate	

Note. Poverty rate = ratio (number of times one value contains or is contained in another) of the number of people in a given age group whose income falls below the poverty line.

such issues as colonization[1] (United Nations, 2016), fear of starvation, human rights violations, natural disasters, religious persecution, or international wars (Delgado Wise, 2013; Martinez & Marquez, 2014; Sorrellis, 2016; United Nations Refugee Agency [UNHCR], 2017). Refugees are involuntary migrants.

To best understand current society in the United States, it is important to keep in mind that the United States is also a nation that established itself through the "subjugation" and genocide of the original inhabitants (First Nations people), and "prospered" using slave labor (Martin & Nakayama, 2012, p. 8). In the 15th, 16th, and 17th centuries, colonizers from Spain and Portugal conquered territory in the Americas (as well as in Asia and Africa). These colonizers, called *Conquistadors*, were warriors who were not part of an army but went to the Americas on their own accord in search of the rich resources (e.g., gold, slaves, sugar) in that region of the world (Elliott, 2002; Restall & Fernández-Armesto, 2012). Although they were not technically working for the King of Spain, they did have a "document being a license to invade and conquer" (Restall & Fernández-Armesto, 2012, p. 8). Well before the English, the Spaniards "reached the Appalachians, the Mississippi, the Grand Canyon and Great Plains . . . sailed along the East Coast as far as Bangor Main and up the Pacific Coast to California and as far as Oregon" (Schmid, 2013, p. 155). Their goal of expanding their wealth and empire brought them to territory that is now known as the southwest United States, specifically Arizona, California, New Mexico, and Texas (Kessell, 2003). During the 16th and 17th centuries, Spaniards, primarily from the southern regions of Spain, immigrated to

---

[1] There are still areas under colonial rule; specifically, there are 16 non-self-governing territories (NSGTs) where over 1.6 million people are still living. These NSGTs are Western Sahara, Anguilla, Bermuda, British Virgin Islands, Cayman Islands, Falkland Islands, Montserrat, Saint Helena, Turks and Caicos Islands, U.S. Virgin Islands, Gibraltar, American Samoa, French Polynesia, Guam, New Caledonia, Pitcairn, and Tokelau (United Nations, 2016).

the United States in search of farmland, and among these immigrants were Sephardic Jews and Iberian Moors (Schmid, 2013).

In the 1600s, people from England protesting the Church of England colonized what is now known as the east coast of the United States (Taylor & Foner, 2001). In 1787, the U.S. Constitution was written and then ratified in 1788 and became operationalized in 1789 (Channing & Joyce, 1993). By 1795, the United States had constructed a Naturalization Act to determine who would be/could be a citizen of the United States. There were requirements for being a citizen, but the act was only applicable to "free-born white persons," unless you were a person from a country that was at war with the United States (Gerber, 2011, pp. 19–20; Third Congress Session II[2]). In that case, you could not become a citizen, even if you were "free" and "white." In the 17th through 19th centuries, Africans were forcefully enslaved and brought to the U. S. and Caribbean.

Immigration has always been part of the history of the United States; it experienced constant immigration since its inception. In the 19th century, Irish, Germans, Dutch, Polish, people from Spain, and Italians immigrated to the United States with unequal responses from the people in the United States (Gerber, 2011). For example, the nativists (i.e., those opposed to immigration due to religious, cultural, or political differences of those immigrating into a country), contrasted the Irish who immigrated to the United States before the Great Famine in 1845 with those who immigrated to the United States after the famine. The Irish migrating during and after the Great Famine were characterized negatively (i.e., poor, not smart, and without skills) (Gerber, 2011), which was not a true characterization, of course, but one made from fear by those who opposed the traditions and reli-

gion (Catholicism) that the Irish brought with them to the land known now as the United States (Poxon, 2012). Germans who immigrated to the United States around this time, were being pushed toward the United States by civil unrest at home. They were opposed by the nativists in the United States because the Germans maintained their own culture and language through German language schools (Gonzalez, 2008). In addition to the Naturalization Act mentioned earlier, other legislation was implemented to regulate or discourage immigration. Such acts and events included the Chinese Exclusion Act of 1882, following the immigration of Chinese persons to work on the U.S. railroads in 1868. This act served to prevent Chinese persons from immigrating into the United States, and those who were already in the United States from becoming U.S. citizens (Soennichsen, 2011).

Regardless of why people came, come they did to the United States. Over the years, immigration has altered the demographic landscape of the United States because the diversity of immigrants has changed over the years (Martin & Nakayama, 2012). In the 1890s, significant numbers of immigrants from Europe came to the United States. Since the 1970s, immigrants have been arriving in the United States from Asia and Latin America (Zong & Batalova, 2017). In 2015, many immigrants to the United States were from Mexico (Table 12–2), and in 2016, there were approximately 84.3 million immigrants in the United States (Zong & Batalova, 2017). It is important to note here that current immigration does not match the numbers of European immigrants who came to the United States in the 1800s and 1900s (Martin & Nakayama, 2012).

Also, in the United States of late, there is the perception that there is an increase in Mexican immigrants in the United States. The "Mexican immigrant" is often a phrase that

---

[2]Third Congress Session II, ch. 19, 20, 1795. Retrieved from http://legisworks.org/sal/1/stats/STATUTE-1-Pg414a.pdf

TABLE 12–2. Top 10 Countries Immigrants Were From in 2015

Countries	Percent of immigrants this year (%)
Mexico	27
India	6
China	5
Philippines	5
El Salvador	3
Vietnam	3
Cuba	3
Dominican Republic	2
Korea	2
Guatemala	2
	58% of U.S. immigrant population in 2015

Source: Adapted from Zong and Batalova (2017).

is erroneously used to refer to all immigrants from Latin America, which would include people who have cultural backgrounds quite different from each other, such as persons from Cuba, Puerto Rico, and the Dominican Republic, as well as from Mexico. "Mexican immigrants" were vilified by a U.S. presidential candidate in 2015. A presidential candidate in the United States who won the presidential race in 2016 made the following statement about Mexican immigrants when he announced his candidacy, "When Mexico sends its people, they're not sending their best. . . . They're sending people that have lots of problems, and they're bringing those problems with us. They're bringing drugs. They're bringing crime. They're rapists. And some, I assume, are good people." (Ye He Lee, 2015) This was a blanket statement made about all Mexicans, which was a gross mischaracterization of this ethnic group and promoted mis-

conceptions of and negative perceptions about this group. It is dangerous to have a "single story" about any cultural, ethnic, or racialized group or nationality.

Read and reflect on the following summary of a TED Talk given in 2009 by Chimamanda Ngozi Adichie, a Nigerian novelist. The talk is called "*The Danger of a Single Story*" and can be heard at this link: https://www.ted.com/talks/chimamanda_adichie_the_danger_of_a_single_story. In fact, do not settle for reading the summary below—go to the link and hear her powerful message for yourselves.

Box 12–1

Chimamanda Ngozi Adichie begins the TED talk by telling the story of her life growing up in Nigeria. As a child, she heard from her mother over and again how difficult life was for the young man working in their home. Because Chimamanda only heard one story about his family's impoverishment and misfortunes, she was shocked to learn that the young man's brother had the ability to make beautifully woven baskets. She states,

> I was startled. It had not occurred to me that anybody in his family could actually make something. All I had heard about them was how poor they were, so that it had become impossible for me to see them as anything else but poor. Their poverty was my single story of them.

She then gives another example of her first year in the United States as a college student. Chimamanda's roommate wondered how she was able to speak English, did not believe Chimamanda could cook, and she asked Chimamanda if she (the roommate) could listen to Chimamanda's "tribal music." Chimamanda reports that her roommate was "very disappointed when I produced my tape of Mariah Carey." Chimamanda goes on to say that her roommate,

[F]elt sorry for me even before she saw me. Her default position toward me, as an African, was a kind of patronizing, well-meaning pity. My roommate had a single story of Africa: a single story of catastrophe. In this single story, there was no possibility of Africans being similar to her in any way, no possibility of feelings more complex than pity, no possibility of a connection as human equals.

What do you think about the "danger of a single story"? Do you have a single story about cultural, ethnic, or racial groups in your own country or in other countries? What is the danger of having a single story about a group or groups of people? A single story is what develops when the history, culture, and character of a people are not known and/or are misrepresented. We believe this is what happened when "Mexicans" and by proxy all immigrants from Latin America were disparaged in the press by a person wielding a great deal of power over some segments of the U.S. population. It is important to note here that Mexican immigration to the United States has decreased, and return migration—that is, movement from the United States back to Mexico—has increased between 2009 and 2014 (Pew Research Center, 2015).

The population of people from African countries has doubled in the United States every 10 years since 1970 (Pew Research Center, 2017). This population is largely from Nigeria, Ethiopia, Egypt, Ghana, and Kenya, although other African countries are represented (i.e., South Africa, Somalia, Morocco, Liberia, Cameroon, Sierra Leone, Cape Verde, Sudan, Eritrea, Democratic Republic of Congo [DRC], Tanzania, Senegal, Zimbabwe, Algeria, Togo, and Uganda) (Anderson, 2017). Refer to Figure 12–1.

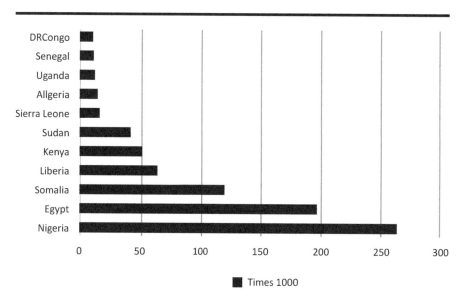

FIGURE 12–1. Number of immigrants to the United States from African countries. Adapted from Anderson, 2017. Illustrated by Severin Provance.

Understanding and being prepared to address international issues and a global population has been addressed in the American Speech-Language-Hearing Association (ASHA). As of 2017, ASHA has an International Issues Board that was started in the mid-2000s, a Special Interest Group (SIG 17) since 2010 that focuses on global issues in communication sciences, and a director of International Programs since 2011. The International Issues Board is charged with developing, monitoring, and recommending "Association policies and actions related to international issues" and facilitates strategic planning and collaborating with speech, language, and hearing organizations around the world (ASHA, 2017a). The coordinating committee for the SIG 17 focuses on promoting "research, networking, collaboration, education and mentoring for affiliates, students, and other service providers" locally and globally (ASHA, 2017b).

ASHA also collaborates with international organizations such as the Pan American Health Organization (PAHO) (ASHA, 2017a), interacts with the World Health Organization (WHO) around the Global Disability Action Plan (http://www.who.int/disabilities/actionplan/en/), the International Classification of Functioning, Disability, and Health (ICF)—you learned about this framework in Chapter 3—and the International Classification of Diseases (http://www.who.int/classifications/icd/en/). ASHA has been collaborating in PAHO priority countries that have indicated a need to address communication disorders. These countries include El Salvador, Guyana, Honduras, Paraguay, Cuba, and Ecuador. The goal of this collaboration is on sustainable growth, which is to "strengthen and build capacity" in these countries focused on speech, language, swallowing, and hear-

ing (ASHA, 2017c). Furthermore, ASHA is one of the founding organizations of the International Communication Project (ICP), along with Speech Pathology Australia (SPA), Speech-Language and Audiology Canada (SAC), Orthophonie et Audiologie Canada (OAC), New Zealand Speech-Language Therapists Association (NZSTA), Irish Association of Speech and Language Therapists (IASLT), and the Royal College of Speech Language Therapists (RCSLT) (ICP, 2014–2017). ICP was founded in 2014 and following is a quote about this initiative:

> The International Communication Project (ICP) is an advocate for those with communication disabilities, as well as their families, caregivers and communication professionals. The ICP highlights the importance of human communication and how communication disabilities significantly impact every aspect of life . . . the ICP is built on the premise that communication is vital to life; yet is largely ignored as a disability. (ICP, 2014–2017, http://www.internationalcommunica tionproject.com/about-icp/)

The authors of this text have both served as the coordinator for the ASHA SIG 17, Global Issues in Communication Sciences and Related Disorders. We have noted that since 2006, increasingly more information about SLPs and audiologists working in countries other than their home country, and about global and international issues pertaining to these professions have been presented at the annual ASHA conventions. A gross search of the ASHA Web page (http://www.asha.org) on April 10, 2017, using the word "international," and another search using the terms "global NOT aphasia,"[3] showed that there was a combined total of 2,679 presentations made during ASHA conventions since 2006 focusing

---

[3] There is a severe language disorder called *global aphasia*, which is composed of several comprehension and expressive language deficits. If we did not include "NOT aphasia" in this search, we would have acquired sources about global aphasia rather than international/global practice.

on international/global issues. Of these 2,679 presentations, none were made prior to 2006, approximately 175 were made in 2006, and 216 were presented in 2015. The most presentations were made in 2011 ($N = 402$), the year that the WHO and the World Bank Group (WBG) published the *World Report on Disabilities* (WHO, 2011). More about this report and other documents and policies is presented later in this chapter. Additionally, Hyter and colleagues (Hyter, Roman, Staley, & McPherson, 2017) recently published an article proposing competencies for effective global engagement.

There are greater opportunities now, than ever before, for a SLP or audiologist to travel abroad and provide services to individuals, families, and communities with communication impairments. The professions of speech-language pathology and audiology can be found across the world on every continent. Dr. Yvette Hyter has worked in Senegal, a country located in West Africa, every summer since the year 2002. She has engaged in collaborative research with professors and SLPs located in Senegal, and had the opportunity to guest lecture about African American English in classes at the national university. Dr. Hyter provides services using cultural reciprocity and a consultation model to a school educating children who are Deaf, Hard of Hearing, and who have language and speech impairments, using the conceptual framework described in Chapter 3 of this text (Hyter, 2014). Much of these collaborations have focused on phonological and literacy development, as well as classroom-based literacy interventions. Additionally, Dr. Hyter co-teaches a study abroad course in Senegal with a professor from special education and another with specialization in political economy and the African Diaspora. This study abroad course is interdisciplinary and focuses on the consequences of globalization on systems, including health, linguistic, educational, political, and ecological systems. She has written more about this course in the ASHA *SIG 17 Perspectives* (Hyter, 2012).

Dr. Marlene Salas-Provance has served as a member of an international medical team that performs surgery for cleft lip and palate around the world since 2004. She has worked with in-country SLPs in China, the Philippines, El Salvador, Venezuela, the Dominican Republic, and for the past 10 years, in Peru. In these countries, she has made professional presentations to medical and professional staff either in Spanish or working with an interpreter in China. She has facilitated community connections to continue the work of the medical team. Her work has been focused in Lima, Peru, since 2007 where she has developed professional relationships. She is involved in the training of medical professionals (ENT physicians/SLPs) to conduct endoscopic studies, radiologists and SLPs preparing the speech protocol for patients to complete videofluoroscopic examinations, constructing speech bulbs with the orthodontist, identifying appropriate feeding methods and bottles for babies with cleft palate, and working with parents and SLPs regarding speech therapy protocols and home therapy. In addition, Dr. Salas-Provance has provided opportunities for graduate students in speech-language pathology to have an international clinical experience in the Lima clinic. There are now two Peruvian SLPs and an orthodontist who follow all cases and provide continuation of services. Dr. Salas-Provance and two of her medical colleagues partnered on an article of their experience in Lima, Peru (Salas-Provance, Escobedo, & Marchino, 2014). Beyond Drs. Hyter and Salas-Provance, there are many SLPs and audiologists working outside of their home countries.

As of December 2016, ASHA had 504 international affiliates from 60 different countries, resulting in 36 more affiliates than were reported in 2015 (ASHA, 2016). International affiliates are ASHA members but live and work in other countries. These members are not necessarily U.S. citizens, but they could be, and they are also citizens of other countries.

It is commendable that there is so much interest in speech, language, and hearing sciences in providing services outside of one's home country. The models of international engagement exhibited by both Hyter and Salas-Provance are only two of the myriad ways that one can engage globally. All of us are at different places on the culturally responsive and globally sustainable continuum as illustrated in Figure 12–2; that is, some of us are at the beginning stage of figuring out how to be culturally responsive, and others are at a different location on that continuum trying to determine how our interactions abroad can result in sustainable transformation. Still, there are those of us yet on another location on the continuum who are engaged in culturally responsive and globally sustainable prac-tice, while also continuing to engage in critical self-reflection.

Undoubtedly, you have heard about the "ugly American" phenomenon. These ugly behaviors occur when people from the United States show a lack of respect for cultural values and practices in other countries. For example, this disrespect might include such things as any or all of the following:

- wearing a spaghetti-strapped blouse without a bra when being invited to the home of a devout family that practices Islam, stating, "They know I'm not Muslim. It doesn't matter what I wear";
- sitting outside on the porch of a hotel in Europe singing so loud that your voice can be heard a block away;

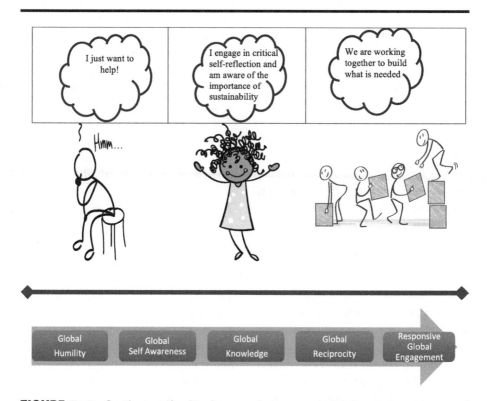

FIGURE 12–2. Continuum of cultural responsiveness and global engagement mapped onto the pathway to responsive global engagement. Based on Hyter, 2014. Dronathan/Siridhata/Trueffelpix/Shutterstock.com

- deciding that you "do not have to learn how to greet people in the local language, because I speak English," and because "everyone should know that language"; and
- believing that you know what people in a country need better than they know for themselves, as in, "I just want to go there to help those poor people, so they can learn how to be better."

Although we are sure being "ugly" or "disrespectful" is not anyone's intent, it can happen, particularly if we are not constantly implementing some of the tools and developing some of the skills being discussed in this chapter.

Review and reflect on the following case. While reading the case, think about what questions and/or concerns you would have if you were the person featured in the case in Box 12–2.

Box 12–2

[*You—Insert your name here*]
You are a graduate student at a university in the United States. You learned about a unique opportunity to travel to a country on one of the six habitable continents (Asia, Africa, North America, South America, Europe, or Australia[4]) during spring break. You learned that there were preschools, schools, hospitals, and clinics that were looking for people to volunteer their time and expertise. You remember talking with an acquaintance last year about her or his abroad experience, and she or he learned so much and was so excited about that opportunity. You, of course, are interested in gaining experience learning about another country, working abroad, and "helping out."

In groups of two or three persons, discuss the following questions. Be sure to incorporate the concepts, methods, and theories you have learned about throughout this text.

- Think about the frameworks presented in Chapter 3. What framework or frameworks might be useful in helping you be most prepared for working in the preschool, school, hospital, or clinic abroad?
- Think about the relationship between culture and language (Chapter 5) and hearing (Chapter 6). What might you need to know about these relationships before working in the preschool, school, hospital, or clinic abroad?
- Think about ethnographic practices discussed in Chapter 7. What ethnographic tools might be helpful to you while you are abroad?
- Think about the social structures that may affect the families of the children attending the preschool. What might you be prepared to consider when working with the children and families enrolled in the preschool, or with others with communication disabilities in schools, hospitals, or clinics? If you plan to engage in research, how can you implement research that is culturally responsive and sustainable (as discussed in Chapter 8)?
- Think about Chapter 9 (Working With Interpreters), Chapter 10 (Culturally Responsive Assessment), and Chapter 11 (Culturally Responsive Intervention). What skills should you possess to be effective in the preschool, school, hospital, or clinic?

In addition to being familiar with the information provided in this text so far, it is equally as important to be familiar with international goals, frameworks, and organizations.

---

[4]Note that Antarctica is not listed here because it is not currently inhabited or inhabitable.

INTERNATIONAL DOCUMENTS, GUIDELINES, AND POLICIES

Before you become globally engaged, it is important to be familiar with some international reports, documents, organizations, and policies that should be used to contribute to a framework for global engagement in speech, language, and hearing sciences. In this section, we discuss the UN Convention on the Rights of Persons with Disabilities, Millennium Development Goals (MDGs), Sustainable Development Goals (SDGs), the WHO Report on Disabilities (WHO, 2011), and the African Health Observatory (AHO). Another organization that we want to remind you of is the Pan American Health Organization (PAHO), mentioned earlier in the chapter.

UN Convention on the Rights of Persons With Disabilities

The United Nations is an international organization that was created in 1945 after World War II. Its members are 193 sovereign countries. Its role in the world is to "maintain international peace and security, protect human rights, provide humanitarian aid, promote sustainable development, and uphold international law" (United Nations, 2016). The UN *Convention on the Rights of Persons with Disabilities* (UN, 2006, 2016) adopted by the United Nations in 2006, is the first comprehensive human rights plan of the 21st century (United Nations, 2016). This document has 173 signatories and focuses on identifying the rights of persons with disabilities, and on implementing policies that facilitate these persons to gain and exercise these rights. It is composed of 50 articles; the titles are presented in Table 12–3, and the full text of the convention can be read here: https://www.un.org/development/desa/disabilities/convention-on-the-rights-of-persons-with-disabilities/convention-on-the-rights-of-persons-with-disabilities-2.html

Although the convention is signed by 173 nation-states, the convention was ratified (confirmed/approved) by all the signatories except for 14, of which one is the United States (United Nations, 2017). U.S. government officials who are in favor of the United States ratifying this convention believe that it would be meaningful in continuing to protect the rights and dignity of persons with disabilities. Those who oppose ratifying the convention state that it would give the United Nations jurisdiction over U.S. laws (PBS, 2014). Table 12–4 lists some of the protections in the treaty.

UN Millennium Development Goals (MDGs; 2000–2015)

The UN Millennium Development Goals (United Nations, 2015) were targeted by the United Nations between 2000 and 2015. There were eight goals that the 189 UN countries were to address over that 15-year period. These eight goals were to

1. eradicate extreme poverty and hunger;
2. achieve universal primary education;
3. promote gender equality and empower women;
4. reduce child mortality;
5. improve maternal health;
6. combat HIV/AIDS, malaria, and other diseases;
7. ensure environmental sustainability; and
8. develop a global partnership for development.

The UN Millennium Development Goals (MDGs) Report 2015 indicates that "with targeted interventions, sound strategies, adequate

TABLE 12–3. Titles of the Articles of the Convention on the Rights of Persons With Disabilities

Article Number	Article Title	Article Number	Article Title
Preamble		Article 26	Habilitation and rehabilitation
Article 1	Purpose	Article 27	Work and employment
Article 2	Definitions	Article 28	Adequate standard of living and social protection
Article 3	General principles		
Article 4	General obligations	Article 29	Participation in political and public life
Article 5	Equality and non-discrimination	Article 30	Participation in cultural life, recreation, leisure, and sport
Article 6	Women with disabilities		
Article 7	Children with disabilities	Article 31	Statistics and data collection
Article 8	Awareness-raising	Article 32	International cooperation
Article 9	Accessibility	Article 33	National implementation and monitoring
Article 10	Right to life		
Article 11	Situations of risk and humanitarian emergencies	Article 34	Committee on the Rights of Persons with Disabilities
Article 12	Equal recognition before the law	Article 35	Reports by States Parties
Article 13	Access to justice	Article 36	Consideration of reports
Article 14	Liberty and security of person	Article 37	Cooperation between States Parties and the Committee
Article 15	Freedom of torture or cruel, inhuman, or degrading treatment or punishment	Article 38	Relationship of the Committee with other bodies
Article 16	Freedom from exploitation, violence, and abuse	Article 39	Report of the Committee
		Article 40	Conference of States Parties
Article 17	Protecting the integrity of the person	Article 41	Depositary
		Article 42	Signature
Article 18	Liberty of movement and nationality	Article 43	Consent to be bound
Article 19	Living independently and being included in the community	Article 44	Regional integration organizations
Article 20	Personal mobility	Article 45	Entry into force
Article 21	Freedoms of expression and opinion, and access to information	Article 46	Reservations
		Article 47	Amendments
Article 22	Respect for privacy	Article 48	Denunciation
Article 23	Respect for home and the family	Article 49	Accessible format
Article 24	Education	Article 50	Authentic texts
Article 25	Health		

Source: From https://www.un.org/development/desa/disabilities/convention-on-the-rights-of-persons-with-disabilities/convention-on-the-rights-of-persons-with-disabilities-2.html, by Division for Social Policy and Development Disability, ©2017 United Nations. Reprinted with the permission of the United Nations.

TABLE 12–4. Some of the Protections in the UN Convention on the Rights of Persons With Disabilities

Article 4	• Develop and implement policies and laws securing the rights in the convention • Abolish laws, regulations, customs, and practices that discriminate against persons with disabilities
Article 6	• Ensure equal rights and advancement of women and girls with disabilities
Article 7	• Protect children with disabilities
Article 8	• Improve the situation of persons with disabilities by combating stereotypes and prejudices and promote awareness of the capabilities of persons with disabilities
Article 10	• Guarantee that persons with disabilities enjoy their right to life equally with others

Source: Based on United Nations (n.d.). *The convention in brief.*

resources, and political will, even the poorest countries can make dramatic and unprecedented progress" (p. 4). Table 12–5 shows the MDGs and the progress made as of 2015. Unfortunately, persons with disabilities were not included in the MDGs (International Disability and Development Consortium [IDDC], 2015).

Although there has been a great deal of success with the MDGs, the poorest countries and most vulnerable populations are still not having their needs met (United Nations, 2015, p. 8). Specifically, gender inequality persists, large economic disparities between rural and urban households exist, climate change and environmental degradation negatively affect impoverished persons the most, conflicts and war have significant negative impacts on development, and impoverishment endures. Specifically, the United Nations (2015) reports that "about 800 million people still live in extreme poverty (i.e., living on less than $1.25 per day) and suffer from hunger. Over 160 million children under age five have inadequate height for their age due to insufficient food" (p. 8). At the end of 2015, the UN

countries developed and implemented Sustainable Development Goals (SDGs). These goals, designed to build on the successes of the MDGs, are discussed in the next section.

UN Sustainable Development Goals (2015–2030)

As of 2015, the United Nations developed the SDGs, which build on the success of the MDGs and are composed of 17 transformative goals to be achieved by 2030. These goals were adopted by 193 member states of the United Nations at the UN Summit in September 2015 (United Nations, 2016). Sustainable development refers to meeting the needs of all people in ways that are long-standing, that include economic growth, social inclusion, environmental protection, and integrated ecosystems in ways that are equitable (Sachs, 2015). Also, Sachs stresses that sustainable development occurs when, "economic progress is widespread; extreme poverty is eliminated; social trust is encouraged through policies that strengthen the community; and the environ-

TABLE 12–5. Outcome of the Millennium Development Goal, 2015

Millennium Development Goal	2015 Outcome
Goal 1: Eradicate extreme poverty and hunger	Global number of people living in extreme poverty has declined by more than half; the proportion of undernourished people in the developing regions has fallen by almost half since 1990 (p. 4)
Goal 2: Achieve universal primary education	Primary school net enrollment rate in the developing regions has reached 91% in 2015, up from 83% in 2000; literacy rate has increased globally from 83% to 91%; and the gender gap has narrowed (p. 4)
Goal 3: Promote gender equality and empower women	Gender disparity in primary, secondary, and tertiary education has been eliminated in developing regions; women have gained parliamentary representation in nearly 90% of the 174 countries (p. 5)
Goal 4: Reduce child mortality	The number of deaths of children under the age of 5 has reduced from 12.7 to 6 million globally (p. 5)
Goal 5: Improve maternal health	Global maternal mortality ratio (deaths per 100,000 live births) has declined by 45% worldwide; use of contraceptives among married women increased from 55% in 1990 to 64% in 2015 (p. 6)
Goal 6: Combat HIV/AIDS, malaria, and other diseases	Global antiretroviral therapy treatment has increased from 0.8 million in 2003 to 13.6 million in 2014 (p. 6)
Goal 7: Ensure environmental sustainability	1.9 billion more people have gained access to piped drinking water, an increase from 2.3 billion in 1990 to 4.2 billion in 2015
Goal 8: Develop a global partnership for development	Assistance from developed countries increased by 66% between 2000 and 2014, reaching $135.2 billion

Source: Based on United Nations (2015).

ment is protected from human-induced degradation" (p. 3). In short, sustainability is a set of goals to which all of us in the world should aspire. The SDGs are depicted in Figure 12–3.

The International Disability Development Consortium has determined that persons with disabilities are explicitly referenced in six SDGs (i.e., 4, 6, 7, 8, 10, and 11) (IDDC, 2015), and that 13 of the SDGs are particularly related to persons with disabilities. Further, IDDC has indicated the need for disaggregated data for persons with and without disabilities. The IDDC provide some guidance as to what achieving the SDGs will look like for persons with disabilities:

- SDG Goal 1: No poverty
  - This goal will be achieved for persons with disabilities when "all are lifted out of extreme poverty, empowered, active contributors to society and enjoy equal rights" (p. 42)

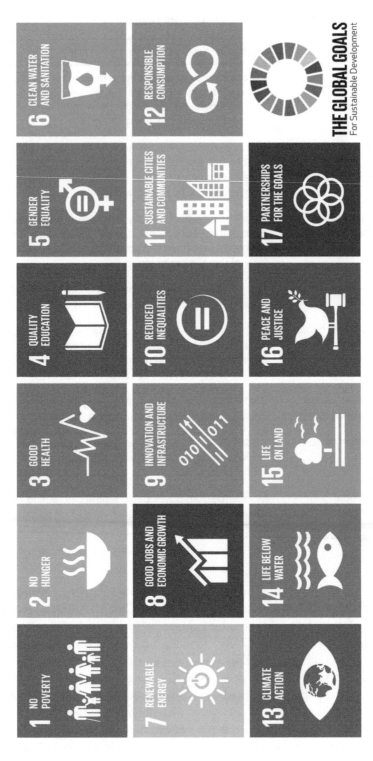

FIGURE 12–3. Sustainable development goals. Reprinted with permission from United Nations, 2017. Sustainable development goals kick off start to new year. Retrieved from http://www.un.org/sustainabledevelopment/blog/2015/12/sustainable-development-goals-kick-off-with-start-of-new-year/

- SDG Goal 2: Zero Hunger
  - □ Food security is realized for persons with disabilities everywhere (p. 44)
- SDG Goal 3: Good Health and Well-being
  - □ Access to universal health coverage and health care services is realized including for health costs related to disability (p. 46)
- SDG Goal 4: Quality and Inclusive Education
  - □ Inclusive, accessible, and quality education for children and persons with disabilities is realized at all levels of education, leading to relevant and effective learning outcomes (p. 48)
- SDG Goal 5: Gender Equality
  - □ End violence and discrimination toward girls and women with disabilities or toward women with children with disabilities, to ensure that both are not excluded from society (p. 50)
- SDG Goal 6: Clean Water and Sanitation
  - □ Access to safe drinking water and sanitation is provided
- SDG Goal 7: Energy
  - □ Households with persons with disabilities have access to electricity (p. 54)
- SDG Goal 8: Employment
  - □ The expansion of antidiscrimination provisions in labor and labor-related laws
  - □ The realization for reasonable accommodation and creating more inclusive mainstream initiatives to promote full and productive employment for persons with disabilities
  - □ Access to training and vocational education courses
  - □ Access to bank loans and micro-finances to start-up businesses (p. 56)
- SDG Goal 9: Industry, Innovation, and Infrastructure
  - □ Realize access to credit and establish enabling public policy environments to enhance possibilities for persons with disabilities

- □ Ensure that built, transport, and communications infrastructure are inclusive and accessible to persons with disabilities
- □ Provide increased access to public services to promote full and equal inclusion into society through information and communication technologies for persons with disabilities (p. 58)
- SDG Goal 10: Reduced Inequalities
  - □ Participate equally in political activities
  - □ All national laws and policies are disability inclusive and seek to eliminate discrimination and provide for reasonable accommodation
  - □ Have equal access to all social, cultural, economic, and political opportunities and that can access all services on equal basis with others
  - □ Achieve social protection and essential public services for persons with disabilities (p. 60)
- SIG Goal 11: Sustainable Cities and Communities
  - □ Cities and human settlements are livable, inclusive, accessible with universal design principles that can lead to a safer, more resilient world for all
  - □ Inclusion and meaningful participation of persons with disabilities in all disaster risk reduction and disaster risk management programs (p. 62)
- SDG Goal 13: Climate Change
  - □ Provision of food, water, and shelter security for people with disabilities and their families
  - □ Ensuring that people with disabilities are front and center in seeking to create awareness, understanding, and solutions (p. 64)
- SDG Goal 16: Peace, Justice, and Strong Institutions
  - □ Reduce all forms of violence
  - □ End abuse, exploitation, and trafficking
  - □ Promote the rule of law and ensure equal access to justice for all

□ Effective, accountable, and transparent institutions

□ Responsive, inclusive, participatory, and representative decision making

□ Legal identity for all

□ Public access to information

□ Nondiscriminatory laws (p. 66)

■ SDG Goal 17: Partnerships for the Goals

□ Enhancing the use of technology for persons with disabilities to ensure accessibility

□ Collect data, disaggregated by disability with regard to partnerships with organizations of people with disabilities (Disability Rights Funds, 2016)

□ Bringing together governments, the private sector, civil society, the UN system and other actors including the poorest and most vulnerable (p. 69)

Now that you have read through the SDGs and how they are designed to meet the needs of persons with disabilities, make a list of the other ways that individuals with communication disabilities can be better represented in the SDGs. Examine Table 12–6, which shows the relationship between the SDGs and the Convention on the Rights of Persons with Disabilities (CRPD; Global Disability Rights, 2017). On the left side of a piece of paper, write your list, and on the right side of the same paper, match up your list with the CRPD.

World Health Organization World Report on Disabilities (2011)

The WHO has been in existence since 1948 and includes staff that work in 150 different countries. The main function of the WHO is to work on health systems, communicable and noncommunicable diseases, promotion of health throughout the life span, emergency responses during a health crisis (such as the Ebola[5] pandemic in 2014), as well as other services with governments to "ensure the highest attainable level of health for all people" in the world (WHO, 2017a). In 2011, the WHO joined with the World Bank and developed a World Report on Disabilities (WHO, 2011). The goal of this report was to provide a comprehensive description of the state of disabilities in the world, and to make recommendations for national and international action (WHO, 2011, p. xxi).

You will remember from Chapter 3 that we introduced the WHO International Classification of Functioning, Disability and Health (WHO-ICF) (2001). This model put an emphasis on the impact of contextual factors (e.g., environmental and personal factors) on health functioning and outcomes. The ICF categorizes functioning in three domains, impairments (e.g., problems in body functions such as hearing loss), activity limitations (e.g., difficulty carrying out activities such as walking), and participation restrictions (e.g., employment discrimination). Disability refers to the interface between health conditions and contextual factors. In the World Report on Disability it is estimated that 15% of the world's population (about 1 billion people) has a disability; however, individuals with communication disabilities (e.g., hearing loss, Deafness, and speech, language and literacy impairments) were significantly underrepresented in the data (Wylie, McAllister, Davidson, & Marshall, 2013).

In a special issue of the *International Journal of Speech-Language Pathology*, a series of articles was written about work in this profession in various countries, and SLPs were challenged to "take a broader view on communication disability" (Wylie et al., 2013, p. 1). Working across disciplines will be important

---

[5]See http://www.who.int/mediacentre/factsheets/fs103/en/ for more information on this disease.

TABLE 12–6. Relationship Between Sustainable Development Goals (SDGs) and Articles of the Convention on the Rights of Persons With Disabilities (CPRD)

Articles of the Convention on the Rights of Persons With Disabilities	Sustainable Development Goals
Article 1: Protect fundamental freedoms	16
Article 4: Representative decision making	10, 11, 16
Article 5: Equality and non-discrimination	1, 2, 4, 5, 6, 8, 9, 10, 11, 13, 16
Article 6: Women with disabilities	1, 2, 3, 4, 5, 6, 8, 9, 10, 11, 13, 16
Article 7: Children with disabilities	1, 2, 3, 4, 5, 6, 9, 10, 11, 13, 16
Article 8: Awareness-raising	5, 10
Article 9: Accessibility	1, 2, 3, 4, 5, 6, 7, 8, 9, 10, 11, 13, 16, 17
Article 10: Right to life	1, 3, 16
Article 11: Risk and humanitarian emergencies	1, 3, 6, 10, 11, 13
Article 12: Equal recognition before the law	1, 2, 5, 8, 9, 16
Article 13: Access to justice	16
Article 14: Liberty and security of the person	16
Article 15: Freedom from torture	16
Article 16: Freedom from exploitation, violence and abuse	4, 5, 8, 10, 11, 16
Article 18: Liberty of movement and nationality	16
Article 20: Personal mobility	9, 11
Article 21: Access to information and communication	5, 9, 17
Article 23: Respect for home and the family	3, 5
Article 24: Inclusive education	4
Article 25: Accessible health	3, 5
Article 27: Work and employment	4, 8, 9
Article 28: Adequate standard of living and social protection	1, 2, 5, 6, 7, 10, 11
Article 29: Participation in political and public life	5
Article 31: Statistics and data collection	1, 2, 3, 4, 5, 6, 7, 8, 9, 10, 11, 13, 16, 17
Article 32: International cooperation	1, 2, 3, 4, 6, 7, 9, 10, 11, 13, 16, 17

continues

TABLE 12–6. *continued*

Sustainable Development Goals	Articles of the Convention on the Rights of Persons with Disabilities
1. End poverty	5, 6, 7, 9, 10, 11, 12, 28, 31, 32
2. Zero hunger	5, 6, 7, 9, 12, 28, 31, 32
3. Good health and well-being	6, 7, 9, 10, 11, 23, 25, 31, 32
4. Quality education	5, 6, 7, 9, 16, 24, 27, 31, 32
5. Gender equality	5, 6, 7, 8, 9, 12, 16, 21, 23, 25, 28, 29, 31
6. Clean water and sanitation	5, 6, 7, 9, 11, 28, 31, 32
7. Affordable and clean energy	9, 28, 31, 32
8. Decent work and economic growth	5, 6, 9, 12, 16, 27, 31
9. Industry innovation and infrastructure	5, 6, 7, 9, 13, 20, 21, 27, 31, 32
10. Reduced inequalities	4, 5, 6, 7, 8, 9, 11, 16, 28, 31, 32
11. Sustainable cities and communities	4, 5, 6, 7, 9, 11, 16, 20, 28, 31, 32
12. Responsible consumption and production	
13. Climate action	5, 6, 7, 9, 11, 31, 32
14. Life below water	
15. Life on land	
16. Peace, justice and strong institutions	1, 4, 5, 6, 7, 9, 10, 12, 13, 14, 15, 16, 18, 31, 32
17. Partnerships for the goals	9, 21, 31, 32

Source: Adapted from Global Disability Rights Now (2017), Disability, human rights, and sustainable development. Retrieved from http://www.globaldisabilityrightsnow.org/infographics/link-between-sustainable-development-goals-and-crpd

for providing services using a "broader view" or perspective. For example, in addition to collaborating with families, Dr. Hyter interacts with community members, economists, special education teachers and personnel, NGOs around services and meeting the needs of persons with communication disabilities. Dr. Salas-Provance interacts with physicians, orthodontists, and radiologists.

A "broader view" could be one that shifts from service provided to individuals to service provided to populations—a population-based focus (Barrett & Marshall, 2013; McAllister, Wylie, Davidson, & Marshall, 2013; Wickenden, 2013; Westby, 2013; Wylie et al. 2013). Population-focused care concentrates on groups of people (i.e., populations) rather than individuals, and includes understanding the effects of globalization in different parts of the world (Hyter, 2014), and includes the process of addressing social, political and environmental structures that may facilitate or hinder a population's health (Willis, Biggins, & Donovan, 2003). This strategy, which is widespread in the nursing literature, is typically not addressed in speech, language and hearing sciences curricula in the U. S. This approach to service requires knowledge about populations, understanding of common needs among populations, and an understanding of the demographic, political, economic, and health factors affecting the population (Lundy & Barton, 2016).

Another "broader view" is to work to make policies and services more equitable, and to develop culturally appropriate and relevant services for local populations in the Global South or majority world countries[6] (McAllister et al., 2013). In this way, populations being served should "be at the centre of defining needs, determining appropriate approaches and operating services" (McAllister et al., 2013, p. 120). These authors also strongly warn against importing service delivery models, materials, and procedures from the Global North or minority world countries into the Global South. Importing Global North practices to the Global South may not be culturally responsive and may not address population level needs. Also, this action may not support the participation of local actors in decision making, (McAllister et al., 2013), which makes the services less sustainable.

Below, we review how some have conceptualized population-based SLP services and how this "broader view" of SLP services might look in real life. Carol Westby (2013) describes the PRECEDE-PROCEED model (Green & Kreuter, 2004) in relationship to service to First Nations communities; Helen Barrett and Julie Marshall (2013) describe a program to develop resource capacity in Uganda for meeting needs of persons with communication disabilities; and Mary Wick-

enden (2013) suggests that SLPs should take a human rights approach to providing services to persons with disabilities.

PRECEDE-PROCEED Model

The PRECEDE/PROCEED model was developed as a model for developing, implementing, and evaluating public health programs (Green & Kreuter, 2004). Public health is designed to address structures that affect the health of the public, such as ecological, economic, political and systemic processes (Turnock, 2016). PRECEDE stands for Predisposing, Reinforcing, and Enabling Constructs in Educational Diagnosis and Evaluation, focusing on a pre-assessment of societal or community factors, such as "knowledge, attitudes, beliefs, personal preferences, and existing skills." (Westby, 2013, p. 97). This work is done before intervening. PROCEED refers to Policy, Regulatory, and Organizational Constructs in Educational and Environmental Development, focusing on identifying outcomes of the program implemented in a community or society. The PROCEED part of the model uses the findings of the PRECEDE part of the model to implement a culturally responsive intervention. Data for PRECEDE are collected using participatory action research, which is based on the premise that those who are affected by the research or intervention should be at the center of designing the questions, methods, and interpretations of the analyses. This type of data gathering is consistent with our suggestion to identify implicit information about cultural traditions, values, and goals when engaged in an ethnographic interview with families before an assessment (refer to

---

[6]Global South, and majority world countries are ways of referring to countries that have lower incomes, and where the majority of the people in the world live. The opposite of Global South is the Global North or minority world countries where a minority of the people in the world live, and countries that have high incomes such countries in North America, Europe, and some parts of Asia.

Chapters 7 and 10). Participatory action research primarily emerges from the theories within the "critical" tradition (e.g., Karl Marx, Antonio Gramsci, Paulo Freire, bell hooks, Patricia Collins), with premises underscoring the necessity of critical reflection for change to occur, the importance of collective engagement for addressing unequal power relations, and the significance of including perspectives that have typically been ignored, devalued, and erased (McIntyre, 2008, p. 3). Westby (2013) provides an example of how this method was used with First Nations communities in the U.S. This model has seven phases:

1. Using Participatory Action Research the SLPs and persons with communication disorders and their families and community members collaborate to develop a program. Westby (2013) goes into details about how that information can be gathered including community forums and focus groups (p. 98).
2. Identify the issues that might affect the desired outcomes, such as contextual factors discussed in the WHO-ICF (Westby, 2013, p. 98). Such issues could be the practice of tribal healing ceremonies or needing to receive the approval of tribal elders before taking part in Westernize intervention activities.
3. Identify administrative and policy factors, such as access to resources and allocation of funding, that can influence program implementation (Westby, 2013, p. 98). The policy issues need to be addressed prior to the implementation of an intervention.
4. Design and conduct the intervention based on what was learned in the first three phases.

5. Evaluate the process of the intervention; that is, determine if it is being conducted in the way it was planned.
6. Conduct an impact evaluation to determine if the intervention is having the effect that the community had hoped.
7. Evaluate the outcomes to determine if the desired result is being achieved (Westby, 2013).

As described, the PRECEDE-PROCEED model was designed to be used at the population/community level, and is one that has been used by SLPs. Next, we will describe a program designed to build resource capacity in Uganda for serving persons with communication disabilities as another real-life example of population-level care.

Building Resource Capacity in Uganda

In Uganda, SLP services have been available since 1986; however, those delivering the services were short-term volunteers working with non-governmental organizations (NGOs). Unfortunately, this type of service delivery is not sustainable (Barrett & Marshall, 2013). A degree program was developed in Uganda keeping in mind that there was a need for a "completely different skills set" than the skills taught in programs in the Global North (Barrett & Marshall, 2013, p. 49). SLPs in Uganda contend with issues that are not faced in the Global North such as "limited access to therapy materials and lack of supervision from experienced clinicians" (Barrett & Marshall, 2013, p. 49). SLPs in Uganda have been educated to not only treat impairments but to also transfer their knowledge to others such as, "community-based rehabilitation[7] workers,

---

[7] Community-based rehabilitation (CBR) was implemented by the WHO in the 1970s to increase access to care for individuals with disabilities. The current role of CBR has expanded to also consist of helping people with disabilities be included in society and have equal opportunities for education and advancement (WHO, 2017b).

teachers, nurses, doctors, and family members (Barrett & Marshall, 2013, p. 49).

A Human Rights Approach to SLP and Audiologist Services

Wickenden (2013) suggests that SLPs and audiologists should be focused on the ICF (WHO, 2001) and the UN Conventions on the Rights of People with Disabilities (United Nations, 2006), and a reconceptualized version of community-based rehabilitation to meet the needs of people with disabilities around the world. In the ICF, the multiple aspects of disability are addressed separately and together (p. 15). The UN Convention focuses on the rights of individuals with disabilities, which should be the rights and privileges available to all humans (Wickenden, 2013). Wickenden (2013) also discusses the reconceptualized model of CBR. As mentioned earlier, the focus of CBR is no longer only on ensuring persons with disabilities get access to care, but it also emphasizes the importance of people with disabilities being involved in decision making about their own care (WHO, 2010).

What is being addressed by these authors, Barrett and Marshall (2013), McAllister et al. (2013), Westby (2013), Wickenden (2013), and Wylie et al. (2013), is ethical and sustainable practice. Ethics refers to a set of principles that can be used to guide how one lives and how one engages in professional practices. Ethics is about behaving in ways that are right (differentiated from behaviors that are wrong) (Sekerka, 2016), as well as behaving in ways that are just and beneficial to society. Hoffmann-Holland (2009) suggests that human rights are a formalized version of ethics. He goes back to the *Universal Declaration of Human Rights* (United Nations, 1948), where Article 1 of that declaration states that "All human beings are born free and equal in dignity and rights. They are endowed with reason and conscience and should act towards one another in a spirit

of brotherhood." (United Nations, 1948, Article 1) These words are ever more important to remember now, as the world becomes "smaller." Being ethical requires critical and dialectical thinking and critical self-reflection to make sure that our standards of practice are based on sound principles.

Additionally, we should all be familiar with the standards of practice promoted by ASHA and other professional organizations such as the American Academy of Audiology (AAA) (AAA, 2017; ASHA, 2016). (You can find them at http://www.asha.org/Code-of-Ethics/ or http://www.audiology.org/publications-resources/document-library/code-ethics). The overall principles within the ASHA professional ethics standards are:

1. to provide services responsibly, to value the wellbeing of those being served, and to treat animals participating in research in a benevolent manner;
2. to gain and maintain the highest level of knowledge and skills;
3. to advocate for those with communication and swallowing concerns and provide accurate information about the professions of speech-language pathology and audiology; and
4. to uphold the dignity and autonomy of the professions, to maintain collaborative relationships within and across professions, and to work within the standards of the profession (ASHA, 2016).

These are the ethical principles of speech, language, and hearing sciences. To engage in ethical global engagement, we require additional principles or competencies that will address the ways to uphold the above ethical standards when serving populations outside of one's own country context.

One way to engage globally and ethically is to acquire practices that take the global context into considerations. Think about the Salas-Provance (2010) Hierarchy of Cultural

Knowledge model. To be most effective, it is essential to be open to learning from others and to continue to move along the hierarchy.

- Where are you now on the Hierarchy of Cultural Knowledge?
- What experiences outside of your home country may help you move further on the hierarchy?

Revisit Hyter's (2014) conceptual framework that will facilitate one becoming globally engaged in a more responsive and responsible way. One aspect of that framework is "responsive global engagement, . . . the collaborative or bilateral and sustainable interaction with communities . . ." (Hyter, 2014, p. 115). Responsive global engagement includes the following components:

- global humility,
- global self-awareness,
- global knowledge, and
- global reciprocity.

One important reminder is that movements along the Pathway of Cultural Responsiveness or the Hierarchy of Cultural Knowledge are not destinations but are processes. The goal is to continue to move along those continua with every experience and opportunity to learn. Next, we review the components of responsive global engagement.

Global humility is knowing that there are cultural practices, beliefs, and values that are different than your own, and that are as valuable as your own. If you can approach intercultural and intercountry relationships with humility, you are more likely to be in a position to learn from the people living in the country to which you are traveling, working, and contributing (Hyter, 2014; Ortega & Faller, 2011). This is an essential element to being able to engage in sustainable practices. Read the story about Scott in Box 12–3.

Box 12–3

Several years ago, a student (whom I will call Scott), traveled to a developing country and complained to me that the local archeologist (who was a person who had two doctorates in his field) "did not know his field." I was shocked at Scott's attitude. In retrospect, what may have happened was that Scott did not exercise global humility. Scott assumed that his own knowledge of archeology was: (a) superior to the professional's knowledge, and that (b) the professional's knowledge in this developing country would mirror the knowledge and information to which Scott had access. The professional in the developing country not only had two doctorates in his field as mentioned before, but he had command of the field, and access to the research in the field in at least four different languages.

Rewrite this interaction with Scott in a way that would demonstrates his ability to employ global and cultural humility. In addition to global humility, another important skill for globally responsive practices is critical self-reflection. Being humble facilitates self-awareness and self-reflection (Hyter, 2014).

Critical self-reflection is being able to deconstruct (or examine or judge) your long-held assumptions and beliefs, determine where those assumptions and beliefs come from, why you hold them, and in what other ways you could have thought or responded (Freire, 1998; Mezirow, 1990). To engage in critical self-reflection, one must think critically and dialectically. Critical thinking is the ability to identify underlying assumptions, analyze those assumptions, examine them from a range of perspectives, and then take "informed actions" (Brookfield, 2012, pp. 1, 12). Assumptions, as we mentioned earlier in the text, are uninformed and unquestioned beliefs. Let's apply critical thinking to the case of Scott, mentioned in Box 12–3, using the following guidelines adapted from Brookfield (2012, p. 89). Work with two or three others to respond to the following questions. Keep in mind there is no one right answer to the questions.

1. Identify the assumptions that may have been driving Scott's behavior or thinking. These assumptions can be implicit (indirect; not overt or stated) or explicit (clearly stated; direct). Here, we are trying to identify what beliefs Scott has that support his behavior and thinking.

For example, it seems like Scott assumed that his own knowledge about archeology in the developing country surpassed the knowledge of the professor living and working in the developing country. It also seems like Scott assumed that archeology practiced in the developing country should have mirrored the way archeology was practiced in Scott's country. Can your group identify at least two other assumptions driving Scott's behavior?

2. Which of the assumptions you identified could Scott verify? Are these assumptions valid? If so, based on what context, what experience, and what information?

For example, Scott could read more about research and archeology in parts of the world with which he might not be familiar to verify or refute his assumptions. Also, unless Scott was able to verify his assumptions about archeology in the developing country, his assumptions may not be valid. Your group members should now think together about which assumptions listed for question 1 may be verifiable and valid.

3. Provide alternative interpretations of the scenario involving Scott—"a version of what's happening that is consistent with the events described but that you think 'Scott' would disagree with or has not noticed" (p. 89). In other words, what are other assumptions that could be held about the same events described by Scott?

Perhaps an alternative interpretation of Scott's behavior is that he assumed that the professional in the developing country was not intelligent, or did not know archeology. Could Scott have a single story about the developing country and the people in it and find it difficult to believe that people living in that developing country can have initiative, and their own ideas? Discuss with your group other interpretations of the above scenario.

Keep in mind that this exercise is only an introductory example of beginning to think critically. There are additional exercises on the PluralPlus companion website that can be employed to help you strengthen your critical thinking skills. Let us now turn our attention to dialectical thinking.

Dialectical thinking requires critical thinking, meaning that it includes identifying underlying assumptions and identifying alternative perspectives. It also, however, requires the additional steps of integrating or synthesizing divergent perspectives (Sternberg, Grigorenko, & Jarvin, 2015) and gaining an understanding of the whole system (Santiago-Valles, 1997). Freire (1998) says that "critical understanding leads to critical action" (p. 44); therefore, once you have a new understanding of the whole system (totality), collectively engage in critical action to transform reality—the current situation or problem. This critical action is also called *praxis*—acting together, critically reflecting on the actions, revising, acting, reflecting, revising—with the goal of transforming reality (Freire, 1998, 2003;

Santiago-Valles, 1997). Praxis has been called the "transition from critical thought to reflective intervention in the world" (Giroux, 1981, p. 117).

Keep in mind that dialectical thinking is an iterative and continuous process. As more knowledge is produced, positions toward certain issues may change. Dialectical thinking involves looking for contradictions (Orland-Barak, 2010). It is the ability to negate what we think we already know or believe is true; imagine a different idea, reality, or outcome; and then synthesize the divergent ideas, which helps us have a better understanding of totality or of the whole. With this understanding of totality, we can transform reality (Freire, 2003; Marcuse, 1991).

Totality is the interdependence of social structures that reproduce inequalities within the global system (Bottomore, 1983; Granter, 2016; Marshall, 2016; Santiago-Valles, 1997). In other words, totality refers to the whole global system. Social structures, as discussed in Chapter 3, are interconnected systems that form and organize society (Agger, 2006; Dillon, 2010; Farmer, Nizeye, Stulac, & Keshavjee, 2006). With a better understanding of totality, we have the collective ability to change unequal power relationships. The point of dialectical thinking "is to arrive at the truth" (Macey, 2000, p. 96), and then act on that truth. The truth is always much more complicated than one narrow point of view. Reality is "characterized by a tension between conflicting forces . . . which will be solved as a new synthesis is achieved" (Macey, 2000, p. 96). In this current context of globalization, the conflicting forces play out in daily life as the exercise of power (i.e., politics), and how this exercise of power is enacted through these three interconnected social structures—cultural marginalization or exclusion, economic exploitation, and state sanctioned violence (Hyter, 2014; Santiago-Valles, 1997).

Cultural marginalization or exclusion can occur when some racialized or gendered groups, for example, are kept from fully participating in society by overt actions of others, or it can occur implicitly through institutionalized policies or practices. A White woman being paid less for the same job and experience of a White man is an example of institutionalized marginalization based on gender. The gender pay gap is a form of institutionalized marginalization of women. This pay gap is not just a gender pay gap, it is also racial, where women of color make less than their White female counterparts (Patten, 2016).

Economic exploitation is usually discussed in the literature in terms of labor—that is, the use of someone's labor without paying them complete compensation for their work. It can also mean that one part of society or the world is relegated to producing (working) and another segment of society consumes what the other part of society produces. For example, countries in the Global South are paid "a fraction of the cost" for their natural resources, which are consumed primarily by wealthier countries in the Global North (Chiras, 2001, p. 629).

State-sanctioned violence refers to physical or symbolic violence committed with the blessing of the government, such as the violence of the military tacticians (Howie, 2012) or the police force engaged in abuses of the public without punishment (Barton & Johns, 2014). Examples of state-sanctioned violence are evident throughout the history of the United States, such as redlining[8] in neighborhoods from the early 1930s until the early 1960s (Hannah-Jones, 2012). More recent examples are the killings of unarmed Black

---

[8]Redlining was a provision of the Federal Housing Administration that prevented certain properties from being occupied by people of color. Neighborhoods were divided based on the income and the race of the people who lived in a neighborhood.

men and women by police. In 2016 alone, 34% of the unarmed people killed by the police were Black males, who make up only 6% of the U.S. population (Craven, 2017).

Dialectical thinking helps us synthesize the parts of a problem resulting in an explanation that surpasses the individual parts, and helps us explain the interdependent relations (the connections) among social structures (Kellner, 1989; Santiago-Valles, 1997). Figure 12–4

provides a graphic of the whole global system or totality—the outer square, the interconnected social structures—the smaller squares with bidirectional arrows between them, and the role politics (the exercise of power) plays in the system.

Let's try another exercise. A topic that has been in the news quite frequently this year (2017) is a debate about which public restrooms should be used by people who are

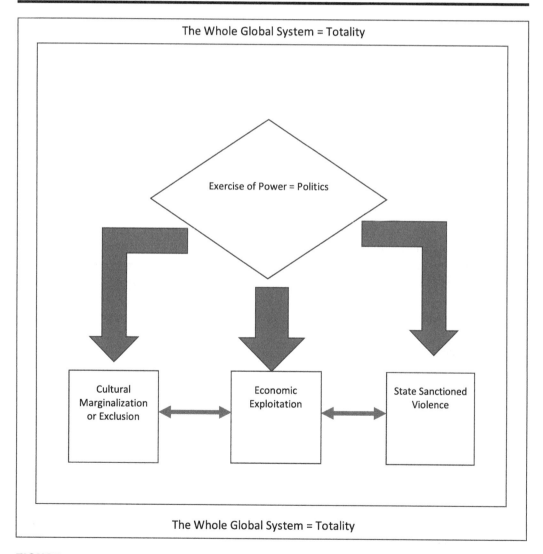

FIGURE 12–4. Totality and interconnecting social structures. Based on Santiago-Valles, 1997.

transgender. We follow the steps below to try to find the synthesis to this problem, which has strong opposing views, and then let our new understanding of this issue guide our next steps. The steps, while working in groups of three or four, to thinking dialectally about the rights of persons who are transgender are as follows:

1. Identify shared problems by asking questions such as what do we have in common and about which issues are we mutually concerned? The issue has already been selected for you so move on to Step 2.
2. Put the issue in historical and global perspectives. For example, ask questions such as, What historical events lead to the current point or situation? Have other countries faced similar issues? If so, how did they respond? You need to do some research to be able to respond to these questions.
3. Examine the relationships among social structures regarding this problem. For example, you would ask questions such as How is politics (i.e., the exercise of power) being enacted in this case? Is it being represented through cultural marginalization or exclusion, by economic exploitation, and/or state-sanctioned violence? Keep in mind there may also be other factors playing a role, such as race, gender, and religion (Kellner, 1999).

Let's think about these questions together. People who are transgender are currently not allowed in some states to use the restroom with which they feel most comfortable—cultural marginalization or exclusion seems to be at play here. Also, the current federal government sanctions this exclusion—state-sanctioned violence (symbolic, not physical violence but violence nevertheless). What other social structures may be involved in

this case? What are other ways that cultural marginalization and exclusion and state-sanctioned violence might manifest regarding this issue? Remember that culture as a social structure includes race, gender, media, schooling, and religion (Hoare & Nowell Smith, 1971; Hyter, 2014).

1. Once you understand totality, which is a holistic view of an entire issue, you are prepared to identify and synthesize each side of the issue. The synthesis is a solution that is better than either opposing side alone.

One synthesis could be that all public restrooms in the United States should be made into gender neutral restrooms. There may be precedence for these types of restrooms in other countries. What are the benefits and challenges with this synthesis? What are other ways to bring the two divergent views about restroom use by people who are transgender into a synthesized whole?

2. Engage in praxis by moving from critical thought to reflective action to transform reality—to transforms things from how they currently are to a more developed idea or course of action. Engaging in praxis (reflective action with others) is one way to gain global knowledge.

Global knowledge is produced collectively. Fleck (1981), a microbiologist, wrote about thought collectives, which are groups of people who engage around and with information, learn from each other, solve problems together, and produce new knowledge together. Knowledge comes from collective engagement with others, and not necessarily others who are just like you. Global knowledge is produced by engaging with others around the topic of global issues or about a region of the world. Learning global knowledge is acquired by constantly striving to produce, learn, and utilize valid information about cultural groups and cultural practices in home and abroad countries (Hyter, 2014). Learning, however, is not an individual endeavor but one that is collective.

Reciprocity is important to effective global engagement and culturally responsive practices because it requires us to think in bidirectional terms, rather than in unidirectional terms. When traveling abroad we take on humility knowing that there are other ways of knowing, other knowledge, other practices that are valuable and effective in the other national or cultural context. Also, we gain knowledge through reading, discussing what we have read, and engaging in conversations with others, about the country and cultural context in which we will be working. Using the perspective of global engagement and intentional culturally responsive practice, prepares individuals to make a global impact in a positive way. For our profession, making a positive impact is through speech, language, and hearing services or research, and advocacy for policies, legislation, and practices that support persons with disabilities. There can be attempts (known or unknown) to bypass this rigorous preparation before taking the journey to "make a difference" in another country. A common misunderstanding is that to go abroad as a "volunteer" is to be in a position to engage in the provision of services. There is a continuum of growth that must occur, from being a volunteer to being able to make global contributions in a responsible manner. We address this issue next.

"VOLUNTOURISM" OR EFFECTIVE VOLUNTEERING?

Voluntourism is a concept that refers to traveling to another country to volunteer on a short-term project without taking into consideration the local needs or culture, and without engaging the local population in the development or planning of the work (Guttentag, 2009; Hickey, McKenna, Woods, & Archibald, 2012; Kushner, 2016). Voluntourism can create dependence and take jobs away from local actors (Guttentag, 2009; Hyter, 2014; Low, 2016). Sometimes this happens, and often it is a first step in beginning to work on a global level, but we wanted you to be aware of problems with volunteering without sufficient information about the history, context, and needs of the country or community in which you will be volunteering. Engaging in global work from positions of humility, self-reflection, knowledge, and reciprocity, and engaging in sustainable practices can be useful for avoiding the pitfalls associated with voluntourism. One can, however, volunteer and work toward sustainable practice and partnerships. Salas-Provance et al. (2014) state that when there are bidirectional exchanges between service providers and communities, the path to sustainable services has begun to be developed. Sustainable services are essential for long-term changes and effectiveness in a community. It is important for volunteers to work with community members to "identify the social capital . . . which will sustain their services once they return to their respective countries" (Salas-Provance, 2014, p. 71). We discuss sustainable practice next.

Sustainable Practice

Sustainability is when communities receive long-term benefit from a practice or service (Stringer, 2017). Over the years, several definitions of sustainability (or concepts that mean sustainability) have emerged (Hanson, Salmoni, & Volpe, 2009). Table 12–7, adapted from Hanson et al. (2009), shows a range of definitions for sustainability.

TABLE 12–7. Some Definitions of Sustainability in the Research Literature

Authors	Year	Definition Provided
Steckler & Goodman	1989	*Institutionalization:* the integration and long-term viability of a new program within an existing organization
Bracht et al.	1994	*Incorporation:* the transfer of responsibility from the external initiating agency to the incorporating agency where the incorporating agency assumes complete responsibility
Brown	1998	*Sustainability:* conversion of institutional capacity into the performance required for continued effectiveness
O'Loughlin, Renaud, Richard, Sanchex Gomez, & Paradis	1998	*Sustainability:* the extent to which a new program becomes integrated or embedded into an organization's normal operations
Olsen	1998	*Sustainable health service:* the long-term ability of an organizational system to mobilize and allocate appropriate and sufficient resources for public health activities
Shediac-Rizkallah, & Bone	1998	*Sustainability:* the notion of continuation of a program that is able to be dynamic rather than inflexible
Glasgow, Vogt, & Boles	1999	*Institutionalization:* when a practice or policy becomes routine and part of an organization's everyday culture and norms
Crisp, Swerissen, & Duckett	2000	*Capacity building:* to improve community health practices that are sustained after the limited period of external resources
Evashwick & Ory	2003	*Sustainability:* a program that endures from its inception
Mancini & Marek	2004	*Sustainability:* a program's continuous response to community issues
Pluye, Potvin, & Denis	2004	*Sustainability:* produced by programs that are routinized within organization where the program intended to be sustained is based up by an organization
Nilsen, Timpka, Nordenfelt, & Lindqvist	2005	*Sustainability:* the maintenance of a level of activity so the program will provide continuous management of a health problem
Pluye, Potvin, Denis, Pelletier, & Mannoni	2005	*Sustainability:* the continuation of a program
Humphreys, Wakerman, & Wells	2006	*Sustainability:* the ability to provide ongoing access to appropriate quality care in a manner that is both cost efficient and health effective

Source: Reprinted from Hanson, Salmoni, & Volpe (2009, p. 305).

An important aspect to consider in sustainable practice is the relationship between the receivers of a service and those implementing it. Specifically, Stringer (2017) promotes a model of service that focuses on "collaboration, training and distribution of resources" (p. 3) rather than on direct service provision by people outside of the country or culture. These collaborations can also help to build capacity in the community or country (Stringer, 2017), and when they are not present, sustainable practices and programs may not materialize (Dent et al., 2016).

As an example, the work that Dr. Hyter does in Senegal is largely focused on collaboration with orthophonistes (SLPS) around providing services to children who are Deaf and hard of hearing, and those with language and speech disabilities, supporting and building capacity with service providers through the delivery of in-services, providing literature and research (that the service providers in Senegal have requested), and facilitating the acquisition and distribution of material resources. One year, teachers at a school for Deaf and hard of hearing children, asked for ideas about ways to help the children differentiate "wh" questions. In French, "wh" questions begin with "qu," and there is very little differentiation between the questions in terms of lip movement (e.g., "what" is "quelle" [kɛl], "who" is "qui" [ki], and "when" is "quand" [kã]). Dr. Hyter and her students developed some suggestions using cued speech; discussed those suggestions with the staff, teachers, and administrators; and taught a class using the suggestions with the staff, teachers, and administrators observing. Then the teachers took the suggestions and lesson developed by Dr. Hyter and her students, modified them so that they were more accessible to the students, and now that is a strategy that is used in the school to help students differentiate "wh" questions.

Building capacity is an important concept to understand. The UN Development Programme (2006) defines capacity development as "the ability to perform functions, solve problems, set and achieve objectives" at three levels: individual, institutional, and societal (p. 7). Central to capacity is to ensure that people can use the knowledge they have gathered along with their personal skill sets to pave their own futures. In the national discussion of sustainability (UNV, 2011), it is described from a framework of "livelihood sustainability," which is described in the following way:

> A "sustainable livelihood comprises the capabilities, assets, (which include both material and social resources) and activities required for a means of living. A livelihood is sustainable when it can cope with, and recover from, stresses and shocks and maintain or enhance its capabilities and assets" (both now and in the future, while not undermining the natural resource base). (Chambers & Conway, 1991, p. 6)

For example, Dr. Salas-Provance has been involved in building capacity in the area of cleft palate in Lima, Peru. Numerous children receive surgical repair for their clefts through a volunteer medical team. However, after the medical team departs the country, the families must continue the work to develop their children's speech. In one example, three mothers of 2-year-old children received training on how to continue speech and language development at home. These three mothers also were introduced to a local SLP who then arranged continued treatment for the three children. The mothers immediately planned their transportation schedules to make their therapy appointments. They felt empowered and were now able to advocate for their children's speech therapy needs. These mothers were provided information that allowed them to incorporate the continued treatments for their children into their everyday lifestyle. The resources that were currently in their country were made accessible to them, along with their newly acquired skills.

Volunteers have a great responsibility to identify the social capital (i.e., host community), which will sustain their service once they return to their respective countries (Woolcock & Narayan, 2000). Terms used to describe this type of community support or joint effort include *mutirao* in Brazil; *batsiranai* in Zimbabwe; *bayanihan* in the Philippines; *gotong royong* in Indonesia; *harambee* in Kenya; *shramadama* in Sri Lanka; *tirelosetshaba* in Botswana; *taka'ful* in Arab States; *minga* in Ecuador and Peru; and *neighboring* or *barn raising* in the United States (Post, 2005). It may be necessary to assist families in developing self-help groups in their communities to sustain efforts. This earlier example shows how in addition to building capacity, sustainable practices require economic and social development, availability of training, as well as the availability of information. Solomon (2005) focused on strategies such as closing the information-utilization gap, which is: (a) the gap between *having* information about a problem and then *utilizing* that information to address the problem; and (b) situating services in the economic, political, social, and cultural needs of the community, as identified by the community (Solomon, 2005).

As more and more SLPs and audiologists desire to have an abroad experience, or more experiences with individuals whose diverse cultures and language backgrounds differ from the service providers, we need to be humble enough to remember that people often know exactly what they need but frequently lack the material resources to put what they need in place. One notable study interviewed 40 stakeholders from three different communities about their definition of sustainable (Hanson et al., 2009). These stakeholders focused more on how to create sustainable programs rather than on how to define a sustainable program. It is important to take note of the suggestions

made by those stakeholders regarding how to build a sustainable program or practice. These suggestions include:

- raising awareness of the program or issue being addressed by the program;
- determining ways that the program can fund itself;
- educating the public/community about the program;
- planning continuously; and
- creating varied partners (Hanson et al., 2009, p. 308).

There is an activity on the PluralPlus companion website that will help you think more systematically about ethical and sustainable global engagement.

CHAPTER SUMMARY

One of the consequences of globalization is the forced or voluntary movement of people from one region of the world to another. Additionally, there are increasing opportunities for SLPS and audiologists to travel abroad, outside of their own countries, to volunteer and/or deliver services to individuals or groups in other countries. Because of these reasons, it is imperative to consider the next logical step in the development of culturally responsive practices, which is to also prepare yourself to serve populations from and in countries other than your own. You learned that you cannot/ should not just jump into international work but should prepare for that journey systematically. One place to start in your preparation is to familiarize yourself with global agreements, documents, and organizations such as the United Nations and the Millennium Development Goals and the Sustainable Development Goals, World Health Organization, Pan American Health Organization, and others.

Additionally, as you prepare for global speech-language and hearing services, it is important to keep in mind the importance of learning as much as possible about the populations you plan to serve. Novelist Chimamanda Ngozi Adichie provided an important lesson of what could happen if we have only a "single story" about other groups. Additionally, you learned about the knowledge, skills, and attitudes necessary to be effective in global practice including humility, knowledge, critical self-reflection, critical thinking, and dialectical thinking. Be wary of *voluntourism*, but build on opportunities to *volunteer* so that the work becomes sustainable and useful to the communities abroad for a long time to come.

New Zealand, you may want to identify a program in Germany. The point is to identify a community problem regarding communication disabilities where solving the problem will require skills and knowledge beyond which you alone have access to in your environment. Develop a plan for developing a sustainable solution to that problem:

a. What steps should be taken?
b. Who are the stakeholders?
c. What should/could your role be in relationship to the stakeholders?
d. What activity/planning and programming may be effective?

EXTENDED LEARNING

1. Identify a current and contentious issue in speech, language, and hearing sciences. Think about these issues critically and dialectically. Identify a synthesis to the problem and how if the synthesis was implemented, it might look in real practice. Here is a starter list of topics, but it is not exhaustive:
   a. requiring bilingual language assessment and intervention,
   b. requiring teachers to learn African American English in order to support children proficient in AAE in learning another linguistic code,
   c. considering total communication versus sign language only, and
   d. determining schooling budgets based on property value and taxes.
2. Identify a speech-language pathology and/or an audiology program in a part of the world different from where you live. For example, if you are living in the United States, identify a program in Mali, perhaps. If you are living in

FURTHER READING

Hyter, Y. D., Roman, T. R., Staley, B., & McPherson, B. (2017). Competencies for effective global engagement: A proposal for Communication Sciences and Disorders. *SIG 17 Perspectives on Global Issues in Communication Sciences and Related Disorders, 2,* 9–20.

International Association of Speech-Language Pathology. (2013). Volume 15, Issue 1.
- Special issue on the implications of the world report on disabilities
- Karen Wylie (Ed.)

Sustainable development goals (United Nations, 2015)
- Hanson, H. M., Salmoni, A. W., & Volpe, R. (2009). Defining program sustainability: Differing views of stakeholders. *Canadian Journal of Public Health, 100*(3), 304–309.
- United Nations. (2015). Transforming our world: The 2030 agenda for sustainable development. General Assembly resolution 70/1. Retrieved from https://sustainabledevelopment.un.org/post2015/transformingourworld

Topics in Language Disorders. (2014). Volume 34, Issue 2
- Special edition on global issues in language disorders: Frameworks, processes, and policies
- Yvette D. Hyter and Dolores Battle (Eds.)

United Nations. (2006). *Convention on the rights of persons with disabilities and optional protocol*. Retrieved from http://www.un.org/disabilities/documents/convention/convoptprot-e.pdf

REFERENCES

Agger, B. (2006). *Critical social theories* (2nd ed.). Boulder, CO: Paradigm.

American Academy of Audiology. (2017). *Code of ethics*. Retrieved from http://www.audiology.org/publications-resources/document-library/code-ethics

American Speech-Language-Hearing Association (AHSA). (2016a). *Highlights and trends: Member and affiliate counts year-end 2016*. Retrieved from http://www.asha.org/uploadedFiles/2016-Member-Counts.pdf

American Speech-Language-Hearing Association (ASHA). (2016b). *Code of ethics*. Retrieved from http://www.asha.org/Code-of-Ethics/

American Speech-Language-Hearing Association (ASHA). (2017a). *International programs*. Retrieved from http://www.asha.org/Members/international/

American Speech-Language-Hearing Association (ASHA). (2017b). *About Special Interest Group 17, Global issues in communication sciences and related disorders*. Retrieved from http://www.asha.org/SIG/17/About-SIG 17/

American Speech-Language-Hearing Association (ASHA). (2017c). *ASHA and the Pan American Health Organization*. Retrieved from http://www.asha.org/Members/international/PAHO/

Anderson, M. (2017, February 14). African immigrant population in U.S. steadily climbs. *Pew Research Center: Fact tank news in the numbers*. Retrieved from http://www.pewresearch.org/fact-tank/2017/02/14/african-immigrant-population-in-u-s-steadily-climbs/

Barrett, H., & Marshall, J. (2013). Implementation of the World Report on Disability: Developing resource capacity to meet the needs of people with communication disability in Uganda. *International Journal of Speech-Language Pathology, 15*(1), 48–52.

Barton, A., & Barnes, N. (2014). Engaging the citizen. In J. Brown (Ed.), *The future of policing* (pp. 417–428). London, UK: Routledge.

Bottomore, T. (1983). *A dictionary of Marxist thought* (2nd ed.). Oxford, UK: Blackwell.

Bracht, N., Finnegan, J., Rissel, C., Weisbrod, R., Gleason, J., Corbett, J., & Veblen-Mortenson, S. (1994). Community ownership and program continuation following a health demonstration project. *Health Education Research, 9*(2), 243–255.

Brookfield, S. D. (2012). *Teaching for critical thinking: Tools and techniques to help students question their assumptions*. San Francisco, CA: Jossey-Bass.

Brown, D. R. (1998). Evaluating institutional sustainability in development programmes: Beyond dollars and cents. *Journal of International Development, 10*(1), 55–69.

Chambers, R., & Conway, G. R. (1991, December). *Sustainable rural livelihoods: Practical concepts for the 21st century*. IDS Discussion Paper 296, IDS, Brighton, UK.

Channing, E., & Joyce, D. D. (1993). *The history of the United States*. Lanham, MD: University Press of America.

Chiras, D. D. (2001). *Environmental science: Creating a sustainable future*. Sudbury, MA: Jones and Bartlett.

Craven, J. (2017, January 1). More than 250 Black people were killed by police in 2016: Too many [updated]. *Huffington Post*. Retrieved from http://www.huffingtonpost.com/entry/black-people-killed-by-police-america_us_577da633e4b0c590f7e7fb17

Crisp, B. R., Swerissen, H., & Duckett, S. J. (2000). Four approaches to capacity building in health: Consequences for measurement and accountability. *Health Promotion International, 15*(2), 99–107.

Delgado Wise, R. (2013). The migration and labor question today: Imperialism, unequal development and forced migration. *Monthly Review, 64*(9). Retrieved from https://monthlyreview.org/2013/02/01/the-migration-and-labor-question-today-imperialism-unequal-development-and-forced-migration/

Dent, E., Hoon, E., Kitson, A., Karnon, J., Newbury, J., Harvey, G., . . . Beilby, J. (2016). Translating a health service intervention into a rural setting: Lessons learned. *BMC Health Services Research, 16*(62). doi:10.1186/s12913-016-1302-0

Dillon, M. (2010). *Introduction to sociological theory: Theorists, concepts, and their applicability to the twenty-first century*. West Sussex, UK: John Wiley & Sons.

Elliott, J. H. (2002). *Imperial Spain*. London, UK: Penguin Books.

Evashwick, C., & Ory, M. (2003). Organizational characteristics of successful innovative health care programs sustained over time. *Family Community Health, 26*(3), 177–193.

Farmer, P. E., Nizeye, B., Stulac, S., & Keshavjee, S. (2006). Structural violence and clinical medicine. *PLoS Medicine 3*(10), 1686–1691.

Fleck, L. (1981). *Genesis and development of a scientific fact*. Chicago, IL: University of Chicago Press.

Freire, P. (1973). *Education for critical consciousness*. New York, NY: Continuum.

Freire, P. (2003). *Pedagogy of the oppressed: 30th anniversary edition*. New York, NY: Continuum.

Gerber, D. A. (2011). *American immigration: A very short introduction*. Oxford, UK: Oxford University Press.

Giroux, H. (1981). *Ideology, culture and the process of schooling*. Philadelphia, PA: Temple University Press.

Glasgow, R. E., Vogt, T. M., & Boles, S. M. (1999). Evaluating the public health impact of health promotion interventions: The RE-AIM framework. *American Journal of Public Health, 89*(9), 1322–1327.

Gonzalez-Barrera, A. (2016, November 19). Chapter 1: Migration flows between the U.S. and Mexico have slowed—and turned toward Mexico. *Pew Research Center: Hispanic trends*. Retrieved from http://www.pewhispanic.org/2015/11/19/chapter-1-migration-flows-between-the-u-s-and-mexico-have-slowed-and-turned-toward-mexico/

Gonzalez, J. M. (Ed.). (2008). *Encyclopedia of bilingual education*. Los Angeles, CA: Sage.

Granter, E. (2016). *Critical social theory and the end of work*. New York, NY: Routledge.

Green, L., & Kreuter, M. (2004). *Health program planning: An educational and ecological approach*. New York, NY: McGraw-Hill.

Guttentag, D. A. (2009). The possible negative impacts of volunteer tourism. *International Journal of Tourism Research, 11*(6), 537–551.

Hannah-Jones, N. (2013). *Living apart: How the government betrayed a landmark civil rights law*. Audible Audiobook, Unabridged.

Hanson, H. M., Salmoni, A. W., & Volpe, R. (2009). Defining program sustainability: Differing views of stakeholders. *Canadian Journal of Public Health, 100*(3), 204–309.

Hickey, E., McKenna, M., Woods, C., & Archibald, C. (2012). Ethical concerns in voluntourism in speech-language pathology and audiology. *Perspectives in Global Issues in Communication Sciences and Related Disorders, 2*(2), 40–48.

Hoare, Q., & Nowell Smith, G. (1971). *Selections from the prison notebooks of Antonio Gramsci* [Edited and translated]. New York, NY: International Publishers.

Hoffmann-Holland, K. (2009). Ethnics and human rights in a globalized world: An interdisciplinary approach. In K. Hoffmann-Holland (Ed.), *Ethics and human rights in a globalized world: An interdisciplinary and international approach* (pp. 1–12). Tübigen, Germany: Mohr Siebeck.

Howie, L. (2012). *Witnesses to terror: Understanding the meanings and consequences of terrorism*. New York, NY: Palgrave Macmillan.

Humphreys, J. S., Wakerman, J., & Wells, R. (2006). What do we mean by sustainable rural health services? Implication for rural health research. *Australian Journal of Rural Health, 14*, 33–35.

Hyter, Y. D. (2014). A conceptual framework for responsive global engagement in communication sciences and disorders. *Topics in Language Disorders, 34*(2), 103–120.

Hyter, Y. D., Roman, T. R., Staley, B., & McPherson, B. (2017). Competencies for effective global engagement: A proposal for communication sciences and disorders. *Perspectives of the ASHA SIG 17, 2*(1), 9–20.

International Communication Project. (2014–2017). *Founding organizations*. Retrieved from http://www.internationalcommunicationproject.com/about-icp/who-we-are/

International Disability and Development Consortium (IDDC), & International Disability

Alliance. (2015, September 25). *The 2030 agenda: The inclusion of persons with disabilities*. Retrieved from http://www.international disabilityalliance.org/sites/default/files/docu ments/2030_agenda_comprehensive_guide_ for_persons_with_disabilities_comp.pdf

Kellner, D. (1989). *Critical theory, Marxism and modernity*. Baltimore, MD: John Hopkins University Press.

Kessell, J. L. (2003). *Spain in the Southwest: A narrative history of colonial New Mexico, Arizona, Texas, and California*. Norman, OK: University of Oklahoma Press.

Kushner, J. (2016, March 22). The voluntourist's dilemma. *New York Times Magazine*. Retrieved from https://www.nytimes.com/2016/03/22/ magazine/the-voluntourists-dilemma.html

Low, R. (2016). *Good intentions are not enough: Why we fail at helping others*. Hackensack, NJ: WS Professional.

Lundy, K. S., & Barton, J. A. (2016). Community and population health: Assessment and intervention. In K. S. Lundy & S. Janes (Eds.), *Community health nursing: Caring for the public's health* (pp. 33–68). Burlington, MA: Jones and Bartlett Learning.

Macey, D. (2000). *Dictionary of critical theory*. London, UK: Penguin Books.

Mancini, J. A., & Marek, L. I. (2004). Sustaining community-based programs for families: Conceptualization and measurement. *Family Relations, 53*(4), 339–347.

Marcuse, H. (1991). *One dimensional man* (2nd ed.). Abingdon, UK: Routledge.

Marshall, P. (2016). *A complex integral realist perspective: Towards a new axial vision*. New York, NY: Routledge.

Martin, J. N., & Nakayama, T. K. (2012). *Intercultural communication in contexts* (6th ed.). New York, NY: McGraw-Hill.

Martinez, M., & Marquez, M. (2014, July 16). What's the difference between immigrant and refugee? *CNN*. Retrieved from http://www .cnn.com/2014/07/15/us/immigrant-refugee-definition/

McAllister, L., Wylie, K., Davidson, B., & Marshall, J. (2013). The World Report on Disability: An impetus to reconceptualize services for people with communication disability. *Inter-national Journal of Speech-Language Pathology, 15*(1), 118–126.

McIntyre, A. (2008). *Participatory action research*. Los Angeles, CA: Sage.

Mezirow, J. (1990). How critical reflection triggers transformative learning. In J. Mezirow (Ed.), *Fostering critical reflection in adulthood* (pp. 1–20). San Francisco, CA: Jossey-Bass.

Naturalization Act of 1795, 3rd Congress, Session II, 1 Stat. 414-415. (1795). Retrieved from http://leg isworks.org/sal/1/stats/STATUTE-1Pg414a.pdf

Ngozi Adichie, C. (2009). *The danger of a single story: TED Talk*. Retrieved from https://www .ted.com/talks/chimamanda_adichie_the_dan ger_of_a_single_story

Nilsen, P., Timpka, T., Nordenfelt, L., & Lindqvist, K. (2005). Towards improved understanding of injury prevention program sustainability. *Safety Science, 43*, 815–833.

O'Loughlin, J., Renaud, L., Richard, L., Sanchez Gomex, I., & Paradis, G. (1998). Correlates of the sustainability of community-based heart health promotion interventions. *Preventive Medicine, 27*, 702–712.

Olsen, I. T. (1998). Sustainability of health care: A framework for analysis. *Health Policy Plan, 13*(3), 287–295.

Orland-Barak, L. (2010). *Learning to mentor-as-praxis: Foundations for a curriculum in teacher education*. London, UK: Springer.

Ortega, R. M., & Faller, K. C. (2011). Training child welfare workers from an intersectional cultural humility perspective: A paradigm shift. *Child Welfare, 90*(5), 27–49.

Patten, E. (2016, July 1). Racial, gender wage gaps persist in U. S. despite some progress. *Pew Research Center Fact Tank*. Retrieved from http:// www.pewresearch.org/fact-tank/2016/07/01/ racial-gender-wage-gaps-persist-in-u-s-despite-some-progress/

PBS. (2014, March 13). *PBS News Hour: What prevents the U.S. from signing the U.N. disabilities treaty?* Retrieved from http://www.pbs.org/ newshour/bb/un-treaty-disability/

Pew Research Center. (2017, March 4). *Migration*. Retrieved from http://www.pewresearch.org/ topics/migration/

Pluye, P., Potvin, L., & Denis, J. L. (2004). Making public health programs last: Conceptualizing sustainability. *Evaluation and Program Planning, 27,* 121–133.

Pluye, P., Potvin, L., Denis, J. L., Pelletier, J., & Mannoni, C. (2005). Program sustainability begins with the first events. *Evaluation and Program Planning, 28,* 123–137.

Post, S. G. (2005). Altruism, happiness, and health: It's good to be good. *International Journal of Behavioural Medicine, 12*(2), 66–77.

Poxon, M. K. (2012). *Irish Philadelphia: Images of America.* Charleston, SC: Arcadia.

Restall, M., & Fernandez-Armesto, F. (2012). *The Conquistadors: A very short introduction.* Oxford, UK: Oxford University Press.

Salas-Provance, M., Escobedo, M., & Marchino, M. (2014). Volunteerism: An anchor for global change through partnerships in learning and service. *Perspectives on Global Issues in Communication Sciences and Related Disorders, 4*(2), 68–74.

Santiago-Valles, W. F. (1997). *Memories of the future: Maroon intellectuals from the Caribbean and the sources of their communication strategies, 1925–1940* (Unpublished doctoral dissertation). Simon Fraser University, British Columbia, Canada.

Schmid, C. L. (2013). Spanish and Spanish Americans, to 1870. In E. R. Barkan (Ed.), *Immigrants in American history: Arrival, adaptation, and integration* (pp. 155–160). Santa Barbara, CA: ABC-CLIO.

Sekerka, L. E. (2016). *Ethics is a daily deal: Choosing to build moral strength as a practice.* New York, NY: Springer.

Shediac-Rizkallah, M. C., & Bone, L. R. (1998). Planning for community-based health programs: Conceptual frameworks and future directions for research, practice and policy. *Health Education Research, 13*(1), 87–108.

Soennichsen, J. (2011). *The Chinese Exclusion Act of 1882.* Santa Barbara, CA: Greenwood.

Solomon, N. M. (2005). Health information generation and utilization for informed decision-making in equitable health service management of Kenya Partnership for Health program. *International Journal for Equity in Health, 4*(8). doi:10.1186/1475-9276-4-8

Sorrellis, K. (2016). *Intercultural communication: Globalization and social justice* (2nd ed.). Los Angeles, CA: Sage.

Steckler, A., & Goodman, R. M. (1989). How to institutionalize health promotion programs. *American Journal of Health Promotion, 3*(4), 34–44.

Sternberg, R., Grigorenko, E., & Jarvin, L. (2015). *Teaching for wisdom, intelligence, creativity, and success.* New York, NY: First Skyhorse.

Stringer, P. (2017). Issue of sustainability in global humanitarian programs. *SIG 17 Perspectives on Global Issues in Communication Sciences and Related Disorders, 2*(1), 3–8.

Taylor, A., & Foner, E. (2001). *American colonies.* New York, NY: Penguin.

Turnock, B. J. (2016). *Public health: What it is and how it works.* Burlington, MA: Jones and Bartlett Learning.

United Nations. (n.d.). Convention on the Rights of Persons with Disabilities and Optional Protocol. Retrieved from http://www.un.org/disabilities/documents/convention/convoptprot-e.pdf

United Nations. (1948, December 10). *Universal Declaration of Human Rights.* General Assembly resolution 217 A. New York, NY: Author.

United Nations. (2015). *The Millennium Development Goals Report 2015.* Retrieved from http://www.un.org/millenniumgoals/2015_MDG_Report/pdf/MDG%202015%20rev%20(July%201).pdf

United Nations. (2016). *Working papers on non-self-governing territories* (NSGTs). Retrieved from http://www.un.org/en/decolonization/nonselfgovterritories.shtml

United Nations. (2017). *Sustainable development goals kick off start to new year.* Retrieved from http://www.un.org/sustainabledevelopment/blog/2015/12/sustainable-development-goals-kick-off-with-start-of-new-year/

UN Development Programme (UNDP). (2006). *Definition of basic concepts and terminology in governance and public administration.* UNDP Policy Document. New York, NY: Author.

UN Refugee Agency (UNHCR). (2017). *What is a refugee?* Retrieved from http://www.unrefugees.org/what-is-a-refugee/

UN Volunteers. (2011). *State of the World's Volunteerism Report: Universal values for global wellbeing.* Retrieved from https://www.unv.org/sites/default/files/2011%20State%20of%20the%20World%27s%20Volunteerism%20Report%

20-%20Universal%20Values%20for%20 Global%20Well-being%20Overview.pdf

Wearing, S., & McGee, N. G. (2013). *International volunteer tourism: Integrating travellers and communication*. Oxfordshire, UK: CAB International.

Westby, C. (2013). Implementing recommendations of the World Report on Disability for Indigenous populations. *International Journal of Speech-Language Pathology, 15*(1), 96–100.

Wickenden, M. (2013). Widening the SLP lens: How can we improve the well-being of people with communication disabilities globally. *International Journal of Speech-Language Pathology, 15*(1), 14–20.

Willis, E. M., Biggins, A. L., & Donovan, J. E. (2003). Population focused practice. In J. E. Hitchcock, P. E. Schubert, & S. A. Thomas (Eds.), *Community health nursing: Caring in action* (2nd ed., pp. 302–320). Clifton Park, NY: Thomson Delmar Learning.

Woolcock, M., & Narayan, D. (2000). Social capital: Implications for development theory, research and policy. *The World Bank Research Observer, 15*(2), 225–249.

World Health Organization (WHO). (2001). *International classification of functioning, disability and health*. Geneva, Switzerland: Author.

World Health Organization (WHO). (2010). *Community based rehabilitation guidelines*. Retrieved from http://www.who.int/disabilities/cbr/guide lines/en/

World Health Organization (WHO). (2011). *World report on disability*. Geneva, Switzerland: Author.

World Health Organization (WHO). (2017a). *About the World Health Organization*. Retrieved from http://www.who.int/about/en/

World Health Organization (WHO). (2017b). *Community-based rehabilitation (CBR)*. Retrieved from http://www.who.int/disabilities/cbr/en/

Wylie, K., McAllister, L., Davidson, B., & Marshall, J. (2013). Changing practice: Implications of the World Report on Disability for responding to communication disability in underserved populations. *International Journal of Speech-Language Pathology, 15*(1), 1–13.

Ye He Lee, M. (2015, July 8). Donald Trump's false comments connecting Mexican immigrants and crime. *The Washington Post Fact Checker Analysis*. Retrieved from https://www.washington post.com/news/fact-checker/wp/2015/07/08/ donald-trumps-false-comments-connecting-mexican-immigrants-and-crime/?utm_term=. 16d322bb06b1

Zong, J., & Batalova, J. (2017, March 8). Frequently requested statistics on immigrants and immigration in the United States. *Migration Policy Institute*. Retrieved from https://www. migrationpolicy.org/article/frequently-request ed-statistics-immigrants-and-immigration-united-states

INDEX

Note: Page numbers in **bold** reference non-text material.